NATURAL HEALING WITH HERBS

NATURAL HEALING WITH HERBS

Humbart Santillo B.S., M.H.

Edited by Subhuti Dharmananda, Ph.D.

HOHM PRESS

Hohm Press, P.O. Box 2501, Prescott, Arizona 86302

1st Edition Published 1984. 9th Printing 1991.
Printed in the United States of America

Library of Congress Cataloging in Publication Data

Santillo, Smokey
     Natural Healing With Herbs.

     Bibliography: p.
     Includes index.
     1. Naturopathy. 2. Herbs — Therapeutic use
I. Dharmananda, Subhuti, II. Title
RZ 440.S24 1983   615.5'35   84-553
ISBN 0-934252-08-4

The theories and formulae presented in this book are expressed as the author's opinion and
as such are not meant to be used to diagnose, prescribe, or to administer in any manner to
any physical ailments. In any matters related to your health please contact a qualified, licensed
health practitioner.

D E D I C A T I O N

Mom, Dad, and my wife Dawn,

Special love and admiration goes to my Dad for demonstrating so much faith in me and in wholistic methods of healing. He exhibited remarkable faith and courage in his battle with lymphoma. I'll always remember him for the strength and support he gave me while finishing this manuscript.

TABLE OF CONTENTS

This chapter explains causes of disease as being improper diet, poor attitude, stress, etc., which can result in toxemia. Suggestions are given to correct these conditions, such as fasting, proper diet, rest and attitude adjustment.

A mixture of diagnostic methods are presented, correlating both the Naturopathic and the Chinese Yin/Yang methods of analysis. These are simplified for use by both the layperson and the doctor.

A therapy is a method used in treating disease. All diseases, whether acute or chronic can be categorized into one of the ten therapies discussed. This system is original to the author.

This chapter explains the preparations, and methods of applying herbs both internally and externally: capsules, tinctures, decoctions, infusions, poultices, plasters, and more.

This chapter explains the best time to administer tinctures, teas, pills, capsules, etc., as well as how to determine dosages for children and adults during both chronic and acute disease. It also shows how rest periods during the treatment of illness aid in determining dosages of herbs, length of herbal treatment and the intensity of the illness.

The difference between a healing crisis and a disease crisis is thoroughly explained.

This chapter explains how to utilize the individual's energy level during treatment to avoid causing enervation (loss of nerve energy).

This chapter explains how to determine the equivalency between liquid herb preparations and capsules. Also, a complete list of over 120 herbs is given including their suggested dosage and their preparations.

FOREWORD

Fifteen or twenty years ago, during the "Golden Age" of modern medicine, a book with this title would have had little chance of even appearing on bookstore shelves. So strong was the belief in modern medicine's credo—better living through chemistry—that no "responsible" person, professional or otherwise, mentioned the word "herbs."

Today, as the deadly consequences of a modern, artificial civilization are becoming more apparent to both medical professionals and the public at large, *Natural Healing With Herbs* merits and receives center stage.

In the first of my six decades of life, I was treated for colds by my mother with concoctions containing horehound and licorice, although I did not know about concepts like herbs or folk medicine. My second decade, in which I saw an M.D. only upon entry into the U.S. Navy, was followed by my admission in my third decade, into Medical School.

Because of my interest in history, I registered for an elective course in medical history taught by the renowned Professor Ilse Veith. Professor Veith taught me enough about acupuncture and moxibustion so that I was not surprised when President Nixon, newly returned from China, brought the "news" two decades later, about this astounding Oriental healing system to American citizens.

My fourth decade and part of the fifth were spent conscientiously (and unthinkingly) performing on my patients the standard procedures of the medical establishment.

Finally, the last 10 to 15 years has witnessed my own gradual awakening and that of the American public. One doesn't have to read the polls to discover that the confidence level of people in their doctors has plummetted from 88% five years ago to 48% today. The evidence that people are deserting modern medicine and seeking preventative medicine is all around us: from personal conversations, daily radio and TV disclosures, and the growing skepticism of even the most conservative print journalists. But the best evidence of the decline of the medical theocracy comes from my patients' desperate search for alternatives—"What can I do instead of taking valium, inderal, tagamet, thorazine; instead of having surgery; instead of having my child's tonsils removed; instead of chemotherapy for cancer?"

Now, "Smokey" Santillo has provided a powerful response to their pleas. I can now recommend that patients regard the three decades (from the 40's through the 60's) as a radical departure from a natural way of living. I can advise that they closely examine the traditional healing systems not only from ancient Greece and Rome, China, India and Tibet, but even those of my own religious background (the greatest Jewish physician of all times, 13th century Moses Maimonides, wrote not only of chicken soup, but of herbal remedies and cleansing and healing baths)*.

"Natural Healing With Herbs" can give every person an authoritative, detailed, practical, understandable, comprehensive, clear and exciting look into the traditional and modern naturopathic healing methods. It should also be read by every student who intends to practice professionally the healing arts.

Smokey Santillo has given us the first book to set forth a truly contemporary *system* of herbal healing for modern America. He also presents an original synthesis of traditional oriental and western methods that is especially relevant for the people of this country.

The herbs discussed herein are not exotic, hard-to-find specimens, but those available at most health food stores or even around the home. The recommendations for using them are clear and well-founded, based on the author's many years of experience in working with people. By correlating traditional diagnostic and healing methods from East *and* West, he has devised a system that can do more for us than either one alone. This is an original system that addresses not only well-understood and agreed upon issues of naturopathic healing (like the importance of good diet and cleansing to eliminate toxins in the body), but also such questions as transition diets and the development of an appropriate therapy to suit *individual* needs. All of this is made understandable for patients as well as naturopathic (and even allopathic) practitioners in this unique, forward-looking volume. Cross-referencing herbs with the ailments for which they are specific completes the practical, systematic approach. This is a book we have been waiting for for some time.

Those inside the medical establishment—M.D.'s, medical students and house officers—may feel that they need not learn about herbs, that their medical licenses protect them against inroads by naturopaths. Far from regarding the herbal therapists as peers in the healing arts, the M.D. may consider them "quacks" even though their knowledge is extremely beneficial and essential. However, alternative practitioners, your day in the sun is not far off! The growing public recognition that many problems exist within the medical establishment, has resulted in a renaissance of interest in Milton Friedman's 32-year old proposal to delicense medicine.** Just recently, attorney Lori B. Andrews of the American Bar Association published her "deregulating doctoring" (Peoples Medical Society, Emmaus PA 18049, 1983). This landmark document concludes with a call for "replacing the licensing system with a certification system...as a first step toward...assuring people...the choice among a wide range of health care practitioners."

But even measures short of medical delicensure now being considered and implemented in many states will go a long way towards legitimatizing the use of herbs in the management of human health and disease. Concomitantly, these liberating measures will free us all to choose our own method of health care, and experienced herbalists like Mr. Santillo will then have the opportunity, through students, to make herbal and naturopathic healing easily available to every American citizen.

Meanwhile, Smokey Santillo, in Arizona, is personally available only to his own community and to those able to travel long distances, or attend his public lectures. But for everyone else, both healthy and otherwise, this book, the definitive work on herbology, is your avenue to his time-tested, wise advice. For most Americans, *Natural Healing With Herbs* represents the real medicine of the future. For those of you lucky enough to have this book in your hands, the future is today.

Robert S. Mendelsohn, M.D.
February, 1984

*1) *The Medical Writings of Moses Maimonides,* translated and edited by Fred Rosner, M.D. and Suessman Muntner, M.D., J.B. Lippincott, 1969.

2) *The Medical Aphorisms of Moses Maimonides,* translated and edited by Fred Rosner, M.D. and Suessman Muntner, M.D., Yeshiva University Press, 1970.

**Capitalism and Freedom,* Milton Friedman, University of Chicago Press, 1962.

EDITOR'S PREFACE

There are numerous herbal traditions in the world, each emphasizing therapeutic techniques suitable for the predominant disorders of the society at the time the tradition evolved. The firmly rooted traditions of India, Tibet, and China all have an extensive literature describing theory and practice, but the American and European traditions are much more poorly represented as a result of their very erratic course of development. Smokey Santillo has now provided us with a comprehensive work on the American naturopathic approach to herbology.

American naturopathy has its roots in the ancient healing arts of Egypt. The methods of using herbs, diet, hydrotherapy, exercise, and other means of maintaining and restoring health were passed from the Egyptians to the Greeks and largely adopted by Hippocrates (ca. 400 B.C.). In the Golden Age of Western herbology, from 500 B.C. until around 200 A.D., several great physicians and scholars learned and classified hundreds of important plants useful in healing. Information from Galen and Dioscorides is still cited frequently in modern herbals. The scientific names of several important medicinal plants are derived from the mythical figures of the Greeks and Romans.

Unfortunately, Western herbology stagnated, and even declined, during the ensuing twelve centuries (much of the knowledge and progress in Western herbology was transferred to the Arab world, but little of this was recaptured by the Europeans). Poor hygiene, disregard for scholarship and discovery, and many other factors led to horrible conditions including frequent plagues, short lifespan, and extremely high infant mortality.

The Renaissance, with the invention of the printing press, the rekindling of scientific pursuits, and the broadening of international trade brought new interest in herbal drugs. In the 18th century, the great Swedish botanist, Carl Linne, provided the world with an international language of plant names allowing herbs from every nation to be compared and classified. Thus the revival of Western herbology was underway, given a great boost by the importation of efficacious plant drugs from the Americas and from the Far East.

Yet, no sooner had herbology been revived and vitalized then the discoveries of chemical and pharmacological principles in the early 19th century drew this brief period of awakening to a close. By the middle of that century, active ingredients of herbs were being used in place of the whole plant materials and the concerns of the medical profession were turning away from the old theories of physiology and pathology to those of the new. Then came a drastic blow to natural healing: the "patent medicine era" in the U.S., from around 1880 to 1910, turned all home-made remedies into a hoax. The Food and Drug Administration was developed, in part, to deal with this situation. Drugs, herbal or otherwise, were taken out of the hands of the people at large and placed into the hands of a closed medical group of persons who had undergone a specific "orthodox" training.

The decline of herbology was hastened by two subsequent events, both occuring at about the same time: the commercial availability of penicillin and related "wonder drugs" that cured many of the diseases of the day quickly and reliably, and World War II, which cut off supplies of herbs from around the world and gave great stimulus to the synthetic drug industry.

Advocates of herbal remedies persisted through these times, but most were men (very few women) who had little education and whose theories and claims often went completely counter to the accepted modern understanding of human physiology, disease etiology, and treatment. Contrasting concepts are not in themselves problematic, but had these advocates received some training in the more "orthodox" view and had they experienced a wider range of natural healing traditions, they would have made a much better case for their particular views and could have explained their differences from orthodoxy in a meaningful way. Too often, however, they simply by-passed addressing the educated public and sought out those who were more gullible. This is not to say that the herbs and other therapies that they advocated weren't good: in many cases they worked quite well. But both the credibility and the unity of herbology and natural healing suffered greatly as a result of this type of advocacy.

The best known advocates of herbology and naturopathy in the U.S. include Samuel Thomson (the founder of "Thomsonian Medicine"), Jethro Kloss, and John Christopher. Each has provided advice about diet (avoid meat, sugar, processed foods, nicotine, alcohol, etc; fast occasionally), hydrotherapy (use baths and hot and cold compresses as therapy), enemas (use them frequently), and herbs. As a result of the work of these men and others like them, many millions of Americans have been experimenting with herbal remedies and other aspects of naturopathy.

While the basic tenets of American naturopathy have remained fairly constant over the past century, much has changed since the works of Thomson (end of the 18th century), Kloss (early 20th century), and even Christopher (who produced a major work on herbology in the early 1970's that was finally published as *School of Natural Healing* in 1976). New or different diseases have come to our attention, new products for health care have been discovered and developed, new herbs are being used (especially numerous imports from China, but also from India, Africa, and South America), new methods of therapy have been popularized (e.g. acupuncture and reflexology), and new approaches to herbal combining, therapeutic technique, and diagnosis have been integrated into the American model from other cultures, such as Oriental healing arts.

Smokey Santillo, having studied naturopathy for many years at several different schools, and being an experienced practitioner of herbology, has the necessary background to provide an updated expression of American naturopathy. For example, the herb information in this book, compared to other works, has been expanded to include new herbs, the presentation of the knowledge has been much better organized; herbs that are no longer commercially available and those not commonly used by herbalists have been deleted. Hydrotherapy and the use of enemas is explained here in much greater detail. The dietary suggestions in this book are based on the teachings of raw food advocates, many of whom have developed their ideas quite recently — during the past two decades. There are strong recommendations to avoid animal products and to develop a long-term committment to reduce the amount of cooking. This emphasis is drawn from the fact that during the past fifty years the American population has moved further and further away from natural foods and has adopted, as common habit, the use of processed foods high in protein, fat, and sugar, low in fiber and usually overcooked. It also represents a broad concern for the nutritional value of foods, with the recognition that vitamins and other nutritional factors are damaged by cooking. It should be noted here that other herbal traditions, notably the Oriental, advocate just the opposite—avoidance of too much raw food and reliance on cooked foods (but then, these Eastern cultures have not yet suffered under the influence of processed food, excessive meat consumption, etc. for many decades).

New treatment schemes have been developed in this book for many common ailments taking into account the recent experiences of herbalists with new herbs or new combinations. Therapeutic principles presented here are based not only on the long-held theories of naturopathy, but are also influenced by the important contributions of Chinese herbology.

Natural Healing with Herbs develops a very basic thesis about health and disease: living in harmony with nature (eating natural foods, moderation in all activities, adequate rest and exercise, etc.) promotes health, and deviations from this promote the accumulations of toxins in the body ("toxemia") and reduced nerve energy ("enervation"). The toxins, and more importantly, the body's attempts to eliminate them, produce the disease symptoms that most people experience. One thus comes to view most diseases as an uncomfortable feeling resulting from natural healing (cleansing) processes being pushed too hard. To rid oneself of disease, one first stops adding toxins to the body by fasting, resting, and by draining the colon of wastes (using enemas). Then, one promotes the natural detoxification processes by the use of blood purifying herbs, plus various external applications (local changes in temperature using hydrotherapy, or herbal preparations). This simple set of practices is complicated by the fact that each disease has its characteristic set of symptoms and areas of the body that are most severely affected. The bulk of this book, then, tells you precisely how to choose the appropriate herbs to relieve uncomfortable symptoms, strengthen individual organs, and aid the detoxification process at different stages of the ailment. It similarly tells you how to best utilize fasts or specific foods, hydrotherapy, and enemas.

In reading this book, one quickly sees that Smokey Santillo does not advocate a passive approach to treating disease that is so commonly promoted today. One does not simply take some herb capsules, or drink a few cups of bitter tea and then expect to become completely healthy and free of the disorder. In fact, Smokey advocates one of the most aggressive programs of health care in use today: fasting, frequent use of enemas, the combining of several herbs to make a more effective remedy, external applications of herbs, multiple baths or local applications of water, homeopathic remedies, and special diets are all considered in treating any ailment, severe (such as cancer) or mild (such as the common cold). All this may seem too much trouble for some, but in Smokey's view the benefits to health obtained by pursuing a vigorous course of therapy and by following it up with a controlled diet are well worth it. Even if you opt to use only one or two of the many therapeutic techniques in treating an ailment, this book will be very helpful in guiding you step by step in choosing the appropriate therapy and applying it in the proper manner.

As editor, my major concern has been to insure the highest possible degree of interconnection between sections within a chapter and also between one chapter and the next, so that the book presents a unified picture of naturopathy. This represents no easy task: modern American naturopathy is really a conglomerate of several theoretical propositions and several practical approaches that have never been formally linked. It is my hope that this book will lay the groundwork for additional efforts to integrate the American natural healing arts. Naturopathy may then serve as a viable adjunct to the dominant medical system.

Subhuti Dharmananda, Ph.D.
Director, Institute for Traditional
Medicine and Preventive Health Care
Santa Cruz, California 95060
October 1983

ACKNOWLEDGEMENTS

Dr. Thurman Fleet (founder of the Concept-Therapy Institute); Charles Mattox, George Fleet, Warren McKenney (Executive Committee, Concept-Therapy Institute); Mike Santillo; Shelley Benevento (food specialist); Gene Ross; Ed Smith (herbalist); Robert Thomson (author of "Natural Medicine" - McGraw-Hill); Robert Bauman, Naprapath; Dr. Stutzer; Tim Lewis (my work-out partner); Jim Fein (attorney); the Tucson Mountain Beamers; Dr. Phil Zimmerman; Bruce Fairchild; Paul Lee (Chi Herbal Products, Santa Cruz, California); Klark Black, Karl Lifferth, Mike Corrigan (Nature's Way Products, Inc. representatives); Dale Black; Subhuti Dharmananda (editor); Dr. John R. Christopher; Jym Marinakas, Don Hirschi (Myopractors); Linda Forbes (Chinese Herbalist); Victoras Kulvinskas (author of "Survival into the 21st Century"); Dr. Ann Wigmore; Shari Polk, Sandy Morris Snelling, Linda Kapitan (typists); Tom Murr, Rita Friend (Better Health Products); Babes; Dr. Juts-Cheraux; Dan McCue; Gary Heuck; Dr. Bernard Jensen; Michio Kushi; Joe Zuccarello (Hohm Press); Jimi Steinitz (Publicist); Jeff Kinart; John Shay; Jerry Cacciatore; Aaron Scheff, D.C.; Pat Hursey; Mr. and Mrs. Bedell; Kati and Ernie; Dale Bennett (Chamberlin's Natural Foods, Winter Park, Florida); Sandi and Lynn Dostal.

INTRODUCTION

We are facing, late in this twentieth century, the possible destruction of modern civilization. Poised between total annihilation of the human race through nuclear warfare and rapid degeneration of physical and mental condition, mankind is in the midst of the greatest biological crisis ever experienced in written history.

To redirect the human race from its routes of decline, all philosophies and cultures, thoughts and ideas, wisdom and knowledge, and arts and techniques throughout the world must unite regardless of differences in theory and practice.

Now that human existence is at stake, ancient and modern, East and West, must join in cooperation. The contributions and advances of the modern system of allopathic medicine over the past several centuries are well appreciated and recognized, but are not enough to assure the health of people on this planet. In order to preserve and develop health and well-being, it is necessary to bring about the active participation of every individual and family. Towards this aim, the natural healing arts, which have been practiced widely for several thousand years by traditional cultures in various areas of our world, have to be recovered for daily application by all.

Needless to say, the central issue in the creation of healthy society is daily lifestyle. The optimum lifestyle is one within a clean environment—including air, water and soil; it incorporates sound dietary practice, using macrobiotically selected and prepared whole grains, vegetables, beans, sea vegetables, fruits and occasionally animal food. This lifestyle includes having a spirit of gratitude, an appreciation for the universe, nature, society and people.

Along with this common base in daily life, it is also necessary to develop additional methods of health maintenance. These may include such practices as acupuncture, moxibustion, shiatsu massage, yoga, sports, breathing exercises, meditation, chanting, and other physical and mental practices. These are especially appropriate in the alleviation of disorders for which medical attention is not necessarily required.

However, within the scope of health maintenance and relief from disorders lies a huge domain: natural healing with herbs, the origin of modern medication. In the Orient—where even now a large portion of medication and drugs are comprised of natural herbs—and in the West, the history of the use of natural herbs goes back to unknown times. Some of this information has been preserved in the classics, while some has been passed along in families from one generation to the next, or kept within a small circle of people.

Many modern-day people have had experiences with their grandmothers' "prescriptions" for headache, pain, menstrual irregularity, nausea, nosebleed, shoulder pain, and other symptoms. As with grandmother's practical wisdom, the use of herbs—for both internal use and external compresses or plasters—can often achieve rapid solution of a problem.

The underlying principle of herb medicine is twofold. Like conventional medicine and drugs, the chemical compounds in particular herbs have, through time and experience, come to be considered the active agents—stimulants, inhibitors, supplements or synthesizers. This first aspect of herbs spawned the production of chemical compounds. Their extraction from particular herbs later evolved into the form of conventional medicinal drugs.

The second aspect of herb medicine is that of energies. The amount, quality, and degree of forces released and generated from particular herbs contribute to the alteration of energies in various metabolic functions and energy streams through meridians, resulting in the improvement of balance in physical and mental conditions as a whole. However, this facet of herbs has not been utilized in modern conventional medicine simply due to the lack of understanding of energy, vibration, or forces which are more difficult to perceive and measure than material compounds. Yet, the real contribution of herbs to physical and mental recovery is largely in this aspect.

For satisfactory utilization of energies, vitalities, vibrations and forces preserved in particular herbs, extractions of compounds should be avoided. It is recommended, rather, to use the whole or a natural portion of the herb.

It is also important to understand the conditions under which these energies peak in natural herbs, for instance: during summer or winter, under the full moon or new moon, in the mountains or valleys, on dry land or wet muddy soil, in the morning or evening. All of these natural environmental conditions should be carefully considered when herbs are collected.

Furthermore, it is important to consider the appropriate processes for increasing or decreasing the natural energy of an herb. Such techniques as drying, boiling, roasting, powdering, or combining with other herbs of similar or different type of energies, may be utilized in order to create satisfactory results.

Natural healing with herbs is in itself a huge science. It embodies a complex which requires the understanding of nature, the earth, galactic motion, wind, weather, climate, soil, water, as well as the characteristics of plants and conditions of people. The application of herbs for natural healing actually requires unlimited wisdom, insight, and an understanding of the order of the universe, nature and humanity. It also requires varying the kind and combination of herbs, and methods of processing, according to individual circumstance and personal differences.

To our great pleasure, "Smokey" Santillo has compiled this comprehensive anthology on the use of herbs. Here Mr. Santillo has assembled major bodies of traditional knowledge on the usage and effects of herbs. This book is essential for people who wish to develop their understanding of health maintenance.

I am personally grateful to Mr. Santillo for the reason that I have been also concerned with the health and well-being of people in modern society as a biological and psychological ground for one peaceful, healthy world. This is all the more important at this critical time when social trends point towards development of more bionation and psychonation, or artificialization, because of a shortage of wisdom and knowledge with regard to natural approaches to health. These natural approaches, within daily lifestyle itself, can be practiced by any person with common sense.

We sincerely hope that, in a united effort with all modern conventional medical knowledge and technique, traditional and alternative approaches, and with sound dietary practice and healthy natural lifestyles, *Natural Healing With Herbs* may serve as a milestone in opening a new era for health.

January, 1984
Michio Kushi
Brookline, Massachusetts

THE NATURE OF HEALTH AND DISEASE

We are complex beings, functioning on physical, mental, and spiritual levels. It is no easy task to define the "right way" of living in order to maintain health and vigor, yet we all sense that certain types of attitudes and habits improve health while other types are detrimental. I think that it is possible to be healthy, but only when one understands the laws governing man and his environment, and then acts upon this knowledge.

The factors most strongly influencing our health include our emotions and thoughts, our diet, and our rest and exercise. While the individuality of each human confounds any attempt to draw up specific rules for behavior that would insure health and longevity, even a brief period of observation of our society reveals the important changes that could overcome most ailments.

Negative thoughts and attitudes are far too prevalent and produce physiological responses ultimately giving rise to constipation, nutritional imbalance, hyperacid stomach, ulcers, hypertension, and other problems. Fear, worry, anger, anxiety, jealousy, destructive criticism, vanity, hatred, envy, selfishness, and greed are examples of the negative mental attitudes that are so destructive to the body. In contrast, there is strong healing potential in the positive thoughts and attitudes of faith, hope, generosity, aspiration, patience, sympathy, kindness, courage, forgiveness, duty, and love. True health remains an unreachable goal until man gains control over his thoughts and recognizes that they can be healing or disease-causing.

Dietary indiscretion is a clearly established cause of many disorders from stomach ache to heart disease and cancer. Too much meat, dairy products, processed foods, coffee, alcohol, cooked foods, and highly seasoned meals leave a residue of toxins in the body. This strains the body's natural eliminative processes and interferes with other physiological functions. Resistance to disease organisms is greatly reduced, absorption and utilization of nutrients is hampered, and chronic symptoms develop. On the other hand, raw fruits and vegetables, fresh juices, and regular fasting help to cleanse the system of accumulated toxins, reinforce the natural functions and and aid the healing processes. While most people know the value of washing the outside of the body to stay healthy, too few have given recognition to the vital importance of inner cleanliness.

Physical exercise strengthens the heart, lungs, and circulation while toning the musculature. Oxygen and nutrients are efficiently carried to every organ and tissue not only during exercise, but throughout the day as a result of vigorous physical activity. Exercise will regulate the appetite and body weight, help overcome nervousness and insomnia, and improve mental concentration and stamina. The type of exercise chosen should be one which feels rejuvenating and does not cause pain or discomfort. You should feel good when you finish exercising, not exhausted. To sit lethargic day after day destroys the posture, encourages shallow breathing, and reduces the functional capacity of every organ. Even 20 minutes of vigorous activity a day can satisfy most of your body's needs.

Just as one needs physical activity, one also must have adequate rest. It is not good to do any one line of work day in and day out, not even if you love your work. Diverting the concentration in recreation and other enjoyable things of life will renew one's strength and improve efficiency. Resting occasionally during a hectic period will prevent an otherwise inevitable sickness that forces bedrest and a slower pace without the enjoyment of a planned rest period. Fresh air, natural scenery, quiet, and contemplation are all essentials regardless of the lifestyle you have chosen.

According to the views of naturopathy, then, the primary cause of disease is the failure to take into account the importance of positive attitudes, proper diet, and balanced exercise and rest, as well as other factors that may be regarded as natural laws of living. By violating these natural laws, we produce in the body a state of "toxemia," that is, accumulation of poisons and waste products. The toxins may be introduced, as in the case of eating impure foods or smoking cigarettes, or they may be produced by the body, as occurs with severe stress, nervousness, and negative emotion, or they may fail to be eliminated because of lack of exercise, inadequate rest, or inability of the organ to deal with a foreign substance. As a result of this toxemia we also experience "enervation," lowered vital energy due to the poisoning of the nervous system, the blockage of blood flow by accumulated toxins, and the inability of organ systems to properly communicate with one another when the blood supply is polluted.

Most diseases (and chronic or acute symptoms which are not yet identified with specific diseases) are really the result of an overtaxed eliminative system. As the body does its best to purge the poisons from the system, the person suffering from toxemia may experience excessive mucus discharge, vomiting or diarrhea, sweating, skin rashes, and other symptoms. If the eliminative organs are sufficiently exhausted or blocked, the individual may experience pain, constipation, headaches, red eyes, lethargy, swellings, and even mental disturbance. Thus, many sicknesses may be viewed as part of the healing process in which the body is trying to overcome a toxic condition.

If one applies drugs to suppress the symptoms, then one also suppresses the healing and cleansing processes. The disease may appear to be gone, but the toxemia has not been relieved; in fact, the drugs may even make the toxic condition much worse. In a matter of time, the body eventually finds another means of eliminating toxins, and this often manifests as an even more severe disease. The naturopath is thus interested not in stopping the disease, but in helping it run its course in an efficient and more comfortable manner. By using a cleansing diet and short fasts, cleaning the colon by using enemas, aiding eliminative processes and purifying the blood through the proper choice of herbs, and by other methods, the natural physician quickly clears up the disease by clearing up the underlying toxic state.

It is not always easy to overcome sickness. Simply popping a few herb capsules or drinking a bitter tea may not be enough. One usually has to use a vigorous approach, and if the disease is a chronic one, the therapy may be a lengthy one. Some individuals will naturally resist undertaking so many changes in lifestyle and taking the time necessary to apply the essential therapies. They may think that it is not all worth it, yet they rarely weigh the consequences of continuing with lowered vitality, annoying recurrent symptoms, and increasingly severe diseases. Those who cherish life and understand that wonderful rewards await those who pursue true health realize that the efforts are all worth while. Each person must make up his own mind as to whether he wants health and wants to take the effort to achieve health or if he wants disease and the consequences.

We must come to realize the great need for preventive health care programs, accepting responsibility for our health and modifying our lifestyles to minimize disease. To increase health at the individual level will lead to social reconstruction. It was recently revealed for example, that some two million surgical operations, costing four billion dollars and more than ten thousand lives were unnecessary. If the public focuses its attention on healthy living rather than on symptomatic relief and crisis intervention, it will take a tremendous burden off our health care system and our society as a whole.

DIAGNOSIS

Diagnosis is discovering what the nature of an illness is by analyzing the emotions and the symptoms that are manifesting inside and outside of the body. Although diagnosis is mostly determined by a skilled therapist or physician, the simple methods discussed here will aid in determining what the disease is and how to choose the proper therapy. This, of course, is the first step that is taken before treating any disease. I strongly suggest that if there is any question in mind about what the disease is or how to treat it, to seek help from someone who is qualified in this area.

In this chapter we will be discussing a mixture of diagnostic methods. We will be discussing the Chinese methods based upon the yin and yang principles which will aid the reader in getting an overall picture of the disease. Diseases can be classified in Chinese medicine as either hot, cold, yin, yang, excess or deficient, internal or external. In getting a final picture of the disease, there are some naturopathic methods of diagnosis which take the primary and secondary symptoms of a disease into view which we will incorporate into the Chinese approach. Once this is accomplished, the therapy needed for treatment will be easy to choose. The therapies will be discussed in the next section.

The constitution of the individual is considered first by Chinese physicians which basically indicates whether the patient has a yin or yang constitution. This helps to determine which diseases a person tends to gravitate towards and his fundamental tendencies in eating and thinking. People with yang constitutions tend to be in a hurry both in eating and thinking and usually develop develop yang ailments. Yin constitutions seem to be more passive, inactive, slower at making decisions and have tendencies to develop yin diseases. However, this is not always the case. A yang constitution can have yin ailments, and a yin constitution can have yang ailments. In treating these imbalances, diet and herbal therapies are used. More concentrated parts of plants and vegetables would be considered yang, while less concentrated food and plant substances would be yin. Fruits and vegetables would be considered yin foods while seeds, nuts, grains, meats and root vegetables are considered yang. Leaves and flowers of herbs would be yin, while the root seeds and rhizomes of plants are yang. Hence in treating imbalances you use the opposite characteristics. Yin ailments are treated with yang foods and herbs, while yang ailments are treated with yin foods and herbs to bring back the balance. Never use extremes to treat an imbalance. If a person eats only fruit, putting them on 80% grain is shocking to the system. Use slow, gradual changes in bringing an individual back into balance.

To make this chapter easier to understand for people not familiar with the Chinese terms yin and yang, we will substitute the words strong for yang and weak for yin. Here are some basic physical features that divide weak and strong constitutions:

WEAK	STRONG
Inactive individuals	Active individuals
Small bones	Large bones
Negative, shy, timid	Positive, aggressive, outgoing
Slumps over	Stands erect
Large head	Small head
Introspective	Extroverted
Large distance between eyes & mouth	Short distance between eyes & mouth
Nose is long, expanded	Nose is contracted, flat
Eyes are large	Eyes are small
Straight hair	Wavy, curly hair

Those with strong constitutions are usually treated with more vigorous therapies, stronger herbs, longer fasts, and more extreme water temperatures in hydrotherapy. Those with more fragile and weak constitutions are treated with more conservative therapies like milder herbs, short fasts, local hydrotherapies and tonifying therapies.

We will now discuss "differential diagnosis," where we will be using four pairs of opposites, the first being simply weak and strong, which is determined by the constitutions which we have discussed. The three remaining pairs of opposites will tell you whether you have a cold, hot, excess or deficient condition and whether it is internal or external, which is determined by the symptoms.

EXCESS CONDITIONS

Cold/excess: This is excessive cold condition. Excessive liquid intake, cold weather, too many raw foods (raw foodists sometimes tend to overeat raw fruits and leafy green vegetables and not balancing it later with more raw seeds, nuts, carrots, cabbage and other hardy foods), drugs that expand the consciousness and emotions such as fear and sympathy, tend to harm the functions of the organs and cause them to decrease their activity. The symptoms that might manifest are coldness, sluggishness, body aches, diarrhea, digestive disturbances, bloating, darkness under the eyes, low body temperatures, cold hands and feet, muscle cramps and spasms and desire for warmth. The tongue usually has a white coating on it. Cold type ailments are generally treated with cooked foods or broths, warm baths, stimulating and tonifying herbs that have an acrid, aromatic or sweet flavor. This type of an approach to treating cold conditions will help raise body heat and improve circulation, digestion and elimination. The body needs proper heat for the oxidation of nutrients and to burn up toxins.

Heat/excess: This is excessive heat. This can be caused by a diet high in meat, salt, tobacco, coffee and other acid causing foods. Hot weather, excessive excitement and grief, pathogens like bacteria, mucus and excessive toxins and lack of nutrients cause the organs to become overactive and stimulated. Symptoms that you will see are high fevers, thirst, recurrent sore throat, nervousness, painful sores, red face, red eyes, strong body odors, hypertension, gallstones, heart disease, dry skin, inflammations, burning hands and feet, infections and the desire for cool foods and water. The tongue usually has a thick, yellow coating. Hot type ailments are generally treated with raw foods, fruit and vegetable juices, cool baths, anti-inflammatory herbs with a bitter taste, enemas and a calming environment. The main objective here is to reduce body heat and eliminate excessive acid conditions.

DEFICIENT CONDITIONS

These conditions are different than the ones we have been discussing. The symptoms may look similar but the cause is different. In the excess conditions we described, excessive toxins and heavy foods caused the hot condition, and excessive fluids, raw foods and cold weather etc. produced the cold condition. In these deficient conditions, the cold and heat manifests because of inadequate nutrients, poor absorption of nutrients, lack of exercise or due to some deficient metabolic activity. The cause of deficient problems is exactly the opposite of the excess causative factors.

Usually one of the main ways to determine that a deficient condition is present is that the energy is low and the illness is more chronic.

Cold/deficiency: This is when there is deficient body heat and organ activity. The nutrients and fluids feeding the organs are still normal, but the functions of the organs have diminished. Because the activity of the organs is subnormal, there is less activity and inner heat is not produced so we have a cold condition. Injury, not recovering from sickness properly, nutrient deficiency, lack of exercise, drugs, depression and actually any extreme which weakens the body enervates the organs and can result in a deficiency. Some symptoms are low resistance to disease, lethargy, chills, poor circulation, poor eyesight, neuralgia, mucus discharge, frequent urination, weak bladder control, impotence, lower back pain, diminished hearing and weakness etc. The tongue in a cold deficient condition has no coating, is moist and has a pale look to it. Although chronic and acute disease can be caused by deficiencies, all chronic diseases have a deficiency whether in nutrients, organ functions or energy level.

Cold deficient conditions are treated with tonic, astringent, stimulating, nutritive and warming herbal therapy. More nutrients and protein are usually needed in cold deficient problems.

Heat/deficiency: The functions and activities of the organs are normal, but the nutrients and fluids that feed them are deficient. The cause of this condition is lack of protein, vitamin and mineral deficiency, poor blood, low calorie intake and loss of blood.

Heat deficient problems differ from heat excess in that it is not a clear cut hot condition with clear cut symptoms, but rather an alternating hot and cold condition, and with more of a variety of acute conditions, constipation, thirst, dry skin, ringing in the ears, sore throats, skin eruptions, itching and alternating chills and fevers. Premature aging, anemia, allergies and loss of vitality are other possible symptoms. Deficiency with heat illnesses are treated with tonic, cooling (antipyretic) and astringent herbs. Sometimes demulcent herbs like comfrey, mullein and slippery elm are used to treat these conditions when they are accompanied with dry symptoms, such as dry coughs, dry skin, mouth and throat. Avoid astringent herbs during dry conditions because they contain tannic acid which is drying to the internal tissues. No stimulation is used when treating heat deficient conditions because it will only worsen the problem when trying to tone and build the body.

INTERNAL AND EXTERNAL DISEASE

Another way of looking at diseases in Chinese medicine is whether they are external or internal. External refers to conditions in the early stages. These illnesses are usually acute and have not penetrated deeper into the internal organs. External diseases primarily affect body parts like the skin, extremities, head, muscles, sinuses, throat, ears and digestive system. External surface conditions are usually acute ailments of short duration such as colds and flu.

The therapies for surface external ailments are often symptom relieving and for curative effects using diaphoretics (sweating agents), alteratives (blood purifiers), carminatives (which are digestive normalizing), etc. Hydrotherapy, colonics and enemas are also used to reduce the internal toxins.

External cold conditions are characterized by alternating fever/chills, lack of perspiration and a thin, white coating on the tongue. In these cases you would use the same therapy as mentioned above with more stimulating carminative herbs to cause more circulation and heat. External heat conditions are treated with cooling (antipyretic) herbs that will give a calming affect coupled with the detoxification methods mentioned. Noticeable symptoms that help determine external heat conditions are fevers, sweating, a little thirst and a thin, yellow coating on the tongue.

Internal refers to deeper and more chronic diseases which usually affect the major organs as chronic bronchitis or asthma, gastric ulcers, chronic constipation, heart disease, liver/gallbladder diseases, nephritis, cancer, etc. The surface of the body may also be affected by these internal organ disturbances–eczema and other chronic skin diseases, chronic arthritis and neuralgia, recurrent migraines, etc. Internal conditions are treated by taking a special cleansing diet (see cleansing diet in this book) and using herbs that detoxify and remove obstructions and strengthen the organs.

Coldness and heat can also accompany internal conditions. Internal cold conditions are characterized by symptoms of chills, cold limbs, pallor complexion, diarrhea, clear, profuse urine and a pale looking tongue.

In treating internal cold conditions, along with the chosen diet and detoxification methods, warm broths, stimulating and carminative herbs are used. Internal heat conditions have high fevers, thirst, sweating, irritability, red eyes, constipation, yellow urine and a red tongue with a yellow coating. The same detoxification and diet can be used as was suggested in treating internal cold conditions, but cooling (antipyretic) herbs are used without stimulating and carminative herbs. If there is excessive dryness in the mouth, throat and intestines, use demulcent herbs in the treatment.

ANALYZING SYMPTOM INFORMATION

Before a therapy can be chosen or a herbal formula put together, all the symptoms of the disease must be analyzed. Here are a few suggestions that will help in analyzing and determining symptoms.

1. List and analyze body parts that are affected. This will help you determine which herbs you are going to use and which body systems might possibly be disturbed. Determine whether it is an acute or chronic problem. Acute problems are those with a quick onset, strong symptoms, a self-limiting nature and can often be treated simply using one to four herbs. Colds, fevers and flu are examples of acute diseases. The purpose here is to give comfort and to speed the body's defense reactions.

A chronic illness has been present and irritating to the body for a long period of time and could have impaired organic functioning of several body parts.

You will need this information to help you determine the intensity of the treatment and how long you will be treating the condition. Abnormal body secretions are important indications to consider because external fomentations, salves, hydrotherapy, douches and enemas will help counteract these symptoms. Check to see if the symptoms reappear at any particular time. Sometimes if the symptoms appear after meals it could be something the individual ate. If they appear in the mornings, the body may be having difficulty eliminating the toxins from the day before and cleansing herbs and enemas can be used in the mornings to aid elimination. Often symptoms appear at night when the temperature of the body decreases and the metabolism slows down. This means that the constitution is weak and tonification is needed. Infections travel through the body when it is at a low energy level so antibiotic herbs can be given particularly in the evenings. Often there will be fever or chills. This can indicate whether you have a hot or cold condition which will help you determine what therapy to use.

If there are cold extremities, there is trapped heat within the body. Stimulating therapy is needed to circulate the energy and help remove the toxins. Check the blood pressure to see if it is high or low. High blood pressure means that there are toxins and too much sodium in the blood stream. You would design a low sodium, low protein diet. Low blood pressure could mean that the adrenal glands are weak. Kelp and licorice root will help build up the adrenal glands. Is it a disease that is spreading rapidly? If so, the most aggravating symptoms must be treated immediately. Check to see if there are immediate causes such as food allergies, weather or extreme emotions. If so, eliminate them. Ask if it is in the family history. This will help you determine whether it is an acute, chronic or genetic problem. If it is incurable, or curable only by an act of faith, you should know this so as not to make curative promises.

Ask if there have been old symptoms that might have led to the recent illness such as pain, burning areas in the body, constant headaches or constipation. Remember when certain trains of symptoms are present in some organs or apparatus of the body, there are almost always other symptoms present that seem to be unrelated or quite remote and which the person describing the symptoms is not really aware of until their attention is brought to it. Some examples are constant headaches, which can be caused by uterine afflictions. Constipation can cause skin eruptions and toxic blood conditions from the reabsorption of poisons from the bowel and intestines, so look for subjective symptoms.

This will help you determine the cause of the disease and whether the symptoms you are now noticing are a primary (causative) or secondary (brought on by old symptoms not present now, but have manifested other problematic symptoms). In these cases where old symptoms have brought about new ones, the organs have been weakened and you have a chronic condition.

2. Some symptoms are primary, others are reflex. This means that after a chronic disease has become established, which we will consider the primary symptom, other modifications of health take place which might be secondary symptoms. This can confuse the picture. An example would be edema which we will consider the primary symptom. The swelling can be caused by sluggish kidneys and because the kidneys are not eliminating properly, the skin could be eliminating the waste, showing some rashes or other symptoms. So, treating the kidneys would be a proper treatment. Treating the skin is dealing with the reflex symptoms (secondary) which would not be getting to the cause of the illness. One way to avoid this mistake is to question the person about all the earliest symptoms. That will help you find out what preceded the development of the edema. Disease travels certain paths of development and certainly knowledge of pathology would help in these cases. Also study the preceding section on internal and external diseases. By recognizing specific symptoms you can tell whether you have an internal (chronic) or external (acute) illness. If it seems to be an internal problem, then the external symptoms would be secondary symptoms. The primary cause would be internal and your treatment will now be more specific and directional.

The totality of the symptoms must be the sole indication to determine the proper choice of herbs.

3. Primary symptoms are the ones that usually are considered first, these are usually the most acute and aggravating symptoms.

4. The secondary symptoms are less aggravating. They should be listed not only to help give you a full picture of the disease, but to be treated along with the primary symptoms through the choice of herbs used in formulation. (See Herbal Formulation). Secondary symptoms do not need to be the focus of treatment because the primary problems once treated, will not produce the secondary symptoms.

HERBAL THERAPIES AND THEIR APPLICATION

A therapy is a method that is used in treating disease. There are ten major therapies which I have used extensively. Sometimes more than one therapy is used in bringing about a progressive cure. For example, a patient has nausea and a high fever. In this case the stomach might be holding old putrifying food causing the fever. The first therapy would be emesis (vomiting), followed by a relaxing and soothing tea (peppermint or spearmint). For the fever, diaphoresis (sweating) would be my next therapy to stimulate circulation and perspiration. Once the illness is over, I might use tonification therapy to help rebuild the system. So, in this one case, three different therapies were used to bring balance back to the system. Many times only one therapy is needed. Other times, several therapies must follow one another or two or more therapies can be applied at the same time. For instance, a fever may be present with urinary retention. Diaphoresis and deobstruent therapies would be used simultaneously. Diuretics are used as a part of deobstruent therapy. Diaphoretic and diuretic herbs can be combined or used separately.

During all acute or chronic illnesses, always consider using an external treatment (poultices, fomentations, hydrotherapy) in conjunction with an internal treatment (infusions, syrups, tinctures).

The energy level of the patient should be considered before therapy begins. Some therapies are contraindicated during certain illnesses. Emesis and purgation therapies have a tendency to drain energy from the patient. If a weak, debilitated person needs therapy, these two therapies should not be used. More of this will be discussed with each therapy.

Always be ready and observant to determine the best therapies to use during the changing course of the illness. Many times the therapy will need to be changed frequently if the course of disease changes. For example: If when using diaphoresis or purgation, the individual being treated becomes weak and deficient, reducing the dosage or deleting the therapy entirely for a short time may be indicated. Also, switching to tonification therapy to build up the energy level would be beneficial. Then when the individual regains his strength, he may again be treated by diaphoresis therapy or other detoxification methods. Following all therapies, tonification therapy is used to help tone and rebuild the strength of the person that has been treated.

A. Blood Purification Therapy
B. Carminative Therapy
C. Deobstruent Therapy
D. Diaphoresis Therapy
E. Emesis Therapy
F. Heat Dispelling Therapy
G. Purgation Therapy
H. Stimulation Therapy
I. Tonification Therapy
J. Tranquilization Therapy

A. BLOOD PURIFICATION THERAPY

Blood purification therapy is the therapy that is used to purify the blood and lymphatic system if acids and other poisons are causing disease, imbalances and irritations of glands, organs and body tissues.

If the blood and lymphatic system were pure, no disease would exist. The bloodstream is the river of life and during disease and health, the blood is constantly neutralizing poisons and carrying toxins to be eliminated. Air pollution, chemical preservatives, food wastes, the body's natural cellular waste and stress can cause an accumulation of toxins in the body and result in disease at any organ, joint or tissue site.

In aiding blood and lymph cleansing, alterative herbs are used such as burdock root, red clover, echinacea, chaparral, garlic, yellowdock, dandelion, etc. Whenever there is an illness, blood purification, along with bowel cleansing (enemas, colonics) should be considered to assist blood purification therapy. Short fasts using water or vegetable broths, raw vegetable juices like carrot, celery, beet, watercress and citrus juices will help neutralize poisons in the bloodstream and will stimulate the cleansing functions of the liver, bowels and kidneys. Deep breathing and exercise will aid in lung and skin elimination. Dry skin brushing and hydrotherapy help clean the blood and lymph and is very good for elderly people and weak individuals that cannot move around easily and be exposed to more energetic therapies.

Some blood cleansers are diuretics, others are hepatics (liver cleansers), others will influence other organs. Take blood cleansing herbs between meals on an empty stomach. If they cause nausea or stomach upset, adding some licorice root, ginger or other carminatives to the combination usually will help. If this fails, take the herbs with meals or change the formula so it can be taken on an empty stomach.

The kidneys, lungs, liver, bowels and skin are the major eliminatory organs of the body. Always consider herbs that will aid elimination through them to help purify the blood. Stimulating hot and cold alternating fomentations over the weak organs will stimulate cleansing of these body parts.

Blood purification therapy is especially indicated during gout, arthritis, rheumatism, skin diseases, all toxic conditions, during fasts and periodically during cleansing and transition diets, acute and chronic illnesses, infections and low grade fevers.

Blood purification therapy is used to treat heat/excess, cold/deficient, internal and external problems.

In heat/excess the toxins in the blood and lymphatic system have to be removed. Toxins and poisons produce heat in the body. During cold/deficient illness an individual is feeling cold because of the organs not functioning properly. If there is heavy congestion in certain areas of the body, deobstruent therapy is indicated, but if the organs are receiving toxic, poor blood which is hindering the function of them, blood purification is the suitable therapy.

Whether the condition is internal (chronic) or external (acute) the blood needs to be purified. It is one of the main therapies that can be used along with any other therapy needed.

B. CARMINATIVE THERAPY

Carminative therapy aids in bringing warmth, circulation, and stimulation to the deeper parts of the body.

Carminatives are herbs that aid in relieving gas and certain stomach discomforts. Improper food combining, constipation, overeating, eating while sick or uncomfortable, nervousness, junk food eating and eating late at night are some of the things that cause intestinal upset and bring about sickness. The remedy for many of these problems is carminative therapy. When there are chills, bloating caused by gas, a cold feeling in the stomach, constipation (always add a carminative to laxative formulas), poor digestion, slow circulation, colds, fevers, flu, chills and lower back pains are present, carminative therapy is indicated. Carminatives are also added to formulas to help tone and improve digestion.

Some carminatives are: (see carminatives)

Caraway	Ginger	Cardamon
Cayenne	Thyme	Fennel
Garlic	Anise	Cumin

Usually these herbs can be taken as a warm infusion, but they can also be taken in capsule or tablet form along with meals or after eating. Some of them are put into tincture form and can be brought to work or carried while traveling. The tinctures work very well when added to warm water.

This therapy is used to treat cold/deficient, and internal and external problems.

If an individual has a cold/deficient condition it has been a problem for some time, making it more chronic (internal).

The cause could be vitamin, protein or mineral deficiencies, internal congestion, lack of exercise, etc. The therapy will provide heat, circulation, and better absorption of vitamins and minerals, If congestion is hindering the activities of the organs, deobstruent therapy may be combined with carminative therapy. Tonification therapy can also be used if the problem is nutrient deficiency and if the body or specific organs need toning. Often times we will find external symptoms like cold extremities, internal fever but cold on the outside, lack of perspiration and skin itch. This can all be caused by deficient organ functions and inner congestion. Carminatives will work deep and improve circulation, stimulation and heat.

Contraindications. Bleeding bowels and ulcers are contraindications, although in small amounts (10% of a combination) they can be used with demulcent herbs to treat those conditions.

Carminatives are used to break fevers and will produce inner heat. Many times a heavy, robust individual has enough natural heat and carminatives are then contraindicated.

C. DEOBSTRUENT THERAPY

This therapy is indicated whenever there are obstructions or accumulations in the body causing loss of energy and congestion. Overeating, too many dairy products and mucus-causing food, not enough exercise and eating late at night can cause these problems. Always consider a cleansing diet, fasting, hydrotherapy, exercise and bowel cleansing when using deobstruent therapy.

Many times there is a loss of energy flow in the stomach and intestines causing gastrointestinal disturbances resulting in nausea, vomiting, belching and flatulence. Sometimes there is blood stagnation in the abdomen of women causing gynecological problems. An excess of moisture and phlegm can accumulate in the digestive tract causing bloating, pain in the stomach, and heavy mucus conditions. Whether the congestion and blocked energy flow is in the lungs, colon, liver, kidneys, gall bladder, etc., deobstruent therapy is indicated.

The main objective of using this therapy is to break up and stimulate the movement of the built-up waste in these areas and to bring back the proper functions. Deobstruent therapy is used to treat lung congestion, kidney stones, constipation and any area in the body where there is congestion causing lack of blood flow.

There are many herbs that are categorized below that can be used to cleanse and eliminate obstructions for each body part. Choose the proper herb that best fits the symptoms being treated and put them into a formula and decide the best method of application. Study the herbs of your choice in the section on herbs in this book to get an understanding of their healing properties. For example, cascara sagrada is a cholagogue (an herb that decongests the gall bladder). It is also a digestive tonic. It would be a good herb to chose if the person being treated has symptoms such as weak digestion and gall bladder problems.

Most of the time these herbs are taken on an empty stomach or during short fasts until the obstructions are cleared. If a fast is not possible, take the herbs between meals on an empty stomach.

Cholagogue. These are herbs that promote the flow of bile. They are indicated when there are gall stones or congested bile during jaundice, hepatitis and constipation. The following are examples of cholagogues:

Cascara sagrada   Wild yam
Oregon grape root   Gentian

Cholagogues should be combined with antispasmodics or carminatives to ease gas, pain and cramps.

Contraindications. This therapy is contraindicated if bloody stools, large gall stones, hemorrhoids (chronic) are present.

Discutients. These herbs dissolve and remove tumors, abnormal growths, swellings and cysts. They can be used in fomentations and poultices also. Some examples of discutients are:

Garlic   Chaparral
Arnica   Wormwood

Contraindications. See a qualified physician to determine the correct diagnosis before utilizing discutients. Do not rely on discutients alone for malignant tumors, serious infections or growths that threaten the normal function of internal organs.

Expectorants. These herbs facilitate excretion of mucus from the lungs. They are indicated during asthma, colds, flu, lung congestion and coughs.

Elecampane   Comfrey   Lungwort
Yerba santa   Horehound

Contraindications. These herbs are contraindicated when bleeding from the lungs without excessive mucus is present.

Hepatics. These herbs influence and stimulate liver activity. They are indicated for jaundice, hepatitis, gas, poor digestion, liver congestion, gall stones and constipation. Some examples are:

Agrimony   Dandelion
Barberry   Wild yam

Contraindications. If the gall stones are large they may become trapped in the gall bladder duct. X-ray diagnosis may be needed to determine if stones are present.

Lithotriptics. These herbs are agents that dissolve and discharge urinary and bladder stones and gravel. They are indicated for kidney and bladder stones, cloudy urine, urine retention and prostate congestions. Examples are:

Gravel root   Hydrangea   Uva ursi
Parsley root   Corn silk   Dandelion

Anthelmintics. These herbs destroy intestinal worms and parasites. These conditions must be considered as obstructions in the body so they are included in deobstruent therapy (see anthelmintics). They are indicated for the presence of worms and parasites.

Tansy	Black walnut	Garlic
Wormwood	Wood sage	Senna

Contraindications. This treatment is contraindicated when diarrhea, hemorrhoids and bloody bowels are present. If these conditions are present along with worms, add demulcents and astringent herbs combined with anthelmintics.

Deobstruent therapy is used to treat external (surface), internal (deep), heat/excess, and cold/deficient illness. An example in using deobstruent therapy is in the case of high fever (heat/excess) being caused by congestion some place in the body, lungs, stomach, etc. and the body is trying to burn it off. You could use herbs that would be appropriate to clean out those organs of the excess mucus and the fever (heat) would also be reduced. Here, you could combine stimulation therapy (to improve circulation) along with deobstruent therapy.

Cold/deficient means that the organs are not functioning properly. If the cause is congestion, mucus, or toxins, then deobstruent therapy is indicated. If the organs are in a weakened condition, tonification therapy will build up the deficiency.

Deobstruent therapy is used to treat internal problems. This means that there is congestion, mucus, or some type of blockage in the internal body parts. It is also used in cases when there are external symptoms that are caused by internal congestion. An example of this would be constipation. This is internal congestion, but a person could be manifesting skin rashes and body odor caused by reabsorption of waste from the bowel which is being eliminated through the pores of the skin.

D. DIAPHORESIS (Sweating) THERAPY

Diaphoresis therapy increases the circulation at the surface of the body, opening the pores to increase elimination of water through the skin (perspiration). This therapy strengthens the resistance of the surface, dispels internal toxins and relieves surface cold and minor skin conditions. It is almost always employed at the first stages of acute ailments.

When toxins accumulate in the body and cause blockages, the body temperature is elevated to oxidize and burn up these poisons. This is called a fever, which is a natural body defense. The cause of this of course, is related directly to improper diet such as overeating of refined foods, dairy products, meats and constipation and lack of exercise etc. These inner accumulations cut down circulation of blood and nerve energy to the surface of the body, so we have an inner fever and cold extremities. Diaphoresis therapy breaks through these blockages and normalizes circulation causing the poisons to be eliminated through the skin and other organs. Enemas and laxative herbs (purgation therapy) are also considered to move the poisons out through the bowels which assist in normalizing temperature and circulation. A short fast on citrus juice, water or vegetable juice would be appropriate during this therapy.

The herbs used for diaphoretic therapy are usually aromatic and spicy. They have volatile oils which circulate through the body breaking up cold blockages, improving circulation to the surface of the skin and exiting out through the pores. There are warming, stimulating diaphoretics which are used to stimulate sweating and when the person has a history of being cold and has chills. They include ginger, cinnamon, boneset, elder flowers, yarrow, pleurisy root, hyssop and sage. When the patient is in need of sweating therapy but is nervous, there are relaxing diaphoretics such as lemon balm, burdock root or seed, catnip, spearmint, thyme and chamomile. These are also indicated when children and infants need diaphoretic therapy.

Diaphoresis therapy is indicated for illnesses such as colds, flu, chills, neck and shoulder tension, beginning skin conditions, water accumulations in the flesh or joints (rheumatism and arthritis), minor headaches, itching, fevers, etc.

This therapy is also used for those people who have a tendency to be cold. In these cases, a combination of stimulating diaphoretic herbs can be used. More stimulating herbs are used in colder climates, less in warmer weather. Most diaphoretic teas if taken cold, will act as a diuretic.

When there is fever and inner heat, give the person a warm cup of tea made from one or more of the suggested appropriate herbs. Then have them take a hot bath until profuse sweating begins. Next, put them directly to bed without drying, but dressing them in warm bedclothes. Cover with heavy blankets. Herb teas may be administered while the person is in bed. Every few hours rinse them off well and repeat the therapy. See the section on Colds, Fevers and Flu for more detailed instructions.

To increase heat and dispel inner chills, cayenne tincture (5 to 15 drops) can be added to one or more of the teas, or taken alone in warm water. Many times a person may be at work or somewhere they cannot make a tea; in this case carrying cayenne tincture and adding it to warm water would be appropriate.

This therapy is used to treat external (acute) cold/excess and heat/excess conditions. When a person has had acute external symptoms of being cold alternating fever and chills, lack of perspiration, and possibly some minor skin ailments this therapy is used. This therapy is also used to cause sweating while treating fevers (heat/excess).

Cold/excess is treated with diaphoresis therapy only to help bring heat to the surface of the body. Diet plays an important part in treating cold/excess because there is usually too much fluid in raw food causing the cold/excess. Heavy foods such as grains, seeds, nuts, cooked food, etc. will help to stimulate inner heat.

Contraindications. This therapy is not indicated during intestinal disturbances like bleeding ulcers, colitis, inflamed intestines and hemorrhages.

Excessive perspiration and chronic internal ailments such as severe skin problems, cancer, tuberculosis and diabetes are some diseases where an individual should avoid producing excessive inner stimulation and sweating.

E. EMESIS THERAPY

Emesis is the therapy that induces vomiting. In many situations it is better to cause vomiting and get the poison out of the stomach instead of letting it remain in the stomach and travel through the intestines which sometimes takes days, constantly poisoning the blood and causing other symptoms and fevers.

This therapy is indicated when there is a feeling of nausea caused by bad food combinations, excessive eating, food or drug poisoning, excessive mucus during asthma, sinus congestion or food allergies.

Using lobelia tincture (or ipecac, which can be purchased in a drug store), take one teaspoon every ten minutes until vomiting is induced. Follow this therapy with several warm cups of peppermint or spearmint tea to soothe and relax the stomach. These teas will also help neutralize excessive acids in the stomach. Add a little honey or licorice root to these teas if a sweetener is needed. Do not eat for several hours after this therapy.

Emesis therapy is used to treat heat/excess, cold/excess, internal and external conditions. When poisons build up in the stomach area, sometimes this causes fevers and sweating (heat/excess). The reverse can also be seen when there is coldness experienced because the waste build up in the stomach has caused the stomach and intestines to be different in their functions (cold/excess). After vomiting is induced, followed by a soothing mint tea, the fever will usually be reduced and the organ functions back to normal. If not, diaphoresis therapy will aid the situation. Of course, this is considered an internal condition because it is affecting the internal organs. Often external symptoms like cold extremities, sweating, a lack of perspiration, and minor skin ailments can be caused by stomach problems because the energy is trapped in the interior part of the body effecting circulation to the surface. Emesis therapy will release them.

Herbalists many times induce vomiting to treat cold/excess. This is when a person may be very cold and need immediate heat. Vomiting produces warmth and circulation. This method is somewhat obsolete but still can be used. Although, if heat is needed, diaphoresis or carmentative therapy will produce the warmth needed.

Contraindications. This therapy reduces body energy and should not be used in weak, debilitated conditions, severe hypertension and during hemorrhaging. This is an emergency therapy and should not be used on a regular basis.

F. HEAT DISPELLING THERAPY

Heat dispelling therapy is used when there are low grade fevers, acute infections, inflammations, thirst, aversion to heat, fevers, hypertension, minor skin problems and other internal heat problems. The herbs used in this therapy protect the body fluids and internal organs by reducing inflammations. There are several different categories of heat dispelling therapies.

1. Antipyretic therapy is used when there is acute fever (not caused by infections, and when there is no inflammation), facial flushing, sun stroke, persistent inner warmth causing excessive abnormal sweating, heat caused by obesity and thirst. Here we use herbs or fruits called antipyretics such as goldenseal, peppermint, chickweed, sorrel, sumach berries, cleavers, red raspberry leaf tea and plantain or lemon or lime juice, watermelon juice, cranberry juice and prickly pear cactus juice. The herb teas (use full strength) or diluted citrus juice (50% with distilled water) cool, can be used as external washes or fomentations to cool external parts. Use them at temperatures below body temperature (60 to 80 degrees Fahrenheit).

2. Demulcent therapy is using herbs that have mucilagenous qualities that soothe the throat, stomach, lungs, small intestine, and bowels during inflammations. They are used separately or in combinations to counteract inflammations, irritations, ulcers, internal bleeding, and to aid the release of gall and kidney stones.

Demulcents are often used in syrups, concentrates and decoctions. The main objective here is to extract the mucilangenous substance and take it internally to soothe irritation. That is why it should be taken between meals on an empty stomach. If the problem is severe, short fasts are indicated. Sometimes fasts as long as three weeks may be needed in severe cases of ulcers or gastritis. In these cases, raw juice like carrot mixed with apple and cabbage would be suitable. Using enemas and cool baths, exercise and deep breathing will help expel inner heat.

Always use demulcents during kidney and bowel treatments. In most kidney, intestinal and lung formulas you will notice there are demulcents included. This is for inflammations and in case there are deposits or gravel in the kidneys, bladder and gall bladder.

Demulcent herbs include comfrey root, slippery elm, mullein, flaxseed, psyllium seed, marshmallow root (good in kidney combinations) and licorice root.

3. Antibiotic and antiseptic herbs are used when there is a yellow coating on the tongue indicating infections and internal mucus, thirst accompanied with dry lips and fever. In these conditions, with inflammation coupled with infections, antibiotic herbs combined with demulcents are used.

Antibiotic and antiseptic herbs that combat infections are chaparral, myrrh, echinacea, oregon grape root and goldenseal. Demulcent herbs are mullein, licorice root, comfrey root, slippery elm and flaxseed.

Combine three parts antibiotic herbs using one or more herbs, with one part demulcent herb (more if needed) and one-half part of a stimulant antispasmodic herb like fennel, ginger or cumin. For example:

> 2 parts echinacea
> 1 part chaparral
> ½ part fennel
> 1 part flaxseed

Simmer one ounce for ten to fifteen minutes in one ounce of water. Let cool and drink one-half cup every two hours. This combination can be powdered and put in #00 capsules. Take two capsules every two hours until inflammation subsides. Then a maintenence dose of two capsules three times a day may be taken. A short three day fast on vegetable broths, liquid chlorophyll or carrot juice is suggested; then follow the cleansing diet in this book.

4. When there is an internal high temperature accompanied with infected and inflammed throat, surface chills and acute skin ailments (not severe skin ailments like red, hot rashes), then we combine antibiotic herbs (to treat the infection) such as goldenseal, myrrh, etc.; demulcents to treat the inflammation; and antipyretic herbs such as boneset, elder flowers, chickweed, scullcap and seaweeds for the inner heat and surface skin problems.

When combining demulcents, antipyretics and antibiotic herbs, if infection is the most severe symptom, use more antibiotic herbs; if the fever is most severe, use more antipyretic herbs. The severity of the symptoms will help guide you in which property you want emphasized in your combination.

5. If there is internal heat causing severe mental disturbances, combine equal parts antispasmodic herbs like wood betony, scullcap, hops and chamomile with antipyretic herbs such as plantain, chickweed, cleavers, etc. (see part one of this section for antipyretic therapy).

6. In the final stages of infections when there is a low grade fever, the nerves are weak and recovery is slow. Use nervine herbs such as scullcap, hops, wood betony, and mistletoe with refrigerant herbs like chickweed and plantain. Anti-inflammatory herbs like goldenseal and echinacea are also added. The idea here is to tone the nerves to help the energy within to throw off the toxins. For example:

> 2 parts antibiotic   Goldenseal
> 2 parts nervine   Scullcap
> 1 part refrigerant   Chickweed

Nervine herbs can be taken alone in capsule form or as teas between meals if more nerve toning is needed. A short fast using nutritive juices like carrot, parsley and beet (small amounts), or spirulina, bee pollen, green magma (dried barley juice) will be absorbed rapidly without depleting nerve energy through digestive processes.

Because the individual is usually uncomfortable during these problems, short fasts, cool baths and showers and enemas are used along with drinking these teas. Only resume eating when perfectly comfortable again. The teas and juices are usually drunk at room temperature or below body temperature so they will help reduce inner heat. Drink them every one to two hours if need be, or continually sip the liquid throughout the day. Do not over-consume liquids which might cause bloating.

This therapy is used to treat heat/excess, internal or external ailments. The description above gives you an explanation of the type of herbs that are needed. Using heat-dispelling therapy is treating inflammations, infections, and internal irritations. It is using herbs to soothe tissues and neutralize the acids and poisons that may be producing inner heat. This is different than treating heat/excess problems that are caused by heavy congestion where deobstruent and diaphoresis is indicated. When using heat dispelling therapy, you are not trying to move heavy mucus or obstructions out of the body. You are neutralizing and counteracting inflammations and irritations. Often you will combine deobstruent with heat dispelling therapy or follow deobstruent therapy with heat dispelling. If mucus or obstructions are causing the infection, they must be removed first, then the irritations that they have caused are counteracted by heat dispelling procedures.

Often we will see external symptoms like sweating and skin rashes being produced by the inner heat caused by an infection. In cases like these, heat-dispelling can be used to treat these external surface conditions by treating the cause of the problem which is internal. This would be a good example of treating the causes and not the effect (symptoms).

Contraindications. Prolonged use (two to three months) of cooling herbs could possibly weaken inner heat and digestion, causing gas and cramping. Once the inner heat problem is restored to normal, use the tonification therapy.

If there are chills, delicate health, weak digestion, diarrhea and fevers due to a weakened constitution, heat dispelling should be avoided.

G. PURGATION THERAPY

Probably no class of remedies has been so much abused as cathartic herbs. Frequent use and given in too large of quantities will result in greater prostration of the organs. Constipation is a symptom and not a disease. Overeating, lack of exercise, not drinking enough water, lack of bulk foods, fiber, raw fruits and vegetables, too many starches, dairy products and protein foods are some of the causes of constipation. Proper food combinations, adding bulk and fiber to the diet, rest and enough liquids and exercise will usually overcome this condition.

Many times the liver and gall bladder are exhausted and congested, and by using liver tonics and cholagogues (herbs that promote the flow of bile) will help overcome this condition.

Purgation is the therapy that stimulates elimination through the bowel. It is used to relieve constipation, remove excess fluid and eliminate inner heat. Whenever constipation is present, enemas and colonics should be considered along with the herbal therapies. Nerve exhaustion and fatigue can cause the worst forms of chronic constipation. Short fasts and toning therapies would be indicated. Rest, exercise, fresh air, skin brushing and recreation will bring back balance in most cases.

When there is constipation and a cold condition in the body, the person usually experiences chills, abdominal bloating and poor digestion. These conditions are caused by a lack of heat in the body. Exercise is one remedy to produce body heat along with warm baths. Another good suggestion is to add warm spices to the food, for example, ginger, cumin, cardamon, cayenne, nutmeg or cloves. Also, these heating spices may be added to laxative remedies, usually as 10 to 20% of the combination. Teas of ginger, cinnamon and other stimulating herbs can be drank in the morning and between meals to assist body heat.

Purgation therapy is a category which consists of three major types of bowel stimulating herbs. They are aperients, laxatives and purgatives. Some herbs are considered to be more than one category.

1. Aperients are slow acting herbs that can be used alone or in combinations with harsher acting botanicals. If used alone they usually can be used over longer periods of time (two to three months). Seaweeds, bulk seeds like chia, psyllium seeds, flaxweed or natural oils can be used as a constant in most people's diet. Some other aperients are agar agar, turkey rhubarb, olive oil, licorice root, figs, prunes and raisins. If using dried fruit, soak them for four hours in distilled water to reconstitute before using. The seeds I have mentioned can be soaked with dried fruit to bring out their demulcent qualities and eaten before or between meals. Chia seeds, flaxseed and psyllium seeds can be soaked overnight in water or juice in a large jar or kettle. They will swell to three times the amount that is being soaked. Keep in the refrigerator. One tablespoon beween meals will act as an aperient.

For elderly, weakened conditions and children use flaxseed and psyllium seed powders (one teaspoon to a cup of hot water three to four times daily) or one teaspoon of agar agar in one cup of warm water will assist in normality. A decoction may be made from one ounce of freshly grated ginger and two tablespoons of flaxseed. Simmer for fifteen minutes in one pint of water, strain, add honey to taste and drink two cups warm daily. Aperient or laxative herbs can be used in conjuction with the tea. This is a good remedy for children or persons in weakened conditions.

2. Laxatives are herbs which promote bowel activity with mild purgation. These are used when there is blood toxicity, constipation, gall stones, hypertension, insufficient fiber in the diet or when there is a skin condition present caused by constipation where the toxins in the small intestine are being absorbed into the blood and being eliminated through the skin. Laxative herbs

include cascara sagrada, aloe vera, licorice root, senna (small amounts, one cup of the tea daily), psyllium seed, wahoo bark and dandelion root (when there is liver involvement).

During fevers these herbs will promote cooling of the system by eliminating heat from the intestines. They can be combined or taken individually. Laxatives are usually taken before bed. See the section on "Times of Administration." A carminative herb is always added to laxative herbs to prevent cramps and gas.

3. Purgatives are fast acting herbs that will deplete the energy of the body and should not be used during dryness of the bowels, hermorrhoids, bleeding intestines, or prolapse of the intestines, uterus or bladder. These herbs will divert the energy from the outside of the body to the interior. When treating exterior conditions like skin diseases or chills, these are contraindicated.

They will usually work within eight to twenty-four hours and should only be used on robust, strong individuals. Senna, castor oil, buckthorn bark, American mandrake root and jalap are a few. Except for castor oil, these herbs are usually taken in capsule or tablet form combined with a carminative, a demulcent and sometimes other herbs. Whenever the intestines are dry, signified by hard pebbles, tightly packed fecal matter and severe constipation, use demulcent herbs to bathe and lubricate the intestine, along with aperients (see aperients).

Purgation therapy is used to treat heat/excess, internal and external ailments.

When a person is chronically constipated and the toxins are being absorbed into the blood, it can cause infections (heat) any place in the body. Purging and cleansing the bowels would solve the problem. Often people will be cold/deficient because of constipation. When the bowel is full, it can cause mechanical pressure against other organs, hindering circulation. Also circulation through the intestines themselves will be slow. This can cause coldness in the extremities of the body and chills. In this case cleansing the bowels would aid in bringing the normal function back to the organs overcoming the deficient functioning problem and normalizing circulation.

As most of us know, internal problems and external symptoms can be caused by constipation so this therapy can be used to treat internal and external illnesses if the cause is constipation.

If the blood has been absorbing poisons for a long length of time, say one month or more, then blood purification may be added to the treatment. The bloodstream and bowel are two main concerns in most chronic diseases and recurring acute ailments.

Contraindications. Purgation therapy is avoided when there is vomiting, gastrointestinal bleeding and when there is abdominal pain, especially in the area of the appendix. This therapy should also be avoided when severe weakness, weak digestion and chronic diarrhea is present.

Usually purgation therapy is only used in cases of emergency. When severe constipation exists, an enema or colonic can be taken, along with the use of laxative or aperient herbs, and purgatives can be avoided.

H. STIMULATION THERAPY

Stimulation therapy is used to aid the vitality of the system to help overcome acute conditions, and to stimulate internal organs during chronic diseases.

Improper diet, excessive starch, dairy and protein eating, lack of exercise, eating too late at night, stress, constipation and negative emotions are some causes that impede circulation and cause sluggishness. Enemas, acupuncture, hot and cold showers, skin brushing, short fasts, proper food combining and the cleansing diet in this book will help improve circulation and the elimination of toxins.

This therapy increases circulation, breaks up obstructions in the body (heavy mucus conditions) and will produce warmth. It is also used when there is inadequate circulation to the periphery of the body, abdominal chills, weak digestion (use small amounts), low back pains, and the beginning of almost all acute conditions like colds, flus and fevers. Many times toxins are trapped in the blood, lymph, stomach or some other internal organs and stimulation is needed. When low grade fevers are present or infections are slow to cure, stimulation therapy is indicated. Small amounts of stimulants such as ginger, cumin, cayenne and other culinary herbs will help improve slow digestion.

Stimulants are used alone and added to herb formulas to increase the activity of the other herbs and to promote systemic circulation, detoxification, and especially during diaphoresis therapy. Ten percent of most formulas are stimulating herbs.

Ginger, cayenne, angelica, prickly ash, cumin, cardamon, coriander and cloves are excellent stimulants. A good stimulating tea which will help break up mucus conditions and stimulate warmth is:

> 1 ounce freshly grated ginger root
> 1 teaspoon cumin
> ¼ teaspoon licorice root powder
> 1 teaspoon angelica

Simmer for fifteen minutes in three cups of water. Strain, add honey to taste. Drink one-half cup warm every two hours for chills, bad digestion and gas. Stimulation therapy is used to treat heat/excess, cold/deficient, internal and external illnesses. When the organs are not functioning properly, they either need toning (tonification therapy) or cleansing. Many times stimulation therapy is added to the treatment of deficient problems to help raise the energy of these parts. Sometimes stimulation is added to the treatment of heat/excess. Congestion can be causing the high fever and stimulation can help move out the accumulation when used along with diaphoresis or other heat dispelling therapies. Keep in mind that stimulation alone and continued too long without the proper food elements and toning therapies could weaken the body's energy. So stimulation therapy is usually used in adjunct with other therapy or for treating acute external (surface) cold conditions like colds, flu, and fevers.

Deep internal chronic ailments like asthma sometimes need stimulation therapy to aid in detoxification and circulation. While treating circulatory diseases like arteriosclerosis, piles, and hemorrhoids, stimulation therapy can be used along with blood cleansing therapy

I like to call stimulation therapy the in and out therapy because it is seldom used alone but added in with other therapies to accomplish the needs, then taken out.

Contraindications When there is intestinal dryness, intestinal bleeding, hemorrhage, excessive heat caused by obesity or hypertension, chronic high blood pressure and extreme weakness this therapy is not indicated.

Stimulation therapy is usually a short term therapy (two to four weeks). Then it is used occasionally (two to three times weekly) only for acute problems or when warmth is required. This therapy should not be overdone. It can weaken the body and make conditions worse.

I. TONIFICATION THERAPY

Tonification therapy is the means to strengthen blood, organs and vitality of the body. It is indicated when there is low resistance to disease, to improve the functions of the internal organs after injury, after acute diseases, during chronic diseases to build the energy for detoxification, after chronic diseases, to facilitate recovery from injury, miscarriage, childbirth, abortions and to improve sexual energy.

Toning therapy is divided up into several groups.

1. After acute diseases. This is usually a therapy that comprises both food and herbs. Use easily digestible foods like spirulina, sprouts, bee pollen, green magma (dried barley juice), raw vegetable and fruit juices and vegetable broths.

Seaweeds such as kelp, dulse, wakame, hiziki and irish moss are excellent vitamin and mineral supplements which will strengthen the glands, blood and organs.

An acute disease takes energy from the systems of the body, and trying to push the body too fast back to health can be detrimental. Use light herbal tonics like comfrey, nettles, chickweed, watercress and alfalfa in tea form or added to salads. When the energy returns, root herbs like dandelion, ginseng and burdock root will strengthen the whole body. Always use progressive therapy in eliminatory and building therapies.

2. Toning individual organs and systems. This is building specific organs that have been overworked, or are deficient in activity. This therapy is applied after acute or during chronic diseases. Individual tonics are:

HEART

Ginseng
Motherwort
Hawthorn berries

NERVES

Scullcap
Valerian
Lady's slipper
Hops

SPLEEN

Parsley juice
Wheat grass juice
Beet juice
Elecampane

LIVER

Dandelion
Beets
Barberry
Oregon grape root
Carrot juice

BLOOD

All raw vegetables and fruit
   juices
Spirulina
Bee pollen
Wheat grass and parsley juice
Alfalfa
Red clover
Sassafras
Yellowdock

FEMALE REPRODUCTIVE

Dong quai
Red raspberry leaves
Ginseng
Fo-ti
Damiana
False unicorn

GALL BLADDER

Cascara sagrada
Parsley
Goldenseal

STOMACH

Gentian
Agrimony
Elecampane
Wormwood

KIDNEY

Burdock root
Parsley (juice or root)
Kava kava
Pipsissewa

BOWEL

Slant board exercises
Bulk and fiber foods
Running
Massage
Cascara sagrada

PANCREAS

String beans (broth and raw)
Pea pods (broth and raw)
Parsley juice
Jerusalem artichokes
Cedar berries
Brussel sprout juice
Dandelion root
Cascara sagrada

MALE REPRODUCTIVE

Sarsaparilla
Ginseng
Gotu kola
Blessed thistle

3. Vulnerary. These are agents that promote the healing of wounds, cuts and broken bones. During disease you will find times when these herbs will have to be added to formulas to help slow healing wounds. They are:

Calendula flowers	Garlic	Comfrey leaves and
Fenugreek	Hyssop	root
Marshmallow root	Aloe vera	

4. Blood tonic. These are prescribed for persons with anemia, menstrual disorders, after a period of sickness, weak blood and fatigue during infections. See blood tonics in part two of this section.

Tonification therapy is used to treat cold/deficient, heat deficient, internal and external diseases. When we have an internal condition and the body is cold caused by the organs being weakened by injury, long term detoxification, toxins, depression, etc., this therapy will bolster them up to improve their functioning power. If we have a heat/deficient condition, this means that the diet is low in nutrients, or the blood is poor in iron. Diet therapy is indicated and it is considered toning therapy. Sometimes when we have external symptoms showing deficiencies in the skin and hair, this therapy should be used.

It is the therapy that can be used along with any other therapy whenever it is needed. During any treatment if the person being treated weakens, they should be toned up before further detoxification.

Contraindications. Tonification therapy is contraindicated during high fevers, or when there is a lack of energy because of inner congestion and constipation. Always use a progressive tonic therapy. Don't hurry your tonics, they are stimulating and can push the body too fast and cause a weaker condition. If there is any question about using this therapy as to the action, it is better to use small dosages at first and observe the reaction before increasing the amount.

J. TRANQUILIZATION THERAPY

The purpose of this therapy is to calm, relax, arrest, slow down. It is used in trying to bring the body back in balance when hyperactive. It is used whenever necessary before sickness, after or during. When using this therapy, we are considering the hyperactivity of the whole person, the nervous system, individual organs, high blood pressure and all nervous problems whether caused by toxins, deficiencies or strong emotions. This therapy is also used to arrest internal bleeding or hemorrhaging. During other therapies, the person being treated oftentimes develops hyperactivity, pain, etc. and this therapy is used. Skin diseases, diarrhea, sweating excessively and other symptoms can be caused by the nervous system being overtaxed.

Exercise is nature's natural sedative. It helps purify the blood, tones the whole body and relaxes the mind and the body. Don't overdo exercise, but don't do too little either. People who cannot exercise should get plenty of fresh air, deep breathing, have massages and use hydrotherapy (see section on hydrotherapy).

A variety of exercises is important to influence all organs and tissues. Yoga, jogging, weight lifting, swimming, walking, racketball, tai chi, etc. are a few to consider.

If a person is emotionally upset, he should endeavor to seek proper counseling. Courses of study that assist an individual in understanding himself should be pursued. Find one that is suitable and is not offensive to the person in need. I have seen Concept Therapy (a course that has been taught for over 50 years) help thousands of people. The Concept Therapy Institute is located in San Antonio, Texas.

Nerve weaknesses are often caused by the negative thought that influences the nervous system. It can weaken the entire body. A vitamin, herb or drug is no remedy for emotional chaos.

1. Nervines. These are herbs that feed and tone the nerves. They are indicated after acute problems and during chronic diseases. Many times this is a continuous therapy, but it might be used alternately while giving other therapies if the nerves weaken while trying to overcome disease.

As all pain involves nerve tissue, relief will be obtained by normalizing this system. Nervines express their value in painful conditions such as sciatica, neuralgia and sharp shooting pains in the head, legs and spine. Use these herbs to treat specific nerve problems or in combinations with other treatments when there is pain and tension. Usually ten percent of all formulas are nervines or antispasmodic herbs, but they may be used alone. Nervines are specifically indicated in tonification therapy to help rebuild nerve vitality. Use these herbs in fomentations, tinctures, poultices or capsules. Choose whichever herb is appropriate. Some are better for headaches, some for spinal problems, etc.

Scullcap	Wood betony	Valerian
Catnip	Hops	Lady's slipper
Blue vervain		

2. Antispasmodics. These herbs calm nervous tension in the muscles, pelvic area, spine, etc. They prevent the recurrence of spasms and excessive contractions.

These herbs are indicated during tetany, extreme irritability, feebleness, hysteria, intestinal and leg cramps, menstrual cramps, worms in the stomach or intestines which excite spasms, infantile convulsions, cerebral or spinal irritations or irritation caused by stones in the kidney or bladder.

Use these herbs in tincture form to get faster relief. Combine them with other therapies, and use them in external treatment as fomentations and poultices.

Lobelia	Dong quai
Crampbark	Blue cohosh
Skunk cabbage	Black cohosh
Kava kava	Scullcap

3. When there is bleeding internally or externally, styptic and hemostatic properties are indicated.

HEMOSTATICS (internal bleeding)

Bayberry
Tormentil root

STYPTIC (external)

White oak bark
Witch hazel

This therapy is used to treat all internal, external, excess or deficient problems. It is a therapy used to treat symptoms of nervousness, strain, tension and cramping.

During the use of any therapy, nerve related symptoms can appear. If they are severe enough and persistent, this therapy is indicated. Like stimulation therapy, it is used for a short time to accomplish the needed effect, then discontinued.

Contraindications. Sometimes long-term tranquilization therapy can bring on fatigue, slow digestion and slow elimination. This should be considered when treating chronic diseases.

Low blood pressure can be caused by toxins, weak nerves, mental depression etc. Using nervines or antispasmodics can make this situation worse.

This chart will aid the reader in choosing the appropriate herbs for making formulations and in choosing the correct therapy by understanding its effects and contraindications. Once the diagnosis is made and the various symptoms listed, look to the column "Symptoms and Indications" and choose the one that best fits the symptoms. Then follow the chart from left to right. It will indicate the therapy needed, its effects in the body, and its primary action in the body. Next the primary action column, followed by three columns which deal with Chinese diagnosis indicating when the therapy is used to treat internal or external, or excess of deficient diseases.

Under the section "Properties" are listed the properties of herbs that are used in each therapy. The last column, "Contraindications", describes when not to use each therapy. When one becomes proficient in using this chart, it will prove to be of great value in determining the proper therapy and herbs needed to treat symptoms and diseases.

SYMPTOMS AND INDICATIONS	THERAPY	EFFECTS	PRIMARY ACTIONS
All toxic blood conditions, arthritis, skin diseases, low grade fevers, acute and chronic illnesses; during fasting and cleansing diets.	Blood Purification	Cleans the blood stream and lymphatic system.	Detoxification
Relieves gas, stomach discomforts, chills, bloating, cold feeling in stomach, constipation, poor digestion and circulation, colds, flu, fevers, and lower back pain	Carminative	Aids in bringing warmth, circulation and stimulation to the deep parts of the body.	Symptom-relieving
Lung congestion, kidney stones, gall stones, prostate congestion, bloating, all heavy mucus congestion where congestion causes lack of blood flow	Deobstruent	Relieves the body of accumulations and obstructions.	Detoxification
Surface cold and minor skin ailments, colds, flu, chills, neck and shoulder tension, beginning skin conditions, water accumulations in flesh and joints, headaches, itching, fevers	Diaphoresis	Stimulates circulation to the periphery causing warmth and perspiration. Dispells toxins through the pores of the skin. Normalizes circulation.	Symptom-relieving
Nausea, food and drug poisoning, stomach, flu, fermenting food products	Emesis	Induces vomiting, increases warmth and circulation	Symptom-relieving
Acute fevers, facial flushing, sun stroke, abnormal sweating, heat caused by obesity and thirst; irritations of lungs and intestines; infections, inflammations	Heat Dispelling	Dispells heat, soothes irritations and counter-acts infections.	Symptom-relieving

INTERNAL/ EXTERNAL	HEAT/EXCESS COLD/EXCESS	HEAT/DEFICIENT COLD/DEFICIENT	PROPERTIES	CONTRA-INDICATIONS
Internal & External	Heat/Excess	Cold/Deficient	Alteratives Lymphatics	None
Internal & External		Cold/Deficient	Anti-emetics Aromatics Carmina- tives Condiments	Bleeding bowels, ulcers, high fevers
Internal & External	Heat/Excess	Cold/Deficient	Anthelmin- tics, Anti- catarral Chologogues Deobstruent Diuretics Emetics Expectorants Lithotriptics Parasiticides	Diarrhea, hemor- rhoids, Bleeding bowels
External	Heat/Excess		Aromatics Diaphoretics Febrifuges	Intestinal bleeding, ulcers, hemorrages, excessive perspiration, severe skin problems, cancer, tuberculosis, diabetes, when ex- cessive stimulation and perspiration is not needed
Internal & External	Heat/Excess Cold/Excess		Emetics	Debilitated conditions, severe hypertension during hemorrhaging
Internal & External	Heat/Excess		Antacids Antibiotics Antipyretics Antiseptics Demulcents Febrifuges Mucilages	None - as long as the correct herbal prop- erty is chosen. Do not prolong the use of cooling herbs

SYMPTOMS AND INDICATIONS	THERAPY	EFFECTS	PRIMARY ACTION
Constipation, chills, abdominal bloating, fevers, hypertension, minor skin ailments	Purgation	Stimulates elimination through the bowels.	Detoxification
Increase circulation, break up obstructions, produce warmth, increase circulation to the periphery of the body, abdominal chills, weak digestion, lower back pains, onset of acute conditions such as colds, flu, fevers	Stimulation	Aids vitality of the system to help overcome acute conditions, and to stimulate organs during chronic diseases.	Symptom-relieving
Low resistance to disease, improve body functions after injury, following acute diseases, during and after chronic diseases, following miscarriage, childbirth, abortion, and to improve sexual energy	Tonification	To strengthen the blood, organs and vitality of the body.	Building
Cramps, spasms, tensions, nerve weakness, tetany, extreme irritability, menstrual cramps, convulsions, skin diseases, diarrhea, excessive sweating caused by nerve imbalances, and during other therapies when needed	Tranquilization	To bring the body back to normal during hypertension and when there are imbalances in the nervous system.	Symptom-relieving

INTERNAL/ EXTERNAL	HEAT/EXCESS COLD/EXCESS	HEAT/DEFICIENT COLD/DEFICIENT	PROPERTIES	CONTRA-INDICATIONS
Internal & External	Heat/Excess	Cold/Deficient	Aperients Cathartics Laxatives Purgatives	Vomiting, gastro-intestinal bleeding, severe abdominal pain, weak digestion, chronic diarrhea, chronic constipation
Internal & External	Heat/Excess	Heat/Deficient Cold/Deficient	Aromatics Carminatives Condiments Oxytocics Rubefacients Sialagogues	Intestinal dryness and bleeding, hemorrhage, excessive heat caused by obesity, hyperten-sion, chronic high blood pressure, extreme weakness
Internal & External		Cold/Deficient Heat/Deficient	Aphrodisiacs Astringents Cardiacs Emmeno-gogues Galacto-gogues Hepatics Nervines Nutritives Opthalmics Stomachics Tonics Vulneraries	High fevers, lack of energy because of inner congestion and constipation
Internal & External	Heat/Excess Cold/Excess	Heat/Deficient Cold/Deficient	Anodynes Anti-spasmodics Emmeno-gogues Hemostatics Sedatives Styptics	Low blood pressure, mental depression (Use nerve tonics if necessary). Never use this therapy for long periods of time as it can bring on fatigue and slow elimination and digestion

METHODS OF USING HERBS

Through centuries of practice, herbalists have developed several methods of applying herbs in order to satisfy different needs. These methods can be divided into two major categories: the internal and external applications. An internal application is anything which is taken by mouth, swallowed, and then either absorbed and transmitted through the blood or is effective in the gastro-intestinal tract directly. Capsules, tinctures, tablets, pills, teas (infusions and decoctions), syrups, electuaries, are examples of commonly used internal applications. External applications are those which are intended to primarily affect the area to which they are applied and are not swallowed. Poultices, fomentations, enemas, gargles, salves, liniments, and boluses are examples. Often, both internal and external applications are employed to produce a speedy resolution of the disorder. Below, the methods of preparing and adminstering herbs are described.

INTERNAL METHODS

Capsules and tablets. Usually capsules are used to take powdered herbs that are otherwise nauseous to the taste, or for people who cannot drink certain teas. They are also very convenient for individuals who do not have time to make other herbal preparations. The capsules come in different sizes, #0, #00, #000 etc. The average amount of herb in a #0 capsule is 400-450 mg. This varies with the density of the herb and whether the herb is a root or leaf. The average amount in #00 capsules is about 500-600 mg., and in #000 is about 650-850 mg. If there is a problem swallowing the capsules they can be moistened by dipping them in water or a little vegetable oil.

There are advantages to taking capsules instead of tablets. Strong acrid herbs like valerian root or goldenseal are more pleasant to take in capsules because the smell is not noticed as when taken in tablet form. Capsules can also be inserted in the rectum easier than tablets to treat hemorrhoids and other rectal diseases.

Capsules should be stored in a cool, dark place so they will not lose moisture and become brittle. Also, excess heat and moisture will soften the capsules and they will stick together.

Capsules also have disadvantages. Strict vegetarians object to using them because they are made from boiled tissues derived from slaughtered livestock. Tablets would be more preferable for vegetarians.

Tablets on the other hand, do not tend to stick together and will resist a warmer climate than capsules. In certain climates or while traveling on foot or in cars, certainly tablets would be preferable.

It is a controversial subject as to whether some herbs are absorbed better in capsule form or tablet, so the choice is entirely up to the reader based on the information given.

Infusions. An infusion is used when the volatile oils in herbs are needed, as in peppermint and spearmint, or when the constituents are extracted from flowers or leaves. Infusions are used hot or cold (strain and let them cool or keep in the refrigerator). Many times they are made into a "sun tea" which is simple, using the same amounts as described below or more if desired: put the contents in a large glass jar with the cover on and set in the sun for two to four hours. The heat from the sun will do the extraction.

To prepare an infusion, use one ounce of herb to one pint of water. Bring the water to a boil and pour over the herb. Cover the liquid with a tight fitting lid so steam does not escape. Let it stand for twenty minutes, strain and drink.

Pills. Pills are preferred by vegetarians over gelatin capsules which are made from animal products. Some advantages are that no fillers are used and one knows exactly what they are making when preparing home-made pills. They can be made any size for the convenience of smaller children.

The herbal agent is ground fine and a small amount of slippery elm, an herbal syrup, mucilage of gum arabic or other mucilagenous herbs are added (usually 1/10 of the mixture). Add small amounts of water while mixing, keeping the preparation firm. It is then rolled into small pills about the size of a pea. To dry the pills they can be spread out on a pie dish and left to dry at room temperature. Another way is to preheat an oven to 250 degrees, then turn the oven off and place the pie dish in the oven for 15 minutes to a half hour. Check them every five minutes. When they are dry, bottle them and keep them in a cool, dry place. A refrigerator is fine.

When giving them to children, they can be dipped in honey, molasses or peanut butter to help cover the taste.

Tinctures. Tinctures are concentrated herbal extracts that can be preserved over long periods of time. They are usually used when herbs have to be taken over a long period of time because they can be carried around easily and taken in just a little water or under the tongue. Also, they are preferred by many herbalists when treating severe infections because of the rapid absorption and the dosage can be changed easily. Instead of trying to divide up capsules or tablets to change the dosage, drops can be added or subtracted. The course of many infections change rapidly and it is easier to gauge dosages by drops. Another advantage is that they can be added to juices if they are bitter. Tinctures are also easily added to fomentations, infusions, decoctions and poultices to enhance the healing properties. If the patient has an aversion to alcohol or vinegar, the tinctures can be made with glycerine. The medicinal qualities of herbs are extracted in alcohol, glycerine or vinegar to preserve them over a longer period of time.

Combine 4 ounces of powdered herb with 1 pint alcohol (gin, brandy, vodka or glycerine, or apple cider vinegar may be substituted). Combine herbs and alcohol in container with a tight stopper, let stand for 14 days, shaking container twice daily. Strain liquid by pressing through muslin. Pour liquid into bottle (dark glass) and cap it tightly. For long term storage, seal the cap with melted wax.

The final concentration of alcohol in a tincture should not be less than 30%. When buying brandy, gin or other alcoholic beverages to make tinctures, the proof number is twice the amount of alcohol, so if buying liquor at 80 proof, it is 40% alcohol. This would give a 40% alcohol content to the tincture. Tinctures are usually prepared with an alcohol content from 30% to 60% and even higher. If the tincture needs to be diluted, it can be added to a small glass of water.

Fluid extract. In reality, a fluid extract is a concentrated tincture and may be five times as strong as tinctures. This is not always true. It is the opinion of many herbalists that the dosage of fluid extracts should be the same as a tincture or a few drops less, and I have found this to be a good practice. In the chapter on "Herbs for Specific Diseases", the dosages of both tinctures and fluid extracts are given. In many cases they are the same.

Syrup. A syrup is used for coughs, inflammations of the throat and to soothe the stomach and intestinal tract.

Add two ounces of herb or combination of herbs to one quart of water. Simmer with the top off the pot until the volume is reduced to one-half the original amount. Strain and while warm, add two to four ounces of honey or vegetable glycerine to preserve. I often suggest squeezing one-half of a lemon and adding a pinch of cayenne to the finished product to make it more effective.

Licorice root, wild cherry bark, comfrey root, horehound, irish moss and fennel are some herbs used in cough medicines and syrups. See section on asthma, coughs and colds. Syrups can be made by first evaporating approximately half the fluid from decoctions, infusions, expressed juices, etc. and then adding sweetener.

Decoction. To extract the deeper healing qualities of stems, roots and barks, the herbs must be simmered for about 15 to 45 minutes. Many times it is left uncovered during simmering to evaporate some of the water.

Decoctions and infusions must be used before they sour or growth starts (usually within 24 to 72 hours).

Example:
Preparation: One ounce of herb (two ounces if fresh herb is used)
    1 pint cool water
    Simmer for one-half hour (longer if roots are very hard)
If time allows:
    One ounce dry herb or 2 ounces of fresh herb (pulverize for best results)

Soak for 8 to 12 hours in one and one-half pints cool water
Simmer in warm water for thirty minutes.
Strain liquid into clean container. Allow to settle and cool slightly. Drink
liquid while still warm.

Decoction and Infusion Combined. Roots and barks are made into a decoction by simmering for a period of time. Leaves and aromatic herbs are more sensitive to heat and are only steeped so as not to lose the volatile oils. To combine the two, you would first make your decoction, then pour it over your leafy herb, and let it steep for twenty minutes. Therefore, use one more cup of water while making the decoction. Another way is to make the infusion and decoction separately and then combine them. To make infusions and decoctions, use a high grade stainless steel, ceramic or earthenware pot.

Concentrate. Add two ounces of herbs to one quart of distilled water and make a decoction. Strain, then simmer the liquid down to one pint, leaving the top off during simmering. You now have a concentrate. Add one or two ounces of glycerine, honey or blackstrap molasses while the liquid is warm and stir.

Concentrates are very seldom used by modern herbalists. They are usually made to preserve herbs, make syrups or to concentrate nutritional and medicinal constituents so smaller and less frequent dosages have to be taken.

Electuary. An electuary is an herbal preparation mixed with honey, maple syrup, peanut butter or slippery elm to form a paste and then rolled into balls. When children refuse to take capsules, or the herb is too bitter for them to take, mix it with honey, slippery elm, coconut butter or peanut butter. Then have the child swallow it with juice.

Any powdered herb can be mixed with honey, syrup or glycerine and given immediately without preparing in advance. Add honey or syrup to powdered herbs and give in one-half teaspoon dosages. It is best to measure the proper dosage of the powdered herbs first, then add the sweetening agent.

EXTERNAL METHODS

Bolus. A bolus is a suppository inserted into the rectum or vagina to draw out toxins and to treat tumors, swellings, infections, cysts, hemorrhoids and inflammations.

In treating vaginal infections, boluses are only used when douches do not suffice or when a severe infection needs constant attention. Since douches should not be used too regularly, when infections persist boluses can be used to supplement the treatment. Usually, taking antiseptic and antibiotic herbs orally will help clear up the infection without the long term use of douches or boluses.

Astringents, demulcents and antibiotic herbs are used to make up boluses. White oak bark, bayberry and witch hazel are good astringents. Some useful demulcents are comfrey root and slippery elm; good antibiotic herbs are garlic, chaparral, goldenseal and myrrh.

To make a bolus, slowly pour melted cocoa butter over the powdered herbs while stirring. When it becomes a thick dough-like consistency, the mixture is finished. Then roll into strips about one-half inch thick and ¾ inch long. Sometimes it is better to put the mixture in the refrigerator and let it cool a while before rolling it into suppositories. Then put them back into the refrigerator. They will become hard.

Slippery elm can be used in place of cocoa butter. Add 10% of powdered slippery elm to your choice of herbs. This 10% of slippery elm can be volume or weight. Mix in well by putting the herbs in a blender or stirring by hand. Then follow the same directions as given above, except adding water to the mixture instead of melted cocoa butter. Once these are formed into a bolus, let them dry by leaving them exposed to the sun or in an oven under low heat. Be careful not to burn them. As soon as they are dry, put them in a jar and keep them refrigerated.

Before inserting the bolus, let it set at room temperature for 15 to 20 minutes so it will become warm. To help make them easier to insert, dip them in olive oil or warm water and insert immediately. In the evening before bed, or during long rest periods, is the best time to use boluses. The cocoa butter will melt, so take precautions to protect clothing and bedding.

Boluses can become messy. Many times a warm water douche (see douches) has to be used to clean the vagina properly.

Douches. This treatment is used to treat vaginal infections and excessive secretions which are usually sign of a poor diet, too high in protein and starches.

It is prepared by making a strong infusion or decoction using herbs such as goldenseal, myrrh, plantain, slippery elm and white oak bark (for excessive secretions or bleeding). Add one tablespoon of apple cider vinegar to one quart of tea to help maintain an acid pH. Insert the douche carefully while the tea is still warm and retain for three to five minutes.

Douches are usually administered once daily for 5 to 7 days, and only during the infectious period, and once a month for maintenance.

Pregnant women should only use douches when advised by their physician.

Enema or Clyster. For proper use of an enema, see the section on enemas in this book. This is a way of injecting large amounts of water into the bowel to wash out toxins, ease pain during constipation, relax the body and treat headaches, backaches etc. Herbal teas made into a decoction or infusion can have laxative effects, sedative, stimulating, or any other effect you are trying to produce. Choose the herb that has that specific property and use it as an enema. Astringent herbs clean the bowel and are used for bleeding. Add one tablespoon of apple cider vinegar to one quart of liquid when using water or herbal tea enemas.

Fomentation. Fomentations are used to stimulate circulation of blood and lymph, to relieve colic, to warm joints and other body parts, to relieve gas and pain and reduce internal inflammations.

Alternating hot and cold fomentations will stimulate and bring activity to an area. This is a good treatment for urine retention, constipation, sluggish circulation and so forth.

Preparation: soak a cotton towel in an herbal tea infusion or decoction which is as hot as can be tolerated. Fold, wring towel slightly and place on affected area. Place a layer of plastic over the hot towel, then place a thick dry towel or heating pad on top in order to keep the heat in. Resaturate the towel in hot infusion periodically.

Poultice. A poultice is a pulverized or powdered mass of herbs moistened with water, tinctures, infusions, salves, oils or decoctions and applied wet to the surface of the skin. If the fresh herb is to be used, it can be chewed or purverized and applied directly to the skin without moistening. A cloth is then wrapped around the poultice to hold it in place if there will be movement or walking.

Poultices are used to heal bruises, break up congestion, reduce inflammation, withdraw pus, toxins and embedded particles in the skin and to soothe irritation. Once again, herbs are chosen according to the healing properties. Valerian and kava kava made into poultices will ease pain, echinacea and garlic are good for infectious sores. Ginger, prickly ash and cayenne added to poultices will promote circulation.

Clay poultices are excellent when used alone or combined with powdered herbs. At most health food stores you can purchase white, yellow or green clay. Powdered bentonite clay is also very good. Usually clay is mixed with water or an herb tea just enough to make a thick dough-like consistency and applied directly to the surface of the skin. This type of poultice is good for bruises, infections and mixed with pulverized cabbage leaves it is used for boils and tumors. Powdered cayenne or ginger added to a clay poultice is good for sore, arthritic joints.

Cabbage poultice. Pulverize leaves and apply to the skin. This poultice will draw out poisons and pus. Replace it with a new one when it feels hot.

Carrot poultice. Use finely grated carrots or the pulp left over from juicing. Good for sores, bruises, chapped skin and nipples.

Comfrey leaf poultice. Mash the leaves and moisten with comfrey tea, other oils, tinctures or infusions. Good for swellings, open sores and skin openings like cuts and wounds.

Fig poultice. Heat figs for three minutes. Cut open and apply to infected sores to bring them to a head.

Garlic poultice. Pulverize fresh garlic and add warm water and flour. Good for pain, pus and infections.

Oatmeal poultice. Apply cooled outmeal to a soft, natural-fiber cloth. Place poultice over area, cover with dry cloth and apply heating pad. Good for inflammations and insect bites.

Potato poultice. Apply grated raw potato to bruises, sprains or boils.

Tofu poultice. Squeeze out the cake, chop up the tofu and add a teaspoon of ginger and some flour until it thickens. This poultice draws out inflammation and fever.

Oils, tinctures and salves can be added to poultices to give specific results. For example, lobelia tincture gives sedation; cayenne tincture gives stimulation and myrrh tincture is indicated for suppuration and infections.

Plasters. Plasters. Plasters are herbal preparations that are applied externally to snake bites, sores, inflammation and the like.

To make a plaster, the powdered herb is moistened with warm water and spread on a linen, cotton or silk cloth and applied to the skin. It is then covered with a cloth or plastic to keep the moisture in. They are usually applied to the breast, stomach, kidneys or lower back.

Plasters can be made to stimulate or relax certain organs or body parts. Cayenne, ginger and other stimulants can be added to the plaster if a more stimulating effect is needed. Lobelia, hops and other sedative herbs added to plasters will relax and ease pain. Like the rest of the herbal preparations, to produce a certain effect, choose the herb which has the healing property desired. Tinctures, fluid extracts, infusions, liniments, oils and decoctions can also be added to plasters.

Mustard and comfrey root powder are very popular plasters. Mustard should be watched carefully so it is not left on too long to cause blistering. When harsh herbs or stimulants are used, rub the body part first with olive, castor or peanut oil before the plaster is applied. Mustard plasters are harsh.

Salves. A salve is used to treat boils, dry skin and itchy skin conditions. Some salves are used just to moisturize and tone the skin. Astringent herbs like white oak bark and cranesbill will help tone the skin, while herbs with demulcent properties like comfrey will soften and keep the surface moist and healthy looking.

An herbal salve is made by first making an herbal oil and adding beeswax (usually around one and one-half ounces to one pint of oil) to give it a thick consistency. Add a little more beeswax in hot climates (see oils).

Use leaves, flowers, roots, barks, powdered or granulated. Mix them with enough oil to cover (never use mineral oil), bake the solution in a covered pot at 125 to 200 degrees for two to four hours. Follow the same directions here as you would during the oil-making process. When the baking is done, strain. Melt the beeswax and stir it into the oil. Preserve the salve by adding vitamin E oil (one-half teaspoon to a cup of solution, or two drops of gum benzoin tincture to one ounce of salve or oil).

Another basic recipe is to macerate fresh or dried herbs and add to melted pork lard or lanolin. Add lard to just cover the herbs. Simmer on top of the stove or bake in an oven until the herbs become crisp. Strain while hot. The lanolin or lard will harden.

Liniment. This is a fluid herbal extract applied to the skin in cases of strained muscles, sore joints, arthritis, and most any types of inflammation. Stimulating herbs such as cayenne and prickly ash are combined with antispasmodic herbs such as lobelia or wild lettuce. Aromatic oils like wintergreen and eucalyptus are specifics when deep penetration is needed.

Take four ounces of dried herbs, or double the weight if fresh, and add them to one pint of alcohol, vinegar or a good oil (olive oil, peanut or almond oil). Put a tight seal over the container and let it set for 14 days or for 3 to 7 days if needed sooner. Shake a few times daily. Strain, and if desired add ten to thirty drops of an essential oil. Wintergreen and eucalyptus are excellent for deep-rooted problems.

Liniments made with rubbing alcohol or vodka will preserve them. If your base is an oil, add two vitamin E capsules, 200 or 400 units, to one pint, or one tablespoon of glycerine for a preservative to one pint of liquid liniment. Keep all liniments in a dark bottle and out of the sun.

Oil. Some of the properties of herbs are within the oils they contain. Extracting this oil is concentrating the healing essence of the plant. Oils are usually made from mints, spices and aromatic herbs. They are applied externally to treat skin diseases, bring more circulation and warmth to an area, for painful joints, used to give massages, for dry skin and to be rubbed on the surface of the skin before a poultice, hot pack or fomentation is applied to enhance the treatment.

Take two ounces of macerated herb and add one pint of olive oil, linseed or almond oil. Mix carefully and bake in the oven at a temperature of about 115 to 200 degrees until the herbs become crisp. This means you have extracted their oil. It usually takes from two to four hours depending upon the structure of the plant. Strain, and put in a dark bottle. Olive oil usually has a long shelf life before it goes rancid.

Another method is to put the mixture of herbs and oil in a jar and set it in the sun for five days (less in hotter climates). Shake daily. Strain.

For both methods, open a 400 I.U. vitamin capsule and add to preserve the oil. Add one capsule to every cup of oil. Two drops of gum benzoin tincture to one ounce of salve or oil is also an excellent preservative.

When you want the oil to remain on the surface of the skin for long periods of time and to help heal external sores, use oils from sweet almond, avocado, peanut and olive. Sesame, sunflower and wheat germ oil absorb much faster.

Essential oils purchased in a health food store are extracted by a distillation process and are much more concentrated. Ten drops to one ounce of this type is usually added to one cup of oil base to make a therapeutic mixture.

Baths. Herbs and salt are added to water to increase or decrease body activities. When adding herbs to bath water there are two ways of doing so. First, take four to eight ounces of your chosen herb (dry or fresh), fill a stocking or cloth bag which is thin enough to let water absorb into it and back out again. Put the stocking or bag full of herbs in the bath water. In a short time a herb tea will color the water and the bath is ready. The second way is to make a gallon of infusion or decoction and just add it to the bath water. The effect desired depends on the length of time you remain in the tub, the temperature of the water and the herb you choose. The chapter on hydrotherapy should be consulted.

The proper herb is chosen by its healing properties. This simply means if you want a sedative effect, choose a sedative, antispasmodic herb like hops or chamomile. For stimulation, rosemary and thyme are good. Hayflower and oatstraw will help relieve the skin of impurities. One cup of apple cider vinegar added to a bath will relieve poison ivy, overcome fatigue, detoxify and relieve itching or hives. Uva ursi is good for urinary, bladder and prostate problems.

Salt baths will relax the body and help draw out toxins during skin and blood diseases. To draw out poisons, use warmer water (98.6 to 106 degrees) with one to five pounds of epsom salts. The greater the amount of salt, the more perspiration is produced. Colder water (75 to 65 degrees) with just one to two cups of epsom salt will produce a tonic, refreshing effect. The colder the water the more tonic effect produced and less soaking time is indicated.

When taking a hot salt bath, keep a cool towel over the forehead and the back of the neck. This bath is fatiguing and should be done with caution. The time to remain in the warm salt water depends upon the strength of the individual. Usually from 20 to 45 minutes is sufficient.

Gargle. A gargle is an herb tea "infusion" (double strength) made to wash the mouth and back of the throat. Usually goldenseal is used for ulcers or pus in the mouth. Tinctures or volatile oils added to water can also be used as gargles. For example, combine one cup water with four drops tincture of myrrh. A good, stimulating and antiseptic gargle for canker sores, bad breath, bleeding gums or pyorrhea is made by adding one drop peppermint oil to one cup water.

PRINCIPLES OF ADMINISTERING HERBAL THERAPIES

The following are some things to consider before administering herbal therapy.

1. Women usually require smaller dosages than men, due to their lower average weight. Larger persons require larger dosages and smaller or underweight persons require smaller dosages. Children and elderly people also require smaller dosages.

2. During pregnancy, women sometimes respond to herbs differently than when they are not pregnant. Use smaller dosages than normal to start the therapy and observe the response. Sometimes it is best to use mild and nutritive herbs during pregnancy. Some herbs are contraindicated during pregnancy and should be avoided or prescribed only by a skilled herbalist. For example, purgatives, diuretics and emmenagogues are active in the pelvic area and should be avoided or minimized.

3. Sedatives and antispasmodic herbs are usually taken on an empty stomach before bed or whenever needed. They may initiate depression in susceptible subjects in which case you should switch to nutritive herbs or cut the dosage.

4. Highly nervous people require smaller doses of stimulants than do robust or depressed patients.

5. Some individuals have peculiar tolerances to some botanical agents because of:
   a. faulty assimilation
   b. too rapid excretion (diarrhea)
   c. bacteria in the intestinal tract which destroy some medicinal agents

d. habituation of herbs, especially laxatives
e. genetic tolerances
f. prolonged use of some herbs—this may establish a tolerance to plants of the same family
g. impaired eliminatory organs which can cause an accumulation of the botanical
h. allergies to certain plants which can be present or produced after the use of certain herbs.

6. Herbs should be stored in glass jars, covered cans, or other glassware so the freshness and medicinal qualities are not lost. Therapies may be much less effective if the herbs have been exposed to the sun for long periods of time and the healing virtues have been bleached out.

7. Herbal formulas should be properly combined. Some herbs may overpower others or neutralize their effects.

8. Astringent herbs should not be taken along with nutritional supplements high in iron. Then tannins in astringent herbs leach calcium, iron and other important minerals out of the intestines. Astringent therapies are usually of short duration.

9. Slow-acting laxatives should be given in the morning so as not to disturb sleep. Fast-acting laxatives usually take 4-8 hours and slow-acting may take from one to three days. The dosage should not be increased until a three day period is over using the same dosage every day. Then, if the desired results are not noticed, the dosage can be increased. Usually the desired result is two bowel movements daily, unless otherwise indicated by a physician.

10. Blood purifying herbs are taken between meals on an empty stomach.

11. People should be made aware of the different effects and tastes herbs sometimes produce. Strong, bitter herbs can produce nausea if not enough water is taken along with them. Cayenne sometimes gives a burning sensation in the stomach and throat. Astringents like white oak bark and bayberry can leave a dry, scratchy feeling in the throat. Emetics produce nausea and vomiting in large amounts.
Potent herbs can produce toxic effects in large amounts. Poke root, horsetail, juniper berries, aconite, lobelia, mandrake and black cohosh are a few.

12. Persons with a history of high blood pressure should avoid herbs that stimulate the heart or constrict the blood capillaries and arteries, for example, licorice root, ephedra and lily of the valley. Use a sedative type of therapy with a cleansing diet. Cayenne and garlic can be used in normal amounts in high blood pressure cases.

13. Essential oils are usually used externally, added to fomentations, poultices and salves. They are used in gargles, two drops in a cup of warm water or herb tea. Internally, only two to five drops (determined by the oil used) are taken in a cup of tea or with a teaspoon of honey or syrup.

14. In hotter climates many times the medicinal effect of stimulants and purgatives are intensified.

15. Here are some basic rules to follow when administering herbs orally.
   a. For a slow gradual general effect, give substances in small quantities of syrup or milk between meals, to retard absorption.
   b. For a local effect on the stomach or intestines, give the substance in acacia gum or olive oil or in milk, thus lessening absorption.
Remedies should be given before meals for the following effects:
   a. To aid the appetite or to increase the secretion of digestive juices.
   b. For a local effect on the stomach or intestines.
When the substances are irritating they can be given in milk or as a syrup. These substances are soothing to the intestines. The combination of the remedy with the protein of the food lessens the irritation.
Remedies should be given after meals for the following effects:
   a. To neutralize digestive juices (heartburn) when these are present to excess.
   b. To aid absorption of the herbs and produce rapid effects, take one to two hours after meals.
   c. To prevent an irritating effect in the stomach. The irritation is lessened by the combination of the remedy with the protein of the food.
Taste is a very important factor. A person may dislike a remedy because of the bitter, bland or unpleasant taste, but the bitter taste is often necessary for the effect and should not be disguised. If the person experiences strong nausea or vomiting, then the remedy may be taken in a large quantity of fluid or in syrup, wine or honey.
The taste of powders may be disguised by placing the powder in a capsule, or by wrapping it in a small disk of rice paper, but the benefits obtained by the body's reaction to the taste will be missed.
Unpleasant tasting fluids can be given cold, followed by a drink of plain water.

THE COURSE OF HERBAL THERAPY

In using herbal therapy, first choose the preparation that best suits the condition being treated. Make the choice by considering the age of the person, environment in which they live, their lifestyle, whether or not they will have time to prepare a tea and which method of preparation is most convenient.

Tinctures and fluid extracts are very convenient and can be carried with the individual at work or while traveling. When a condition that needs immediate attention is present, a tincture, which is absorbed rapidly, would be a suitable choice. When herbs are strong tasting, a tincture or fluid extract can be added to water to make it more palatable. If herbs have to be taken over a long period of time or if several herbs or herb combinations are being taken, it is easier to use tinctures instead of taking twenty or more gelatin capsules daily.

Capsules are also easy to take, but in warm climates if a person carries capsules with them, they tend to stick together, in which case tablets would be a better choice. Vegetarians prefer tablets over capsules because the gelatin is an animal by-product. Herbal formulas may be purchased already combined in capsules or tablets, which saves time over trying to put powders into capsules yourself. When herbs are to be taken *with* meals, to avoid drinking too much fluid, tinctures, fluid extracts, capsules or tablets are preferred over teas.

Pills can be taken for the same reason as capsules and tablets. An advantage of home-made pills is that you can put your own formula in pill form.

Teas are used if the person has time to make them and when the herb must be tasted to produce an effect on digestion, saliva, etc. When bitter teas are taken they have a tonic effect on digestion and other related organs. Temperature is also important when using teas. A *hot* infusion or decoction is used during sweating therapy. *Cool* teas are used for tonic effect, *warm* teas will creat a feeling of relaxation.

Flowers and leaves usually are made into infusions. A decoction is used when trying to extract healing properties from most roots, barks, twigs and seeds.

Once the proper preparation has been chosen, the dosage is considered.

To determine the proper dosages, study each herb to understand its uses and suggested dosages. Then apply this knowledge, depending upon whether the disease treated is chronic or acute and whether the patient is child or adult. Consider whether the patient is strong, weak, or if pregnancy, lactation or menstruation is present and take into account the age, temperament and sex of the individual. It is always safer to start with smaller or children's dosages even when treating adults if there is any question in mind about the appropriateness of the therapy. Then increase slowly, remaining on each level for two to three days to determine if any unusual reaction manifests. If a child is going to be taking the preparation, first determine the adult dosage and then use the following rule to determine the approximate dosage for the child:

$$\frac{\text{Weight of child in pounds}}{\text{150 (average adult weight)}} = \text{fraction of adult dose to be used}$$

For example:

$$\frac{\text{50 lbs. (child's weight)}}{\text{150 (avg. adult weight)}} = \text{⅓ of the adult dosage}$$

If a translation to capsules from tinctures, teas, fluid extracts or powders is needed, see the chart in this chapter on "Translating Traditional Herb Preparations".

When treating acute diseases like colds, flus, fevers, etc. in children and adults, large doses of the chosen herb or herb formula are given *every two to four hours* until the crisis breaks and the symptoms disappear. Then the same or a decreased dosage of the same herbs is given *two or three times daily* for the next three to seven days. Usually the upper range of the suggested dosage is considered a large dose. The amount can be decreased to the lower range of the suggested dosage after symptoms disappear. Even though the acute symptoms are no longer present, it takes a few days before the remaining waste products such as dead blood cells, mucus, pus and other matter is eliminated from the bloodstream. This stage of disease is known as the "abatement" or "absorption" stage in naturopathic medicine. This is when the healing forces are in the ascendency and the poisons and microorganisms of the disease are gradually absorbed and eliminated and by degree the tissues are cleansed of the waste.

After using the formula in less frequent dosages for three to seven days, another formula is used to help rebuild the body. The herbs chosen should produce more of a tonic, nutritive effect. During this stage of disease called "reconstruction", the body is reconstructing itself and the herbs chosen should promote this function.

Mild herbs should be used when treating children. Avoid using harsh laxatives and strong cleansing herbs. Mild herbs are herbs that can be taken in large amounts, usually one cup of the tea per dose. Peppermint, chamomile, catnip, elder flowers, comfrey leaf, nettles, chickweed, spearmint and alfalfa are examples of mild herbs which are good for children.

Healing crises should be watched very carefully in children. Always consult an experienced physician in cases of infectious disease.

Often you will find that a strong child or an adult experiencing an acute ailment can be treated with mild herbs and a cleansing diet, instead of strong cleansing herbs. If this mild therapy doesn't show positive results in two to three days, switch to stronger herbs. The strength and energy level of the individual being treated will help determine the potency of herbs to use and the amount to apply.

Chronic diseases are treated similarly to acute diseases except there is a long term therapy involved. Cancer, arthritis, asthma and other such diseases affect the whole body and the approach to therapy must be systematic. Short fasts, massage, manipulations, herbs, diet, sunshine, fresh air, sun baths, salt baths, counseling, exercise (if possible) and breathing exercises are used. Of course, these methods are also considered for acute diseases.

The herbs chosen to treat chronic diseases are those that will have an effect on the whole body and bring about a slow, gradual change. The herbs are given frequently (every two to four hours), as when treating acute ailments. Also, use large dosages during the acute flare-up of the chronic disease. If the formula being used brings on a reaction which seems to be negative, cut back on the dosage or skip the treatment entirely for a day or so. If these symptoms immediately disappear during this short rest period, usually this is an indication that the formula is not the proper one or there is an herb that is causing the reaction. The formula should be changed.

While treating chronic diseases, acute symptoms (healing crises) will usually manifest. If in your original formula there are herbs that are specific for the acute symptoms manifested you may not need to use another formula or single herb. But, if the symptoms are severe and persist for two days or more, another formula or herb may be added to the treatment to relieve the symptoms. It is valuable during this time to use enemas, hydrotherapy, spinal manipulations and other therapies to assist the body in cleansing. Once the symptom of the crisis is gone, return to the original treatment and delete the herbs that were used to treat the acute crisis.

This brings us to the most important part of treating chronic dieases, *rest periods*. During rest periods, the person is eating the originally prescribed diet, but does not take herbs internally. A rest period should be taken one day every week. After two to three weeks of treatment, a three day rest is indicated. The rest period gives a true indication of the energy level of the patient. All herbs have some degree of either a stimulating or sedative effect on the body. The three day rest period gives a clear picture of how the treatment is working, what effect it is having, if it should be continued and if the dosage should be increased or decreased. If during the rest period the energy remains low or an infection develops, or if the symptoms worsen, the treatment needs to be continued. On the other hand, if the patient seems to improve during the rest period, extend the rest period a day or so and then continue the treatment with *smaller* doses than were used before. If during the rest period the patient seems to completely recover, the treatment can be changed to a more tonic, nutritive approach. If symptoms that were not present in the original disease condition just prior to treatment keep reappearing continuously during the rest periods, then an herb, formula or therapy should be chosen to treat those symptoms. This situation indicates that the treatment that was originally used was only covering up the lesser symptoms, or that it might have been too aggressive and was pushing the body in a direction not conducive to the course of healing that nature intended.

If during these rest periods the patient seems to be getting stronger and stronger in each period, begin to reduce therapy and extend the rest periods. Gradually, a clear picture of improvement will be noticed and the whole therapy can be directed toward a nutritive, tonic and vitalizing approach (tonification therapy).

HEALING CRISIS

Webster describes the word "crisis" as "the turning point for better or worse in an acute disease or fever". A healing crisis is known in naturopathy as "an acute reaction, resulting from the activity of nature's healing forces in overcoming chronic disease conditions". A crisis is brought about when the body becomes overcrowded with waste and irritating poisons. Cells and tissues begin to throw off the waste and it is carried by the circulating bloodstream to the eliminatory organs, the bowels, kidneys, lungs, skin, nasal passages, ears, throat, bronchi and genito-urinary organs. The organs then become somewhat crowded, irritated and congested. The organs of elimination, heavily laden with waste at this time, produce disease symptoms such as colds, boils, kidney and bladder infections, open sores, perspiration, diarrhea, fevers, etc. All crises are a form of healing and elimination. First the toxins are eliminated, second, the tissues are renewed.

These symptoms and the process of elimination are part of the cure. There is nothing to fear, just work *with* it. *Do not* suppress the symptoms with drugs unless absolutely necessary. In some situations, such as during chronic diseases like cancer, the pain can become severe and drugs sometimes need to be used. Many of the drugs themselves accumulate in the body because our organs were not made to handle them and they are stored in fatty tissue and other parts of the body. The tissues which are imbedded with these foreign elements are actually destroyed or begin a process of degeneration. It has been said by many natural healers that many diseases are actually drug diseases, caused by these inimical elements which only suppress nature's healing forces.

The naturopathic school of thought distinguishes between a "healing crisis" and a "disease crisis". A healing crisis and a disease crisis may look alike by their outward manifestations, but they are taking place under different conditions.

A disease crisis is when the body is loaded to its toleration point with toxins and waste products. The body arouses itself in self-defense and brings forth acute elimination of toxins in the form of a cold, fever, inflammations, etc. The body is on the defense and produces a disease crisis.

If poisons are not eliminated, the body, until it becomes sick, adapts itself to them functioning at a lower energy level. These foreign wastes accumulate and inhibit the organs from performing their normal functions until finally a chronic disease manifests.

On the other hand, a "healing crisis" develops because the healing forces are in the ascending. Through natural living and a frugal diet, the body gets stronger and digs into the tissues and eliminates old chronic waste causing symptoms, which are the healing crisis. During a healing crisis, therapy can be used to a much greater extent because the patient already has endurance and can tolerate cleansing herbs, fasting and advanced water treatments. When people are weaker, building foods, short fasts and tonic herbs are used. Then once the energy returns, more vigorous cleansing methods can be used.

A healing crisis shows that there is enough energy in the body to eliminate unwanted materials. It can take the form of fevers, excessive menstrual discharge, diarrhea, itching, boils, ulcers, hemorrhages etc. Reactions will vary according to how seriously ill the person has been, how much he got abused by the environment he lives and works in.

To be able to differentiate between a healing crisis and a change for the worse during a diease is very important. Whether a person is trying to improve his life by changing his diet and using detoxification methods or not, a crisis, if not watched and understood properly can weaken the individual and last for several days if not treated properly. You can usually see a positive change in a crisis after three days. The most severe symptoms begin to decrease, fevers break, and the person becomes more relaxed and psychologically feels better. If after three days the severe symptoms do not change for the better, then a new course of treatment is indicated.

Many times crises can be avoided if the individual has a strong constitution and proper functioning eliminatory organs. Also, sometimes there are preceding symptoms that show that a crisis is coming and the body is trying to eliminate toxins. Dark urine, sluggishness, fevers, coated tongue, sense of irritability and weakness, headaches and ringing in the ears are a few preceding signs to look for. If therapy is undertaken during these times and the body is assisted by the proper use of herbs, enemas, homeopathy, acupuncture, massage and hydrotherapy, energy blockages that are caused by accumulated waste can be released. The normal energy flow is restored to the eliminatory organs and the poisons are eliminated naturally without a noticeable crisis. Although no person can guarantee that a crisis can be avoided, these natural therapies will always assist nature in re-establishing health and balance.

The body will become stronger after each crisis if a better lifestyle is continued. Each crisis becomes farther apart until the day comes when only health is present and sickness is history. You may experience slight crises once in a while, but they will last for only a short time (one to three days) and will pass and leave you healthier.

Many people ask in what form will the crisis appear and how long will it last. It depends upon the following:

1. The kind of waste (drugs, mucus, uric acid, etc.)

2. The condition of the eliminatory organs.

3. The energy level or vitality of the patient.

Crises will vary according to how seriously ill the person has been. The area of congestion in the body will determine the type of crisis you will have. Constipation can precede diarrhea; lung congestion can precede a crisis in that area, etc. If the mucus is thick, the body will force it out through the mucus membranes producing nasal drip, colds, flu, etc. If the waste cannot be eliminated through natural pathways, the body will burn it off (fevers) or store it as boils and acne. Nature always picks the best adapted organs for elimination. At times we feel pain in our kidneys, bladder or bowels and we believe the organ in question is diseased. On the contrary, it is usually the strongest eliminative organ in the organism and nature is using it for an outlet for the unwanted waste.

Climate plays a great influence on the type of crisis also. If the weather is cold, the pores of the skin are usually covered and contracted so the kidneys, bowels and lungs throw off the excess. In hot climates, the skin can eliminate more acid waste. People wear lighter clothing and the pores are open and elimination takes place. Oftentimes people move to warmer climates and a skin disease develops. In a hot climate the sun drains out the poisons through the open pores where they accumulate and may cause skin diseases such as cancer. It is then said "the sun causes skin cancer" or the "hot weather is bad". Of course, too much sun can cause skin conditions, but this usually is not the problem. The poisons are being drawn to the surface for elimination. If the blood was clean, a great percent of these conditions wouldn't exist.

I have seen people with the worst skin conditions you can imagine. After a thorough cleanse, proper food, rest, exercise and mental attitude, the conditions vanish. They then proceed to enjoy sun bathing after years of not getting the beauty and health-preserving benefits of the sun's rays.

The energy and vitality of an individual also is a determining factor during a crisis. In a robust individual the toxins are eliminated quickly and in a more powerful way. A person who is weak, with low vitality, takes a much longer time to eliminate the toxins. In this case, natural therapy can be of great assistance. When the crisis is over in both weak and strong persons, toning and strengthening the body is a necessity. Exercise, proper diet, toning herbs and hydrotherapy can be used.

A healing crisis usually last from three to seven days. As I mentioned, the most severe symptoms usually decrease around the third day. If the crisis lasts longer than seven days, it is usually because the individual is weak and it is just going to take a little longer, or the treatment was not proper or followed through properly by the sick individual. If there is a question about the length of a sickness or the severity of the problem, consult a qualified physician.

An important thing to remember is never go to extremes in dietary changes. Use a slow transition, educate yourself about diet and normal therapeutics and work with a practitioner who has experience along these lines. Trying to get too pure too fast can be destructive and can postpone your goal.

KEEPING THE DISEASE UNDER CONTROL

Keeping the disease under control is, of course, one of the main objectives to therapy. If excessive stimulation, detoxification or sweating are used, this will deplete the healing integrity of the body.

In the diagram below, the energy level of person is plotted vertically, while the time elapsed during therapy is shown horizontally.

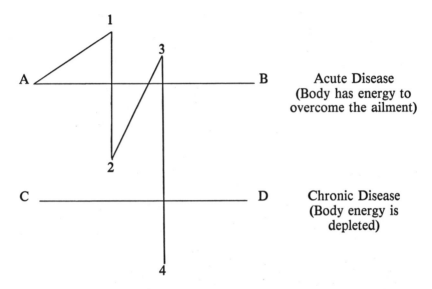

For example, line A to B is a given energy level of a patient. If the person is over stimulated using large amounts of cayenne, ginseng, vitamins, sex, stimulating foods, high protein diet, spices, long-term or too intense detoxification methods, coffee or drugs, they will push the body synthetically up to point 1 where a temporary high and energy level is felt. But because the body was stimulated excessively without adequately nourishing and relaxing of the system, the body will relapse into a fatigued state, down to point 2. When over-stimulation is produced, the body's alkaline reserves, vitamins and nerve fats are being used. This is depleting, and the body must rest to restore these. Yet, because the fatigue is felt, more stimulation is given by the inexperienced therapist or laymen. The body once again is synthetically pushed to point 3, but because of lack of reserves, it doesn't quite reach as high as level 1, but soon falls lower than level 2, down to level 4. If this is continued, the body is too weak to detoxify properly and metabolic toxins are retained in the system, now making the condition worse instead of better. By making this mistake over a period of time, repeating synthetic stimulation, it actually is possible to turn a simple, acute problem (where the energy was present to cure the condition) into a chronic disease with an accompanying low energy level.

This type of problem results from taking excessive amounts of vitamins and herbs that might otherwise produce good results if applied properly and in moderation. Instead of resting, fasting and building, the individual is trying to synthetically produce energy. Recuperation through sleep, fasting and eating small amounts of natural, easily digestible foods will restore normality. It must be remembered that it takes large amounts of energy to digest food, so energy must be present before eating. Never eat while tired. It is better in many cases to sleep your way back to health instead of trying to excessively eat your way back.

By understanding the use of these therapies and closely watching the changing course of the disease with a corresponding change of energy level in the person being treated, one can easily guide a sick individual back to health and sometimes back to a healthier state than before.

TRANSLATING TRADITIONAL HERB PREPARATIONS

Most herb books rarely describe the dosages in terms of number of capsules. Instead, they describe the traditionally used preparations, such as teas, tinctures and fluid extracts. You can translate very roughly the amount of these preparations to the number of capsules as indicated in the following table. Of course, in the case of concentrates, you should be able to rely directly on the instructions found on the package label. This table is for powdered herbs in capsules.

Note: This is for '0' (the small size) capsules, which are the size usually sold pre-filled in bottles. Always begin the first dose smaller to check for sensitivity to the herbs. Note that when taking three doses per day, the number of capsules may be a dozen or more. The numbers given here are approximate since herbal powders vary in their densities and the traditional preparations vary in their strength depending upon the source of herb and the exact method of preparation. Concentrated extracts in capsules are more convenient for the herbs taken in larger doses, since fewer capsules need be taken.

TRANSLATING TRADITIONAL HERB PREPARATIONS
TO HERB POWDERS IN CAPSULES

Traditional Preparation	Number of Capsules/Dose Usually Taken 2-3 Doses/Day
TEAS	
Standard decoction of infusion of one ounce herb per pint of water	
1 fl. oz. (2 tablespoons)	1-2 caps
Wineglass (2-3 fl. oz.)	3-6 caps
Half cup (4 fl. oz.)	6-10 caps

Teaspoon of herb in cup of water, drink all	1-2 caps
Tablespoon of herb in cup of water, drink all	3-6 caps

TINCTURES

Standard tincture of four ounces
herb per pint of alcohol

1-2 drachma (1-2 teaspoons)	3-6 caps

FLUID EXTRACTS

Commercially-prepared by
multiple extraction procedure

1-2 minims (1-2 drops)	1-2 caps
5-6 drops	5-6 caps

POWDERS

Fine powdered herb taken in
a small amount of water

5-10 grains	1-2 caps
10-20 grains	2-3 caps
20-60 grains	3-8 caps

TRADITIONAL PREPARATIONS AND DOSAGE

These instructions indicate the proper dosages for teas with therapeutic properties. Teas are made using one full ounce of dried herb (28 grams) to one pint of distilled water (16 fluid ounces). The teas are made by *infusion* (steeping the herb in boiled water for twenty minutes) or by *decoction* (simmering on low heat for ten minutes to one hour, depending on the hardness of the root). In using these processes, the active ingredients are extracted and the herb absorbs some of the water. After straining the material, about one and one half cups (12 fluid ounces) of the tea will remain, which is consumed as indicated.

COMMON NAME	PART USED	PREPARATION	DOSAGE/FREQUENCY
Alfalfa	leaves	infusion	6 oz. 3x
Aloe Vera	leaves	gel**	2 oz. each time
Angelica	root	decoction	1-2 oz. 3x
Barberry	rootbark	decoction	1 tbs. as needed
Bayberry	rootbark	decoction	1-2 oz. as needed
Black Cohosh	root	decoction	1-2 oz. 3-4x
Black Walnut	leaves	infusion	6 oz. 1-4x

Blessed Thistle	tops	infusion	3 oz. as needed
Blue Cohosh	root	decoction	1-2 oz. 3-4x
Boneset	tops	infusion	3 oz. 3x
Brigham Tea (Ephedra)	stems and branches	decoction	6 oz. 3x
Buchu	leaves	infusion	3 oz. 3-4x
Buckthorn	bark	decoction*	1 tbs. 3x
Burdock	root	decoction	3 oz. 3-4x
Calendula	leaves and flowers	infusion	1 tbs. each hour
Camomile (Chamomile)	flowers	infusion	6 oz. 2-3x
Cascara Sagrada	bark	decoction	1 tsp. 3-4x (before meals)
Catnip	tops	infusion	1 oz. as needed
Cayenne	fruit	infusion	1 tbs. (warm) as needed
Chaparral	stems and leaves	infusion	6 oz. 3x
Chickweed	leaves	infusion	6 oz. 3-4x (between meals)
Cleavers	leaves	infusion	3 oz. 3-4x
Cloves	flower buds	infusion	1-2 tbs. 3x
Coltsfoot	leaves	infusion	6 oz. frequently
Comfrey	leaves	infusion	6 oz. 3x
Comfrey	root	decoction	3 oz. frequently
Crampbark	bark	decoction*	1 tbs. as needed
Damiana	leaves	extract**	15-30 drops 1x
Dandelion	root	decoction	6 oz. frequently
Devil's Claw	root	decoction	6 oz. 3x
Echinacea	root	decoction	1 tbs. 6x
Elder	flowers	infusion	6 oz. 3x
Eyebright	above ground portion	infusion	6 oz. frequently
False Unicorn	root	decoction	6 oz. 3x
Fennel	seed (crushed)	infusion	6 oz. 3x
Fenugreek	seed	decoction	6 oz. 3x
Flax	seed		
Fo-Ti	root	decoction	2 oz. 2-4x
Garlic	bulb	syrup	1 tbs. 3-4x
Garlic	bulb	fresh juice**	½-1 tsp. 3x
Gentian	root	decoction	½ to 1 tsp. 3x
Ginger	root	decoction	6 oz. 3x
Ginseng	root	decoction	½ to 1 oz. 3x
Goldenseal	root (powdered)	infusion	1-2 tsp. 3-6x
Gotu Kola	above ground portion	infusion	3 oz. 3x
Gravel Root	root	decoction	1-2 oz. as needed
Hawthorn	berries	decoction	6 oz. 3x

Hops	fruit	infusion	6 oz. 3x
Horehound	leaves	infusion	6 oz. frequently
Horseradish	root	infusion	6 oz. 1-2x
Horsetail	stem	decoction	2 oz. 3-4x
Irish Moss	whole plant	infusion	3 oz. 2-3x
Juniper	berries	infusion	6 oz. 2-3x
Kava Kava	root	infusion	2 oz. 2x
Kelp	whole plant	powdered**	1 tsp. 2x
Lady's Slipper	root	decoction	1 tbs. in 6 oz. water 3-4x
Lemon Balm	leaves	infusion	6 oz. as needed
Licorice	root	decoction	1 tbs. as needed
Lobelia	tops	infusion	1 tbs. as needed
Lungwort	leaves	infusion	6 oz. at a time
Mandrake	root	decoction	1 tbs. (cold) 2x
Marshmallow	root	decoction	6 oz. 3x
Mistletoe, American	leaves	infusion	3 oz. 2-3x
Mistletoe, European			
Motherwort	herb	infusion	6 oz. 3-4x
Mugwort	leaves	infusion	1 tsp. as needed
Mullein	leaves	infusion	3 oz. frequently
Myrrh	gum (powdered)	infusion	3 oz. 3-4x
Nettles	leaves	infusion	3 oz. frequently
Oat	straw	infusion	6 oz. 3x
Oregon Grape Root	root	decoction	3 oz. 3-4x
Parsley	leaves	infusion	6 oz. 2-3x
Parsley	root	decoction	6 oz. 3x
Passion Flower	plant and flower	tincture**	15-60 drops in water as needed
Peach Tree	leaves	infusion	6 oz. 3x
Pennyroyal	leaves	infusion	6 oz. frequently
Peppermint	leaves	infusion	6oz. 3x
Plantain	leaves	infusion	2-3 oz. as needed
Pleurisy	root	decoction	2-3 oz. as needed
Poke	root	decoction	1-2 oz. 3-4x
Prickly Ash	bark	decoction	1-2 oz. 3-4x
Prince's Pine	tops	infusion	3 oz. as needed
Psyllium	seed	powdered**	1 tsp. in warm water or juice 3x
Queen of the Meadow	root	decoction	1-2 oz. as needed
Raspberry	leaves	infusion	6 oz. frequently
Red Clover	tops	infusion	1-2 oz. 3x
Rose Hips	hips	decoction	3 oz. 3x
Rosemary	leaves	infusion	2 oz. 3x
Safflower	flower	infusion	6 oz. 2x
Sage	leaves	infusion	1 tbs. as needed
Sarsparilla	root	decoction	3 oz. 3x
Sassafras	rootbark	decoction	3 oz. 3-4x

Saw Palmetto	berries	infusion	6 oz. 2-3x
Scullcap	tops	infusion	3 oz. 4-5x
Senna	leaves	infusion	2 oz. 3x
Shepherd's Purse	herb	infusion	6 oz. 2-3x
Slippery Elm	inner bark (powdered)	infusion	6 oz. 3-4x
Spearmint	leaves	infusion	6 oz. 3-4x
Squaw Vine	leaves and berries	infusion	3 oz. 3x
St. John's Wort	tops	infusion	1 oz. as needed
Stone Root	root	decoction	1 tbs. 3x
Thyme	tops	infusion	1 oz. frequently
Turkey Rhubarb	root	infusion	3 oz. 3x
Uva Ursi	leaves	infusion	3 oz. as needed
Valerian	root	infusion	3 oz. 3x
Vervain	flowers and leaves	infusion	3 oz. frequently
White Oak Bark	bark	decoction	3 oz. as needed
White Willow			
Wild Yam	root	decoction	2-3 oz. in water 3-4x
Witch Hazel	bark	decoction	3 oz. as needed
Witch Hazel	leaves	infusion	6 oz. as needed
Wood Betony	tops	infusion	3 oz. 3x
Wormwood	tops	infusion	3 oz. as needed
Yarrow	herb	infusion	6 oz. 3-4x
Yellowdock	root	decoction	1 tbs. in 6 oz. water 3x
Yerba Santa	leaves	infusion	2-3 oz. 3x

*Tea is made using one ounce of herb per quart of water
**Most recommended way to make this herb

Note: 1 fluid ounce = 1 tablespoon (tbs.)

HERBAL PROPERTIES

ALTERATIVES

Alteratives are herbs which alter (purify) the blood. Most herbs for blood purification promote the cleaning action of the spleen, liver, kidneys and bowels. These herbs should be used over a long period of time, allowing gradual detoxification of the entire blood stream which in turn, will improve digestion, assimilation and glandular secretions. Of course, bad habits and poor diet must be corrected to remove the cause of the toxicity of the blood. Infections, cancer, arthritis and skin disease are some of the diseases caused by impure blood.

Alfalfa	Elder	Pipsissewa
Barberry	Eyebright	Plantain
Bayberry	Garlic	Poke root
Black cohosh	Ginseng	Prickly ash
Blessed Thistle	Goldenseal	Raspberry
Burdock root	Gotu kola	Red clover
Cayenne	Kelp	Rhubarb
Chaparral	Licorice root	Sarsparilla
Chickweed	Mandrake	Sassafras
Cleavers	Marshmallow	St. John's wort
Comfrey	Nettles	Uva ursi
Dandelion	Oregon grape root	Wood betony
Devil's claw		Yellowdock
Echinacea		

ANODYNES

Anodynes are herbs that relieve pain by lessening the excitability of the nerves and nerve centers. These are closely allied to the antispasmodics. Most of these herbs can be used externally as fomentations or internally as teas, tinctures or powders.

Chamomile	Lady's slipper	Valerian
Cloves	Lobelia	Vervain
Echinacea	Mullein	White willow
Ginger	Passion flower	Wild lettuce
Hops	Pulsatilla	Wild yam
Juniper berries	Scullcap	Wood Betony
Kava kava		

Anthelmintics

Anthelmintics are herbs which have the capacity to destroy intestinal worms and parasites; there are two categories of anthelmintics:

Vermicides are agents which destroy worms without necessarily causing their expulsion from the bowels. Vermicides should be followed by or combined with laxative or cathartic herbs.

Black walnut	Tansy	Wormwood
Garlic	Thyme	

Vermifuges are agents which expel worms from the bowels, usually having cathartic properties.

Cascara sagrada	Senna	Wormwood
Gentian	Tansy	

Antacids

Antacids is a term applied to agents which correct acid conditions in the stomach, blood and bowels.

Comfrey leaves	Hops	Slippery elm
Comfrey root	Mullein	Wood betony
Flax seed	Red raspberry	

Antibiotics

Antibiotics are agents that inhibit the growth of and destroy viruses and bacteria. These herbs not only destroy germs, but help promote the body's own immunity.

Chaparral	Goldenseal	Myrrh
Echinacea	Hops	Rosemary oil
Garlic	Juniper berries	Thyme

ANTICATARRHALS

These are herbs which eliminate mucus conditions. While ridding the body of catarrh, it is very useful to aid elimination by including laxative herbs for the bowel, or diuretic teas to eliminate excess moisture.

Angelica	Cranesbill	Lobelia
Anise	Cubebs	Lungwort
Bayberry	Elecampane	Marshmallow
Bistort	Figs	Raisins
Cayenne	Flax seed	Tormentil
Coltsfoot	Garlic	Wild cherry
Comfrey	Ginger	Yerba santa
	Horseradish	
	Irish moss	

ANTIEMETICS

These are medicines which have the effect of relieving and suspending sickness of the stomach and thus preventing vomiting.

Anise	Goldenseal	Red clover
Cinnamon	Lobelia (small doses)	Spearmint
Cloves	Peach leaves	Sweet basil
Ginger	Peppermint	

ANTIPYRETICS

Antipyretics are herbs that are cooling to the system and are used to reduce fevers; also called "refrigerants."

Alfalfa	Cranberries	Licorice
Benzoin	Elder flowers	Limes
Boneset	Gotu kola	Oranges
Camphor	Lemon balm	Scullcap
Chickweed	Lemons	Valerian

ANTISEPTICS

These plants have the power to prevent the growth of bacteria.

Anise Oil	Echinacea	Plantain
Barberry	Garlic	Rosemary
Beth root	Goldenseal	Saw palmetto
Bistort	Juniper berries	Thyme
Black walnut	Myrrh	White oak bark

Buchu	Nettles	White willow
Chaparral	Oregon grape root	Wormwood

ANTISPASMODICS

Antispasmodics are herbs to be used for muscular spasms, convulsions and cramps.

Black cohosh	Lady's slipper	Prickly ash
Black haw	Lemon balm	Raspberry
Blue cohosh	Lobelia	Rue
Calendula	Motherwort	Sage
Cascara sagrada	Mistletoe	Scullcap
Cayenne	Mugwort	Skunk cabbage
Crampbark	Mullein	Spearmint
Fennel	Oat	Thyme
Garlic	Passion flowers	Valerian
Hawthorn berries	Peppermint	Vervain
Kava kava	Pleurisy root	Wild yam

APERIENTS

Aperients are herbs that produce mild laxative effects which soften the stools without purging.

Agar-agar	Fruit	Prunes
Figs	Licorice root	Raisins
Flax seed	Olive oil	Rose hips

APHRODISIACS

These are herbs that correct conditions of impotence and impure sex power.

Cloves	Fennel	Kava Kava
Damiana	Fenugreek	Sarsparilla root
False unicorn	Ginseng	Saw palmetto

AROMATICS

Aromatics are herbs which have a fragrant smell and an agreeable, pungent taste. Aromatic herbs have a stimulating effect on the gastrointestinal mucus membrane because of their essential oils. They have a spicy taste and are used to aid digestion and expel wind from the stomach and bowels. They are also used to cover the taste of bitter herbs. If inflammation of the stomach or bowels is present, aromatic herbs should be avoided.

Anise seed	Fennel	Rosemary
Barberry	Ginger	Sage
Buchu	Juniper berries	Sassafras
Cinnamon	Nutmeg	Spearmint
Cloves	Peppermint	St. John's wort
Coriander seed		Wood betony
		Wormwood

ASTRINGENTS

These are herbs which increase the tone and firmness of the tissues and lessen mucus discharge from the nose, intestines, vagina and draining sores.

Bayberry	Fenugreek	Shepherd's purse
Beth root	Gravel root	Slippery elm
Blackberry	Hawthorn berries	Squaw vine
Black walnut	Horsetail	St. John's wort
Bugleweed	Juniper berries	Stoneroot
Calendula	Mullein	Tormentil root
Cayenne	Pipsissewa	Uva ursi
Cleaver	Plantain	Vervain
Comfrey root	Prickly ash	Wild cherry bark
Crampbark	Raspberry	Witch hazel
Cranesbill	Rhubarb	White oak bark
Dandelion	Rosehips	Yarrow
Elecampane	Rosemary	Yellow dock
Ephedra	Sage	Yerba santa
Eyebright		

BLOOD PURIFIERS (See Alteratives)

CARDIACS

Cardiacs are herbs that increase the power of the heart.

Black cohosh	Hawthorn berries	Motherwort
Bugleweed		

CARMINATIVES

Carminatives are herbs containing volatile oils which stimulate the expulsion of flatus (gas) from the gastrointestinal tract. Carminatives also increase the tone of the musculature and stimulate peristalsis. Aromatic herbs are also carminatives.

Angelica	Coriander	Parsley
Anise	Cumin	Pennyroyal
Caraway	Dill	Peppermint
Cardamon	Fennel	Pleurisy root
Catnip	Garlic	Rosemary
Cayenne	Ginger	Sarsparilla
Celery	Juniper berries	Sassafras
Chamomile	Myrrh	Spearmint
		Thyme
		Valerian

CATHARTICS

Cathartics are herbs which cause a rapid evacuation from the upper intestines and the bowels.

Aloe	Rhubarb	Senna
Cascara sagrada		

CHOLAGOGUES

The following are herbs which promote the flow of bile.

Barberry	Dandelion	Olive oil
Beets	Elecampane	Oregon grape root
Bistort	Gentian	Vervain
Boneset	Goldenseal	Wild yam
Cascara sagrada	Hops	Wormwood
Cayenne	Hyssop	Yellow dock
Damiana	Mandrake	

CONDIMENTS

Condiments are herbs used to season foods and to increase digestive activity. Most are good for treating gas and indigestion.

Bay leaves	Coriander	Ginger
Cayenne	Cumin	Nutmeg
Cinnamon	Curry	Pimento
Cloves	Dill	Sweet basil

DEMULCENTS

Demulcents are herbs which soften and relieve irritation of the mucus membranes. They are also used in combination with other powders to bind them in making pills.

Agar-agar
Aloe vera
Burdock root
Chickweed
Coltsfoot
Comfrey root

Corn silk
Fenugreek
Flax seed
Irish moss
Kelp
Licorice root

Lungwort
Marshmallow
Mullein
Peach bark
Psyllium seed
Slippery elm

DEOBSTRUENTS

These herbs remove obstructions. Also see Aperients and Laxatives for treating the intestines.

Barberry (liver, gall bladder)

Culvers root (bowel)

Goldenseal (glands)

Gravel root (kidneys)

Hydrangea root (kidneys)

Plantain (blood, kidneys)

DIAPHORETICS

These are herbs that increase perspiration. The diaphoretics influence the entire circulatory system; there are three categories of diaphoretics:

Stimulating

Angelica
Blessed thistle
Boneset
Buchu
Elder flowers

Ephedra
Garlic
Ginger
Horseradish
Hyssop

Pennyroyal
Peppermint
Spearmint
Yarrow

Neutral

Horehound
Safflower

Sarsparilla

Sassafras

Relaxing

Blue vervain
Burdock root
Calendula
Catnip
Chamomile

Lemon balm
Motherwort
Mugwort
Passion flower
Pleurisy root

Thyme
Vervain
White willow
Wild yam

DISCUTIENTS

These are herbs that dissolve and remove tumors and abnormal growths. These agents are used in poultices, fomentations and taken internally as teas.

Black walnut	Chaparral	Garlic
Burdock root	Devil's claw	Red clover

DIURETICS

Diuretics are herbs that increase the flow of urine. They are usually combined with demulcents to soothe any irritation from acids or gravel. Diuretic herbs can be used in the treatment of backache, prostatitis, sciatica, kidney stones, bladder ache, lymphatic swelling, scalding urine, gonorrhea, skin eruptions, water retention and obesity.

Blackberry	Gotu kola	Parsley
Black cohosh	Gravel root	Pipsissewa
Blue cohosh	Hawthorn berries	Plantain
Buchu	Horseradish	Pleurisy root
Burdock root	Horsetail	Rosemary
Celery seed	Hydrangea	Sassafras
Chaparral	Juniper berries	Saw palmetto
Cleavers	Kava kava	Senna
Corn silk	Kelp	Shepherd's purse
Damiana	Marshmallow	Squaw vine
Dandelion	Mistletoe (American)	St. John's wort
Elecampane	Mistletoe (European)	Stoneroot
False unicorn	Mullein	Uva ursi
Fennel		White oak bark
		White willow

EMETICS

Emetics are substances used to induce vomiting. They are usually administered in tincture and tea form.

Bayberry	Ipecac	Mistletoe (American)
Chaparral	Lobelia tincture	Poke root
False unicorn	Mandrake	
(large doses)	(large doses)	

EMMENAGOGUES

These are herbs which promote menstrual flow.

Angelica	Gentian	Pennyroyal
Beth root	Goldenseal	Prickly ash
Black cohosh	Horsetail	Rue
Black haw	Mistletoe (American)	Safflower
Blessed thistle	Motherwort	Squaw vine

Blue cohosh	Mugwort	Tansy
Chamomile	Myrrh	
Damiana		

EMOLLIENTS

These are remedies that may be applied externally to soften and soothe. They are applied in salves, fomentations and poultices and may be taken internally for their demulcent quality.

Almond oil	Flax seed	Olive oil
Chickweed	Irish moss	Plantain
Coltsfoot	Linseed oil	Slippery elm
Comfrey root	Lungwort	Wheat germ oil
Fenugreek	Marshmallow	

EXPECTORANTS

These are herbs which facilitate the excretion of mucus from the throat and lungs. They usually are combined with demulcents, which are soothing.

Chaparral	Horehound	Nettles
Coltsfoot	Horseradish	Parsley
Comfrey	Hyssop	Plantain
Elecampane	Licorice root	Pleurisy root
Ephedra	Lobelia	Thyme
Fennel	Lungwort	Vervain
Fenugreek	Mullein	Wild cherry
Garlic	Myrrh	Yerba santa

FEBRIFUGES

These are herbs used to reduce fevers.

Boneset	Hyssop	White willow
Catnip	Peppermint	Yarrow
Dandelion	Shepherd's purse	

GALACTAGOGUES

These herbs favor the secretion of milk from the nursing mother.

Anise seed	Dandelion	Raspberry
Blessed thistle	Fennel	Vervain
Cumin	Fenugreek	

HEMOSTATICS

These are herbs that arrest internal bleeding or hemorrhaging. Also see Astringents.

Bayberry	Mullein	White oak bark
Beet root	Nettles	Witch hazel
Blackberry	Tormentil root	Yarrow
Horsetail		

HEPATICS

These are herbs which strengthen, tone and stimulate the secretive functions of the liver. They are useful in the treatment of jaundice and hepatitis.

Aloe vera	Buckthorn	Wild yam
Barberry	Carrot	Wood betony
Bayberry	Dandelion	Yellowdock

LAXATIVES

Laxatives are herbs that promote bowel action.

Agar agar	Flax seed	Peach bark
Boneset	Goldenseal	Poke root
Buckthorn bark	Licorice root	Psyllium seed
Cascara sagrada	Mandrake	Rhubarb
Cleavers	Motherwort	Safflower
Elder	Oregon grape root	Senna
		Yellowdock

LITHOTRIPTICS

Lithotriptics are agents that dissolve and discharge urinary and gall bladder stones and gravel.

Barberry	Dandelion	Marshmallow
Buchu	Devil's claw	Oregon grape root
Cascara sagrada	Gravel root	Parsley
Chaparral	Horsetail	Tormentil
Corn silk	Hydrangea root	Uva ursi
	Juniper berries	

LYMPHATICS

These are herbs used to stimulate and cleanse the lymphatic system.

Black walnut	Echinacea	Poke
Chaparral	Garlic	Yellow dock
Dandelion	Oregon grape root	

MUCILAGES

Mucilages are herbs having mucilaginous properties used to soothe inflamed parts. Also see Demulcents.

Agar agar	Flax seed	Mullein
Chickweed	Lungwort	Okra
Comfrey root	Marshmallow root	Slippery elm

NERVINES

Nervines are herbs which act as a tonic to the nerves. They are used to relieve pain and regulate the nervous system.

Catnip	Lobelia	Peach bark
Celery	Mistletoe	Pleurisy root
Chamomile	Motherwort	Scullcap
Crampbark	Mugwort	St. John's wort
Gravel root	Oats	Vervain
Hops	Parsley	Wood betony
Lady's slipper	Passion flower	

NUTRITIVES

Nutritives are herbs which supply a substantial amount of nutrients and aid in building and toning the body.

Agar agar	Kelp	Rosehips
Alfalfa	Marshmallow root	Slippery elm
Comfrey leaves	Mullein leaves	Watercress
Comfrey root	Nettles	Yellow dock
Horsetail	Red clover	
Irish moss		

Opthalmics

Opthalmics are herbs used for healing diseases of the eyes.

Chickweek	Fennel	Rue
Eyebright	Mullein	

Oxytocics

These are herbs that assist labor and promote easy childbirth.

Angelica	Blue cohosh	Raspberry
Black cohosh	Juniper berries	Squaw vine

Parasiticides

These are herbs that kill and remove parasites from the skin.

Black walnut	Chaparral	Gentian
Cojuput oil	Echinacea	Rue
Cassia oil	False unicorn	Thyme
Cinnamon oil	Garlic	Wood betony

Partrurients (See Oxytocics)

Purgatives

These herbs are agents that have an energetic evacuative effect. Combine these herbs with carminatives to lessen griping.

Buckthorn bark	Mandrake root	Senna
Castor oil		

Resolvents (See Lithotriptics)

Rubefacients

These are agents used as local external applications that stimulate and increase the blood flow to the surface.

Cayenne	Prickly ash	Rue
Mustard seed	Rosemary oil	Thyme oil
Peppermint oil		

SEDATIVES

These herbs are agents which allay excitement of functional activities of an organ or body part. They influence the circulation, reducing nervous expenditure.

All mints	Kava kava	Scullcap
Black haw	Lady's slipper	Sorrel
Bugleweed	Lemon balm	St. John's wort
Catnip	Passion flower	Valerian
Chamomile	Peach bark	Wild cherry bark
Hawthorn berries	Red clover	Witch hazel
Hops	Rue	Wood betony
Hyssop	Saw palmetto	

SIALAGOGUES

These are agents that promote an increased flow of saliva.

Black papper	Ginger
Cayenne	Licorice
Echinacea	Prickly ash

STIMULANTS

Stimulants are herbs which serve as natural agents in assisting the functional activity of the body, increasing energy.

Angelica	Fo-ti	Pennyroyal
Bayberry	Garlic	Peppermint
Black pepper	Ginger	Prickly ash
Blessed thistle	Ginseng	Raspberry
Boneset	Goldenseal	Red clover
Cardamon	Gravel root	Rhubarb
Cayenne	Horseradish	Rosemary
Celery	Hyssop	Rue
Cloves	Juniper berries	Sassafras
Devil's claw	Mandrake	Shepherd's purse
Elder flowers	Mistletoe (European)	Spearmint
Elecampane	Myrrh	Tansy
Ephedra	Oats	Valerian
False unicorn	Onion	Wild cherry bark
Fennel		Yarrow
		Yerba santa

Stomachics

These herbs strengthen the functions of the stomach. They are usually bitter in flavor which promotes and improves digestion and appetite.

Agrimony	Ginseng	Peach bark
Barberry	Goldenseal	Rhubarb
Blessed thistle	Hops	Rosehips
Dandelion	Juniper berries	Rue
Elecampane	Mugwort	Wormwood

Styptics

These herbs arrest bleeding, hemorrhaging and draining wounds. These herbs are usually astringents and may be used externally or internally.

Beth root	Horsetail	White oak bark
Bistort	Plantain leaves	Witch hazel
Blackberry	Tormentil	Yarrow
Cranesbill		

Sudorifics (See Diaphoretics)

Tonics

These are herbs which increase energy and strengthen the body. The effect of tonic herbs is to increase the strength of the muscular and nervous system while improving digestion and assimilation, resulting in a general sense of well-being.

Gall bladder tonics:

Goldenseal	Parsley	Wild yam
Oregon grape root		

Heart tonics:

Bugleweed	Ginseng (Panax)	Motherwort
Hawthorn berries	Mistletoe (European)	

Intestinal tonics:

Barberry	Cascara sagrada	Goldenseal
Blackberry leaves	Cranesbill	Rhubarb

Kidney tonics:

Buchu	Fo-ti	Parsley
Burdock root	Horsetail	Pipsissewa
Celery	Kava kava	Saw palmetto
Cleavers	Mistletoe (American)	Uva ursi

Liver tonics:

Barberry	Dandelion	Goldenseal
Buckthorn bark	Eyebright	Mandrake
Cascara sagrada	Fo-ti	Stoneroot

Lung tonics:

Beth root	Fenugreek	Lungwort
Comfrey	Garlic	Pleurisy root
Elecampane	Irish moss	Wild cherry

Nerve tonics:

Celery	Lady's slipper	Oats
Chamomile	Lobelia	Valerian
Hops	Mistletoe (American)	

Sexual tonics:

Black haw (female)	False unicorn (female)	Sarsaparilla (male)
Damiana	Ginseng	Saw palmetto (male)
(male and female)	(male and female)	
Dong quai (female)		Squaw vine (female)

Stomach tonics:

Agrimony	Gentian	Raspberry
Blessed thistle	Goldenseal	Wild cherry bark
Elecampane	Mugwort	Wormwood

VULNERARIES

These are agents that promote the healing of cuts, wounds and burns by protecting against infection and by stimulating cellular growth.

Aloe vera	Fenugreek	Mullein
Apricot seeds	Garlic	Plantain
Black walnut	Horsetail	Rosemary
Calendula	Lungwort	Slippery elm
Comfrey leaves	Marshmallow	Yarrow
Comfrey root		

In order to help in understanding how to apply herbal therapy, it is important for the reader to learn thoroughly the properties of herbs. All of the properties can be placed into one or more of the three general classifications according to the primary actions they produce in the body. These three categories are detoxifying properties, building and toning properties and symptom-relieving properties.

Detoxifying Properties	Symptom-relieving Properties	Building and toning Properties
Alteratives	Anodynes	Aphrodisiacs
Anthelmintics	Antacids	Astringents
Anticatarrhals	Antibiotics	Cardiacs
Aperients	Antiemetics	Diaphoretics
Cathartics	Antipyretics	Emmenagogues
Cholagogues	Antiseptics	Galactagogues
Deobstruents	Antispasmodics	Hepatics
Discutients	Aromatics	Nervines
Diuretics	Carminatives	Nutritives
Emetics	Condiments	Oxytocics
Expectorants	Demulcents	Stomachics
Laxatives	Diaphoretics	Tonics
Lithotriptics	Emetics	Vulneraries
Lymphatics	Emmenagogues	
Parasiticides	Emollients	
Purgatives	Febrifuges	
	Hemostatics	
	Mucilages	
	Oxytocics	
	Rubefacients	
	Sedatives	
	Sialagogues	
	Stimulants	
	Styptics	

The first classification of properties of herbs is detoxification. When toxins and poisons have accumulated in the body, they must be removed or disease will manifest. To remove these toxins, herbs can be used that have properties that tend to detoxify the system. Herbs have specific properties that influence certain parts of the body and they are chosen accordingly. Herbs that have laxative properties cleanse the bowel, diuretics detoxify the kidneys, herbs that have alterative properties aid in detoxifying the blood and treat constipation, skin diseases, mucus conditions, blood poisoning and lung congestion,which are just a few ailments where detoxification is used.

The second classification we will consider is building and toning. The herbs that have these properties strengthen the body, improving the functions of the internal organs and strengthening the body's resistance to disease. They are used to facilitate recovery from acute ailments, injury, surgery, miscarriage or childbirth. They are also used in the treatment of chronic diseases or after acute disease, anemia, impotence and times of emotional instability.

The third classification of properties is symptom-relieving. The most important activity of the properties listed under this classification are not detoxification or building, but to counteract or relieve specific symptoms. For example, if spasms and tension are the symptoms to be treated, herbs with antispasmodic properties would be used. If bleeding is the symptom, styptics or hemostatics would be indicated to relieve the symptoms.

THE COMMONLY USED HERBS

This chapter provides detailed descriptions of the many herbs in common use, especially those mentioned in other portions of this book. For each herb, the common and botanical names are given, and the part that is usually used is indicated. Major properties are those listed with an initial capital letter, and minor properties are also listed (with an initial lower case letter).

Herbs generally affect the whole body, but there are certain body parts that are most notably affected by each herb. The affected parts are listed in two ways: for each herb, the part primarily affected is mentioned, and then at the end of this chapter, for each body part, a list of herbs affecting it is provided.

There are many different ways that an herb can be prepared for administration, and several of the most common methods for internal use are listed with the usual dosage range for an average adult. Then, under the indications for use of the herb, the most suitable methods of application are listed for each. When the method of application is followed by an asterisk (*), it indicates that the herb is usually used in combination with other herbs when treating the indicated problem. Finally, a brief statement about the properties and use of the herbs consolidates the tables of data and points out the most important aspects.

ALFALFA *(Medicago sativa)*

Part Used: tops

Properties: Alterative, Nutritive; antipyretic

Body Parts Affected: stomach and blood

Preparation and Dosage:

Infusion:	Steep 5 to 15 minutes. 6 oz. three times daily
Tincture:	5 to 15 drops three times daily
Fluid Extract:	½ to 1 tsp. three times daily
Powder:	5 to 10, #0 capsules (30 to 60 grains) three times daily

Indicated Uses:

Internal:	Syrup*, Concentrate*
Arthritis:	Infusion*, Powder
Blood purification	Infusion*, Powder*
Calcium deficiency:	Powder*
Indigestion:	Infusion*, Fluid Extract*
Kidney problems:	Infusion*, Powder*
Rheumatism:	Infusion*, Tincture*, Fluid Extract*, Powder*
Ulcers	Infusion*, Syrup*
Weight loss:	Infusion*, Powder*

Alfalfa was discovered by the Arabs, who called it the "Father of all foods." Its valuable nutritive properties include calcium, magnesium, phosphorus and potassium, plus vitamin K and vitamin P.

It aids in the assimilation of protein, fats and carbohydrates and is an excellent blood purifier. Alfalfa has been substituted for red clover blossoms because of their similar properties. It is good for reducing fevers. Fresh or powdered alfalfa can be added to soups and salads.

AGAR AGAR *(Gelidium amansii)*

Part Used: algae

Properties: Demulcent, Laxative; nutritive

Body Parts Affected: intestines

Preparaion and Dosage:

Infusion:	Steep 5 to 15 minutes. 6 oz. two to three times daily
Fluid Extract:	¼ to 1 fluid oz. two to three times daily
Powder:	10 #0 capsules two to three times daily
Flakes	1 tsp to 1 Tbsp. in juice or warm water two to three times daily

Indicated Uses:

Internal:

Dry intestines:	Powder
Constipation:	Powder*

Agar-agar has the property of absorbing moisture and putrifactive material in the intestinal tract. It swells up into a soft mass and is used for constipation as a mechanical laxative. It is a good remedy when the intestines are dry and the feces are hard. When regularity is needed, use one teaspoon to 1 tablespoon two or three times daily mixed in juice or warm water. This can be taken any time during the day.

Agar can be mixed in breads and cereals for a more laxative effect, or put in other herbal formulas for intestinal lubrication and bulk.

AGRIMONY *(Agrimonia eupatoria)*

Part Used: herb

Properties: Hepatic, Stomachic, astringent, diuretic, tonic

Body Parts Affected: stomach, liver and intestines

Preparation and Dosage:

Decoction:	1 oz. to 1¼ pints water. Simmer down to 1 pint. 3 to 5 Tbsp. three to four times daily
Tincture:	20 to 60 drops three to four times daily
Fluid Extract:	¼ to 1 tsp. three to four times daily
Powder:	5 to 10 #0 capsules (30 to 60 grains) three times daily

Indicated Uses:

Internal

Jaundice:	Decoction*
Skin problems:	Decoction*
Stomach tonic:	Decoction*
Ulcers:	Decoction*, Tincture

External

Vaginal problems:	Douche

An infusion of the leaves has a reputation for the treatment of jaundice and other liver complaints. A strong decoction of the root and leaves is used to treat pimples and skin blotches, ulcers and is used as a stomach tonic.

Externally, a fomentation is used applied to athlete's foot, sores, wounds and insect bites. A douche made from the leaves for excess vaginal secretions works well but should always be combined with a demulcent like mullein or slippery elm.

ALOE VERA *(Aloe vera, var. officinalis)*

Part Used: gel from the leaves

Properties: Demulcent, Emollient, Laxative, Vulnerary; emmenagogue

Body Parts Affected: skin, colon and stomach

Preparation and Dosage:

Gel:	2 oz. each time, up to 1 pint daily
Tincture:	10 to 40 drops three times daily
Fluid Extract:	½ to 1 tsp. three times daily

| Powder: | 4 parts aloe powder with 1 part ginger. Fill #0 capsules. Take 2 capsules three times daily. |

Indicated Uses:

Internal

Chronic constipation	Gel, Fluid Extract
Gastritis:	Gel, Fluid Extract
Hyperacitidy:	Gel, Fluid Extract
Stomach ulcers:	Gel

External

Abscess:	Gel
Burns:	Gel
Infection in wounds:	Gel
Insect bites	Gel
Skin irritations:	Gel
Ulcers:	Gel

The gel of aloe is applied topically to heal severe burns and skin rashes. It can be left on for two days without changing the application.

Aloe acts freely in the lower bowel. It is not to be used in large doses when there are hemorrhoids or when there is irritation in the colon. It should be taken with ginger or fennel tea to inhibit griping. A pint of the gel taken in small doses several times a day has been used for gastric ulcers without any side effects.

Note: The agent is an emmenagogue and should not be used during pregnancy.

ANGELICA *(Angelica archangelica)*

Part Used: root and leaf

Properties: Carminative, Diaphoretic, Emmenagogue, Stimulant; alterative, expectorant, tonic

Body Parts Affected: circulation, heart, stomach, intestines and lungs

Preparation and Dosage:

Infusion (leaf)	Steep herb 15 minutes. Drink 1 to 2 oz. three times daily
Decoction (root)	Simmer 10 to 15 minutes. Drink 1 to 2 oz. three times daily
Tincture:	5 to 15 drops three times daily
Fluid Extract:	½ to 1 tsp. three times daily
Powder:	3 to 5 #0 capsules (15 to 30 grains) three times daily

Indicated Uses:

Internal

Colic:	Tincture, Infusion, Decoction, Fluid Extract
Increase appetite:	Tincture, Infusion, Fluid Extract
Lung congestion:	Infusion
Muscle spasms:	Tincture, Infusion
Nervous headache:	Tincture, Infusion
Relieves flatulence:	Tincture, Infusion, Fluid Extract
Sore throat:	Syrup
Stimulates kidneys:	Tincture*, Infusion*, Fluid Extract*
Stomach cramps:	Tincture, Infusion
Strengthen nerves	Tincture*, Infusion*, Decoction*
Ulcers:	Tincture*, Infusion*, Decoction*
Vomiting:	Tincture*, Infusion*

External

Chest congestion:	Poultice
Muscle spasms:	Fomentation, Liniment, Poultice
Rheumatic pains:	Fomentation, Liniment, Poultice
Stomach cramps:	Fomentation, Liniment, Poultice
Stimulates kidneys:	Fomentation, Liniment, Poultice

Angelica is a good tonic and a remedy for colic, gas, sour stomach and heartburn. It improves circulation, warms the body and relieves spasms of the stomach and bowels. Angelica is a good herb to add to treatments for lung diseases, coughs, colds and fevers. It is equally useful in the form of a tincture or infusion. For a tonic, one to three capsules can be taken each day.

Note: It is a strong emmenagogue and should not be taken by pregnant women. Diabetics should avoid using angelica as it may cause weakness.

BARBERRY *(Berberis vulgaris)*

Part Used: root bark

Properties: Antiseptic, Hepatic, Stomachic; alterative, aromatic, tonic

Body Parts Affected: liver, spleen, digestive tract, blood

Preparation and Dosage:

Infusion:	½ oz. to 1 pint water. Steep 10 minutes. 1 to 4 cups daily before meals
Decoction (root bark):	Simmer 10 minutes. 1 Tbsp. as needed
Tincture:	½ to 1 tsp. as needed
Fluid Extract	½ to 1 tsp. as needed
Powder:	2 to 5 #0 capsules (15 to 30 grains) three times daily

Indicated Uses:

Internal

Anemia:	Tincture, Fluid Extract
Blood purifier:	Tincture*, Fluid Extract*, Decoction*
Boils:	Tincture*, Fluid Extract*, Decoction*
Constipation	Tincture*, Fluid Extract*, Decoction*
Diarrhea:	Decoction*
Digestion:	Tincture*, Fluid Extract*, Decoction*, Powder*
Gall stones:	Decoction*
Heartburn:	Tincture*, Fluid Extract*, Decoction*, owder*
Jaundice:	Fluid Extract*, Decoction*, Syrup*
Swollen and obstructed spleen:	Tincture, Fluid Extract

Because barberry tea is so bitter, it should be taken in small doses. The natural physician uses it chiefly for all sluggish liver conditions. An infusion is also valuable for swollen spleen and chronic stomach problems when taken in tablespoonfuls several times a day, especially before meals.

A combination of barberry with cayenne, goldenseal and lobelia is a specific for jaundice and hepatitis:

> 1 tablespoon of barberry
> 1 tablespoon of goldenseal root powder
> ½ teaspoon of lobelia
> ¼ teaspoon of cayenne

Make a decoction using one pint of distilled water. Take two tablespoons three to five times daily.

BAYBERRY *(Myrica cerifera)*

Part Used: root

Properties: Astringent; emetic, stimulant

Body Parts Affected: circulation, stomach and intestines

Preparation and Dosage:

Decoction (root):	Simmer 10 to 15 minutes. 1 Tbsp. as needed
Tincture:	15 to 30 drops as needed
Fluid Extract:	½ to 1 tsp. as needed
Powder:	4 to 10 #0 capsules (25 to 60 grains) per day

Indicated Uses:

Internal

Canker sores:	Tincture, Fluid Extract, Decoction
Chills:	Decoction, Tincture, Fluid Extract
Congestion of sinus and lungs:	Decoction*
Dysentery:	Tincture, Fluid Extract, Decoction
Hemorrhage (bowels, lungs, uterus):	Tincture, Fluid Extract, Decoction, Powder
Indigestion:	Tincture*, Fluid Extract*, Decoction*
Sore throat:	Tincture, Fluid Extract, Decoction
Weak circulation:	Tincture, Fluid Extract, Decoction

External

Canker sores:	Gargle
Leukorrhea:	Douche
Sore throat:	Gargle
Varicose veins:	Fomentation

Bayberry is a stimulating astringent that raises the vitality of the system. In small doses it improves circulation; in large doses it acts as an emetic. Use as a fomentation over varicose veins to strengthen the blood vessels.

Bayberry is used in all mucus membrane conditions and can be substituted for myrrh.

A douche made with the tea is used to treat prolapse of the uterus, excessive menstrual bleeding and for vaginal infections. The decoction is an excellent gargle for a sore and infected throat or a mouthwash for bleeding gums. Small amounts are used to aid digestion and to treat chronic gastritis, enteritis, diarrhea, leukorrhea and dysentery.

BETH ROOT *(Trillium Pendulum)*

Part Used: root

Properties: Antiseptic, Astringent; emmenagogue, tonic

Body Parts Affected: lungs and uterus

Preparation and Dosage:

Decoction:	Simmer 5 to 15 minutes. 2 to 4 oz. three times daily
Tincture:	1 to 2 tsp. three times daily
Fluid Extract:	½ tsp. three times daily
Powder:	5 to 10 #0 capsules (30 to 60 grains) three times daily

Indicated Uses:

Internal

Coughs:	Decoction*, Syrup*
Bronchial congestion:	Decoction*, Syrup*
Diarrhea:	Decoction
Dysentery:	Decoction
Excessive uterine bleeding (menorrhagia and metrorrhagia):	Decoction, Fluid Extract
Leukorrhea:	Decoction, Fluid Extract

Beth root helps restore normal nerve supply to the organs in the thorax. It is useful in coughs, bronchial problems and hemorrhages from the lungs. It controls excessive menstruation and excessive vaginal discharges. Beth root is an excellent remedy for diarrhea and dysentery.

BISTORT *(Polygonum bistorta)*

Part Used: root

Properties: Astringent, Styptic; antiseptic

Body Parts Affected: bowels, lungs and stomach

Preparation and Dosage:

Decoction:	Simmer 5 to 15 minutes. 1 Tbsp. several times daily
Tincture:	5 to 15 drops several times daily
Fluid Extract	½ to 1 tsp. several times daily
Powder:	1 to 5 #0 capsules (5 to 30 grains) several times daily.

Indicated Uses:

Internal

Diarrhea:.	Syrup*, Powder, Decoction
Dysentery:	Syrup*, Powder, Decoction
Hemorrhages (lungs, stomach, intestines):	Powder, Decoction

External

Hemorrhoids:	Enema with decoction
Mouth (sores)	Gargle with decoction
Sprains:	Poultice*
Tonsilitis:	Gargle with decoction
Wounds:	Poultice*

The ground root of bistort mixed with echinacea, myrrh and goldenseal makes an excellent dressing for wounds and cuts. Mixed with clay and used as a poultice, it is used for sore bruises, strains and sprains.

Bistort is a powerful astringent. A teaspoon of the powdered root in a cup of boiling water, steeped for ten minutes and drunk freely several times a day is a successful treatment for diarrhea, dysentery and hemorrhages from the lungs and stomach.

The decoction is used as a gargle for throat and mouth infections and as a douche for leukorrhea.

BLACKBERRY *(Rubus villosus)*

Part Used: leaves, root bark

Properties: Astringent, Hemostatic, Syptic; diuretic, tonic

Body Parts Affected: stomach and intestines

Preparation and Dosage:

Infusion (leaves): Steep 5 to 15 minutes. (leaves)
    4 oz. three to four
    times daily

Decoction (root bark): Simmer 5 to 15 minutes. 4 oz. three to four
    times daily

Tincture: ½ to 1 tsp. three to four times daily
Fluid Extract: ½ to 1 tsp. three to four times daily
Powder: 2 to 5 #0 capsules (15 to 30 grains) three to
    four times daily

Indicated Uses:

Internal

Diarrhea: Decoction, Infusion, Syrup*
Dysentery: Decoction, Infusion, Syrup*
Poor digestion Decoction, Infusion, Syrup*

A decoction of the root is a good astringent for watery diarrhea, especially in children. The root can be made into a syrup for children. The eclectic physicians used the syrup for children with weak stomachs, no appetite and skin pallor.

The leaves made into an infusion is good for milder cases of diarrhea and for sore throats. The root or leaves are good for poor digestion when caused by deficient glandular secretions of the stomach and intestines.

BLACK COHOSH *(Cimicufuga racemosa)*

Part Used: rhizome

Properties: Antispasmodic, Emmenagogue; alterative, diuretic

Body Parts Affected: uterus, nerves, lungs and heart

Preparation and Dosage:

Infusion:	1 tsp. every 30 minutes to 3 Tbsp. every three hours, according to need
Decoction (root):	Simmer 5 to 15 minutes. 1 to 2 oz. three to four times daily
Tincture:	½ to 1 tsp. three times daily
Fluid Extract:	5 to 30 drops three times daily
Syrup:	½ to 1 Tbsp. three to four times daily
Powder:	1 to 5 #0 capsules (5 to 30 grains) three times daily

Indicated Uses:

Internal

Acute rheumatism:	Tincture, Fluid Extract
Arthritis:Tincture*, Fluid Extract, Decoction*	
Bronchial spasms:	Tincture*, Fluid Extract*, Decoction*
Coughs:	Tincture, Fluid Extract, Decoction, Syrup
Cramps:	Tincture, Fluid Extract, Decoction
Excess uric acid:	Tincture, Fluid Extract
First pains of labor:	Tincture, Fluid Extract
Rheumatic fevers:	Tincture, Fluid Extract

Black cohosh is a powerful remedy in all nervous conditions, fits, convulsions and spasmodic afflictions. Native American women used it for all pelvic conditions, female complaints, uterine troubles, to relieve pains associated with childbirth and menstrual cycles. It will help to bring about menstrual flow that has been retarded by exposure to cold. It is a wonderful remedy to use in high blood pressure formulas to equalize circulation.

Combine in a syrup with wild cherry bark, coltsfoot, yerba santa and elecampane for whooping cough, bronchitis, respiratory spasms and asthma. Black cohosh has also been used for dropsy, rheumatism, snakebites and spinal meningitis.

Note: Black cohosh is a very potent agent and an overdose will produce nausea and vomiting.

BLACK HAW *(Viburnum prunifolium)*

Part Used: bark of the root

Properties: Antispasmodic, Emmenagogue, Sedative, Tonic

Body Parts Affected: uterus, nerves, stomach and intestines

Preparation and Dosage:

Infusion:	Steep 30 minutes. 3 oz. three to four times daily.
Decoction:	1 oz. herb to 1 quart water. Simmer 30 minutes. 1 Tbsp. three to four times daily or as needed
Tincture:	½ to 1 tsp. three to four times daily
Fluid Extract:	½ to 2 tsp. three to four times daily
Powder:	5 to 10 #0 capsules (30 to 60 grains) three to four times daily

Indicated Uses:

Internal

Afterbirth pains:	Tincture, Fluid Extract
Cramps:	Tincture, Fluid Extract
Dysmenorrhea:	Tincture, Fluid Extract, Powder*
Irregular menstrual flow:	Tincture, Fluid Extract, Powder*
Leukorrhea:	Tincture, Fluid Extract, Powder*
Scanty menstrual flow:	Tincture, Fluid Extract, Powder*
Threatened miscarriage:	Tincture, Fluid Extract, Powder*
Uterine inflammation and congestion:	Tincture, Fluid Extract, Powder*

Black haw is a tonic and sedative to the female reproductive organs. It is commonly used to ease cramps and contractions in the pelvic organs. For painful menstruation, whether due to nerve debility or congested tissue, it is excellent. It is good for scanty menstrual flow with a severe bearing-down feeling with intermittent pain. Black haw is equally valuable in chronic uterine inflammation, congested uterus and leukorrhea. It is a good remedy which gives a tonic effect during pregnancy.

BLACK WALNUT *(Juglans nigra)*

Part Used: Leaves and bark

Properties: Antiseptic, Astringent, Vermicide; alterative

Body Parts Affected: blood, intestines and nerves

Preparation and Dosage:

Infusion (leaves):	6 oz. one to four times daily
Decoction (inner bark):	Simmer 10 to 15 minutes. 1 Tbsp three to four times daily
Tincture:	10 to 20 drops three times daily
Fluid Extract	1 to 2 tsp. three to four times daily
Syrup:	1 Tbsp. one to two times daily
Powder:	5 to 10 #0 capsules (30 to 60 grains) three times daily

Indicated Uses:

Internal

Blood purifier:	Tincture, Fluid Extract, Infusion, Decoction
Boils:	Tincture, Fluid Extract, Infusion, Decoction
Cold sores:	Tincture, Fluid Extract, Infusion
Eczema:	Tincture, Fluid Extract, Infusion
Herpes:	Tincture, Fluid Extract, Infusion
Leucorrhea:	Tincture, Fluid Extract, Infusion
Lupus:	Tincture*, Fluid Extract*, Infusion*, Powder*, Decoction*
Mouth sores:	Tincture, Fluid Extract, Infusion
Parasites:	Tincture, Fluid Extract, Infusion
Poison ivy	Tincture, Fluid Extract
Vaginitis:	Tincture, Fluid Extract, Infusion

External

Boils:	Tincture, Fluid Extract, Infusion, Fomentation, Poultice
Herpes:	Tincture, Fluid Extract, Infusion, Fomentation
Leucorrhea:	Douche
Poison ivy:	Fomentation
Vaginitis:	Douche

Black walnut is rich in organic iodine and tannins which provide antiseptic qualities. As an infusion it is good for all toxic blood conditions. The tincture can be used to paint sores and pimples. It may be used for bleeding surfaces or moist skin diseases (apply tincture or powdered leaves). Use the infusion as an injection for vaginitis, bleeding, piles, intestinal worms, dysentery, prolapsed intestines and prolapsed uterus. It is good as a fomentation for ringworm and scabies.

The tincture taken internally over a long period of time will rid the body of warts.

BLESSED THISTLE *(Cerbenia benedicta)*

Part Used: tops

Properties: Emmenagogue, Galactagogue, Stomachic, Tonic; alterative

Body Parts Affected: stomach, heart, blood, mammary glands and uterus

Preparation and Dosage:

Infusion:	Steep 5 to 15 minutes. 3 oz. as needed
Tincture:	5 to 20 drops as needed
Fluid Extract:	½ to 1 tsp. as needed
Powder:	5 to 10 #0 capsules (30 to 60 grains) as needed

Indicated Uses:

Internal

Arthritis:	Tincture*, Fluid Extract*, Powder*, Infusion*
Blood purifier:	Tincture*, Fluid Extract*, Powder*, Infusion*
Cramps:	Tincture, Fluid Extract
Fever:	Tincture, Fluid Extract, Infusion
Female hormone imbalances:	Tincture*, Fluid Extract*, Powder*, Infusion*
Gas:	Tincture, Fluid Extract, Infusion
Headache:	Tincture, Fluid Extract, Infusion
Weak digestion:	Tincture, Fluid Extract, Infusion

This plant is used to improve digestion and circulation and to strengthen the heart. It is useful for all liver, lung and kidney problems. It acts as a brain food and stimulates memory.

The warm tea mixed with equal parts red raspberry leaves and marshmallow root increases mother's milk. As a blood purifier, combine it with yellow dock and burdock root.

Note: Blessed thistle should not be taken alone or in large amounts during pregnancy.

BLUE COHOSH *(Caulophyllum thalictroides)*

Part Used: rhizome

Properties: Antispasmodic, Emmenagogue, Oxytocic; diuretic

Body Parts Affected: uterus, nerves, joints and urinary tract

Preparation and Dosage:

Infusion:	3 oz. three to four times daily
Decoction	Simmer 5 to 15 minutes. 1 to 2 oz. three to four times daily
Tincture:	½ to 1 tsp. three to four times daily
Fluid Extract:	10 to 30 drops (1/6 to 1/2 tsp.) three to four times daily
Powder:	1 to 5 #0 capsules (5 to 30 grains) three to four times daily

Indicated Uses:

Internal

Blood purifier:	Tincture*, Fluid Extract*, Powder*
Childbirth (oxytocic):	Tincture, Fluid Extract

Colic:	Tincture*, Fluid Extract*
Convulsions:	Tincture, Fluid Extract
Cramps:	Tincture, Fluid Extract
Edema:	Tincture*, Fluid Extract*
Epilepsy:	Tincture, Fluid Extract
Heart weakness:	Tincture*, Fluid Extract*, Powder*
Nervous exhaustion:	Tincture, Fluid Extract
Painful menstruation:	Tincture, Fluid Extract
Rheumatic pains:	Tincture, Fluid Extract
Spasmodic muscular pains:	Tincture, Fluid Extract
Whooping cough:	Tincture, Fluid Extract

Blue cohosh is used to regulate menstrual flow and for suppressed menstruation. It was the common remedy among native Americans to ease childbirth and to relieve pains associated with it.

Blue cohosh is used as an antispasmodic in cough medicines and to treat lung problems and all female spasms. It contains potassium, magnesium, calcium, iron, silicon, phosphorous, and helps to alkalinize the blood.

Note: It is not to be used by pregnant women except during the last month of pregnancy.

BONESET *(Eupatorium perfoliatum)*

Part Used: tops

Properties: Diaphoretic, Stimulant; antipyretic, laxative

Body Parts Affected: stomach, liver, intestines and circulation

Preparation and Dosage:

Infusion:	Steep 5 to 15 minutes. 3 oz. three times daily.
Tincture:	10 to 40 drops three times daily
Fluid Extract:	½ to 1 tsp. three times daily
Powder:	4 to 10 #0 capsules (20 to 60 grains) three times daily.

Indicated Uses:

Internal

Bronchitis:	Infusion*, Powder*
Catarrh:	Infusion*, Tincture*, Fluid Extract*
Fevers:	Infusion, Tincture, Fluid Extract
Influenza:	Infusion, Tincture, Fluid Extract
Indigestion:	Tincture, Fluid Extract, Infusion
Jaundice:	Tincture*, Fluid Extract*, Infusion*
Night sweats:	Tincture, Fluid Extract, Infusion
Skin diseases:	Tincture*, Fluid Extract*, Infusion*

Boneset is a specific for treating severe fevers. Use a warm infusion for fevers, flu, and catarrh conditions. Drink four to five cups while in bed to encourage sweating. The cold infusion or tincture is a tonic. One to two tablespoons of the tincture added to hot water can be used for sweating therapy to break fevers.

BUCHU *(Barosma betulina)*

Part Used: leaves

Properties: Antiseptic, Diuretic; diaphoretic

Body Parts Affected: kidneys and bladder

Preparation and Dosage:

Infusion:	Steep 5 to 15 minutes. 3 oz. three to four times daily (do not boil leaves)
Tincture:	½ tsp. three times daily
Fluid Extract:	½ to 1 tsp. three times daily
Powder:	2 to 3 #0 capsules (10 to 15 grains) three times daily

Indicated Uses:

Internal

Bed wetting:	Tincture, Fluid Extract, Infusion
Bladder weakness:	Tincture, Fluid Extract, Infusion, Powder
Diabetes:	Tincture*, Fluid Extract*, Powder*, Infusion*
Gravel:	Tincture*, Fluid Extract*, Infusion*
Prostatitis:	Tincture*, Fluid Extract*, Infusion*, Powder
Rheumatism:	Tincture*, Fluid Extract*, Infusion*, Powder*
Urethral irritation:	Tincture, Fluid Extract, Infusion
Venereal disease:	Tincture*, Fluid Extract*, Infusion*, Powder

Buchu is frequently prescribed in chronic inflammation of the bladder, irritation of the urethra, uric acid problems, diabetes in the first stages, urine retention, nephritis, cystitis, and catarrh of the bladder. It works best when given as a cold infusion. It combines well with uva ursi.

When given warm, it is used to treat enlargement of the prostate gland and burning urine. It can be used in fever remedies. Do not boil buchu leaves.

BUCKTHORN *(Rhamnus frangula)*

Part Used: bark

Properties: Hepatic, Laxative; galactagogue

Body Parts Affected: liver, gall bladder, intestines and blood

Preparation and Dosage:

Decoction:	1 oz. bark to 1 quart water, boiled down to 1 pint.
Tincture:	5 to 60 drops three times daily
Fluid Extract:	½ to 2 tsp. three times daily
Powder:	4 to 10 #0 capsules (20 to 60 grains) three times daily

Indicated Uses:

Internal

Constipation:	Tincture*, Fluid Extract*, Decoction*, Powder
Gall stones:	Tincture*, Fluid Extract*, Decoction*, Powder*
Hemorrhoids:	Powder*
Parasites:	Tincture*, Fluid Extract*, Powder*, Decoction*
Rheumatism:	Tincture*, Fluid Extract*, Powder*, Decoction*
Skin diseases:	Tincture, Fluid Extract*, Powder*, Decoction*
Warts:	Tincture*, Fluid Extract*, Powder*, Decoction*

External

Itching:	Fomentation
Skin diseases:	Tincture, Fluid Extract, Fomentation
Warts:	Tincture, Fluid Extract, Fomentation

Buckthorn is a purgative and acts similar to rhubarb root. It is effective in treating all conditions associated with constipation, liver and gall bladder problems. The decoction will produce sweating when taken hot.

Use as a fomentation for itchy skin problems. Internally, it will keep the bowels regulated, and is used during rheumatism, gout, dropsy and all skin diseases.

Note: Buckthorn should not be used during pregnancy.

BUGLEWEED *(Lycopus virginicus)*

Part Used: whole herb

Properties: Astringent, Sedative; tonic

Body Parts Affected: heart, lungs and circulation

Preparation and Dosage:

Infusion:	Steep 5 to 15 minutes. 6 oz. frequently

Tincture:	½ to 1 tsp. frequently
Fluid Extract:	¼ to 1 tsp. frequently
Powder:	5 to 10 #0 capsules (30 to 60 grains) frequently

Indicated Uses:

Internal

Bronchial congestion:	Infusion*, Fluid Extract, Powder*
Coughs:	Infusion*
Diarrhea:	Infusion*, Fluid Extract*, Powder*
Dysentery:	Infusion*, Fluid Extract*, Powder*
Dyspepsia:	Infusion, Fluid Extract
Excessive menstruation:	Tincture, Fluid Extract
Heart palpitation:	Infusion, Fluid Extract
Hematuria:	Infusion*, Fluid Extract*
Nose bleeds:	Tincture, Fluid Extract

Bugleweed has been used successfully in hemorrhages from the lungs and bowels.

This herb is excellent for heart diseases marked by irregular heartbeat, whether the cause is functional or organic. Bugleweed acts much like digitalis in quieting the pulse, making it useful for treating pericarditis and endocarditis.

In diseases of the respiratory system, it has been used for treating chronic inflammation of the lungs, coughs, and all chest congestive diseases. Bugleweed is considered a sedative and astringent and is used in diseases when the capillary circulation needs to be diminished and the blood flow needs to be reduced in diseases like hemorrhoids, intestinal bleeding or when blood is found in the urine. It is good to use this herb with demulcents when treating the above conditions.

BURDOCK *(Arctium lappa)*

Part Used: root, seeds and leaves

Properties: Root-Alterative, Diaphoretic, Diuretic, demulcent; seeds-Alterative; diuretic, leaves-Tonic

Body Parts Affected: blood, kidneys, and liver

Preparation and Dosage:

Infusion (leaves)	1 cup three to four times daily
Decoction (root &: seeds):	1 oz. root to 1½ pints water, boiled down to 1 pint. 3 oz. three to four times daily
Tincture:	30 to 60 drops three to four times daily
Fluid Extract:	½ to 1 tsp. three to four times daily
Powder (root & seed):	10 to 20 #0 capsules (60 to 120 grains) daily
Powder (leaves)	5 to 10 #0 capsules (30 to 60 grains) three times daily

Indicated Uses:

Internal

Acne:	Tincture, Fluid Extract, Infusion, Decoction
Arthritis:	Tincture*, Fluid Extract*, Infusion*, Decoction*, Powder*
Blood purifier:	Tincture, Fluid Extract, Infusion, Decoction, Powder
Boils:	Tincture, Fluid Extract, Infusion, Decoction
Bursitis:	Tincture*, Fluid Extract*, Infusion*, Powder*, Decoction*
Canker:	Tincture, Fluid Extract, Infusion, Decoction
Chicken Pox:	Tincture, Fluid Extract, Infusion, Decoction
Eczema:	Tincture, Fluid Extract, Infusion, Decoction
Gall stones:	Tincture*, Fluid Extract*, Infusion*, Decoction*
Gout:	Tincture, Fluid Extract, Infusion, Decoction
Itching:	Tincture, Fluid Extract, Infusion, Decoction
Kidney problems:	Tincture, Fluid Extract, Infusion, Decoction
Psoriasis:	Tincture, Fluid Extract, Infusion, Decoction
Ulcers:	Tincture*, Fluid Extract*, Infusion*, Decoction*, Powder*
Venereal diseases:	Tincture*, Fluid Extract*, Infusion*, Decoction*, Powder*

External

Boils:	Fomentation, Salve, Poultice
Eczema	Fomentation, Salve, Poultice
Itching:	Fomentation, Salve, Poultice
Poison ivy and oak:	Salve, Poultice

Burdock root is one of the best blood purifiers for chronic infection, arthritis, rheumatism, skin diseases and sciatica. It provides an abundance of iron and insulin which makes it of special value to the blood. It has volatile oils which makes it a good diaphoretic, and clears the kidneys of excess wastes and uric acid by increasing the flow of urine. It is excellent for gout. Burdock is used for fevers and skin problems such as boils, styes, carbuncles, canker sores, using ½ cup of the decoction three times daily. An infusion of the leaves is used as a stomach tonic and for indigestion. The seeds made into a tincture or extract are good for skin and kidney diseases.

Burdock can be used also as a fomentation for wounds, swellings and hemorrhoids.

CALENDULA *(Calendula officinalis)*

Part Used: flower

Properties: Astringent, Vulnerary; antispasmodic, diaphoretic

Body Parts Affected: blood and skin

Preparation and Dosage:

Infusion:	Steep 5 to 15 minutes. 1 Tbsp. each hour or one cup daily
Tincture:	15 to 30 drops three times daily
Fluid Extract:	½ to 1 tsp. three times daily
Powder:	3 to 10 #0 capsules (15 to 60 grains) three times daily

Indicated Uses:

Internal

Bleeding hemorrhoids:	Tincture, Fluid Extract, Infusion
Cramps:	Tincture, Fluid Extract
Fevers:	Infusion
Hemorrhage:	Tincture, Fluid Extract, Infusion
Skin eruptions:	Infusion, Tincture, Fluid Extract
Small pox and measles:	Infusion
Ulcers:	Infusion*

External

Bee stings:	Fomentation
Earache:	Oil, applied topically
Skin diseases:	Fomentation, Salve
Ulcers:	Fomentation, Salve
Wounds:	Fomentation
Varicose veins:	Fomentation, Salve
Wash wounds:	Infusion

Calendula is non-irritating as a fomentation or salve for sores, burns, bleeding hemorrhoids and wounds. Calendula has been successfully used as a nasal wash for sinus problems. It is also valued in treating vaginal infections, ulcers, pruritis and bleeding. As a warm infusion, it is good for fevers, ulcers and cramps. The oil is put in ears and left overnight for earaches. A strong tea can be used as a sitz bath for bleeding hemorrhoids.

CASCARA SAGRADA *(Rhamnus purshiana)*

Part Used: bark

Properties: Hepatic, Laxative; antispasmodic

Body Parts Affected: colon, stomach, liver, gall bladder and pancreas.

Preparation and Dosage:

Decoction (bark):	Simmer 5 to 15 minutes. 1 tsp. three to four times daily before meals or 1 cup during the day, cold

Tincture:	5 to 20 drops, morning and evening
Fluid Extract:	½ to 1 tsp. at night before retiring
Syrup:	½ to 2 tsp. two to three times daily
Powder:	6 to 12 #0 capsules (10 to 100 grains) daily

Indicated Uses:

Internal

Constipation:	Tincture, Fluid Extract, Powder, Decoction
Cough:	Syrup
Gall bladder diseases:	Tincture*, Fluid Extract*, Decoction*, Powder*
Gall stones:	Tincture*, Fluid Extract*, Decoction*, Powder*
Gastric and intestinal disorders:	Tincture, Fluid Extract, Syrup
Hemorrhoids:	Tincture, Fluid Extract, Syrup
Indigestion:	Tincture, Fluid Extract, Decoction
Jaundice:	Tincture*, Fluid Extract*, Powder*, Decoction*
Liver congestion:	Tincture, Fluid Extract, Decoction, Powder

Cascara sagrada is one of the most valuable remedies for chronic constipation and as a stimulant to the whole digestive system. It is a safe laxative and is known not to be habit forming. It is excellent for intestinal gas, liver and gall bladder complaints, especially enlarged liver.

Cascara is very bitter in tea form and is usually used in tincture or capsule form for a gentle laxative effect.

CATNIP *(Nepata cataria)*

Part Used: tops

Properties: Carminative, Diaphoretic, Sedative; nervine

Body Parts Affected: nerves and intestines

Preparation and Dosage:

Infusion:	Steep 5 to 15 minutes. 1 oz. to 1 cup as needed (do not boil herb)
Tincture:	½ to 1 tsp. as needed
Fluid Extract	¼ to 1 tsp. as needed
Powder:	5 to 10 #0 capsules (30 to 60 grains) three times daily

Indicated Uses:

Internal

Chicken pox:	Infusion
Colic:	Infusion

Colds:	Infusion
Dizziness	Infusion
Fevers:	Infusion
Gas:	Infusion
Headache:	Infusion
Hysteria:	Tincture*, Fluid Extract*, Infusion*
Insomnia:	Infusion
Morning sickness:	Infusion
Mumps:	Infusion*
Smallpox:	Infusion*
Urine retention:	Infusion*

External

Constipation:	Enema
Mumps:	Fomentation
Painful swellings:	Fomentation, Poultice

Catnip is wonderful for children and infants when stomach cramps, spasms, gas and nervousness is present. Make the infusion in large amounts and use as an enema to expel worms, release gas or treat fevers and hysterical headaches. The enema will also increase urination. Mix with chamomile and lemon balm for nervousness in children and adults. Drink the infusion for headaches caused by digestive disturbances. In Europe, it also is used for bronchitis and diarrhea.

CAYENNE *(Capsicum anuum)*

Part Used: fruit

Properties: Carminative, Stimulant; antispasmodic, astringent

Body Parts Affected: heart, circulation, stomach and kidneys

Preparation and Dosage:

Infusion:	1 tsp. to 1 cup boiling water taken in ½ fluid ounce doses. Pour water over cayenne
Tincture:	5 to 15 drops three times daily
Fluid Extract:	10 to 15 drops three times daily
Oil:	For toothache, clean the cavity and place cotton saturated with the oil into the cavity; use sparingly, as it is very potent
Powder (internal):	1 to 2 #0 capsules (1 to 10 grains) three times daily
Powder (external):	For external bleeding,powder may be placed directly on the wound

Indicated Uses:

Internal

Arteriosclerosis:	Tincture*, Powder*

Arthritis:	Tincture*, Powder*
Asthma:	Tincture, Infusion, Powder
Bleeding:	Tincture, Infusion, Powder
Blood pressure (high and low):	Powder*
Bronchitis:	Tincture*, Powder*, Syrup*
Chills:	Tincture, Infusion, Powder
Colds	Tincture, Infusion
Convulsions:	Tincture*, Infusion
Coughs:	Tincture, Infusion, Powder
Indigestion:	Tincture, Infusion, Powder
Infections:	Tincture*, Infusion*, Syrup*
Jaundice:	Tincture*, Infusion*, Powder*, Syrup*
Ulcers:	Tincture*, Infusion*, Powder*, Syrup*
Varicose veins:	Tincture*, Infusion*, Powder*

External

Frostbite:	Tincture, Fomentation, Liniment
Painful joints:	Tincture, Fomentation, Liniment
Swellings:	Tincture, Fomentation, Liniment
Varicose veins:	Tincture, Fomentation, Liniment

Cayenne is effective as a fomentation for rheumatism, inflammation, pleurisy, sores and wounds. It can be used both as an infusion or added to liniments.

Taken as a daily tonic (four days a week) ¼ teaspoon in water or juice, three times daily, it will benefit the heart and circulation. Cayenne can be added to soups and salads. It is excellent when added to formulas to stimulate the action of other herbs. Cayenne is a preventative for heart attacks, flu, colds, indigestion and lack of vitality. It is used in the treatment of the spleen, pancreas, and kidneys and will help heal sores of the stomach.

The powder or tincture can be rubbed on toothaches or swellings. Cayenne will stop bleeding both internally and externally. I have sprinkled powdered cayenne on bleeding cuts and it immediately stops the bleeding. When cooked, cayenne becomes an irritant.

CELERY (Wild) *(Apium graveolens)*

Part Used: root, seeds

Properties: Carminative, Diuretic, Nervine; stimulant, tonic

Body Parts Affected: kidneys, bladder and nerves

Preparation and Dosage:

Decoction (root, seeds): Simmer 5 to 15 minutes. 1 oz. three times daily

Fluid Extract:	10 to 30 drops as needed
Essential Oil	1 to 2 drops three times daily
Powder:	4 to 10 #0 capsules three times daily

Indicated Uses:

Internal:

Dropsy:	Decoction (seed or root), Fluid Extract (seed or root)
Neuralgia:	Decoction (seed or root), Fluid Extract (seed or root)
Rheumatism:	Decoction (seed or root), Fluid Extract (seed or root)
Uric acid (excess):	Decoction (seed or root), Fluid Extract (seed or root)
Urine retention:	Decoction (seed or root), Fluid Extract (seed or root)
Tonic (nerves and kidneys):	Decoction (seed or root), Fluid Extract (seed or root)

A decoction of celery seed is used for incontinence of urine, dropsy, rheumatism, neuralgia and to aid in ridding the body of excess acid. The root can be eaten raw or made into broths to treat the same ailments. The whole plant can be used to treat kidney ailments and rheumatism.

Note: Use moderate amounts during pregnancy.

CHAMOMILE *(Matricaria chamomilla)*

Part Used: flowers

Properties: Emmenagogue, Nervine, Sedative; carminative, diaphoretic, tonic

Body Parts Affected: nerves, stomach, kidneys, spleen and liver

Preparation and Dosage:

Infusion:	Steep 10 to 30 minutes (do not boil flowers). 6 oz. two to three times daily
Tincture:	30 to 60 drops three times daily
Fluid Extract:	½ to 1 tsp. three times daily
Powder:	5 to 10 #0 capsules (30 to 60 grains) three times daily

Indicated Uses:

Internal

Blood purifier:	Tincture*, Infusion*
Cramps:	Tincture, Infusion
Dizziness	Tincture, Infusion
Gas:	Tincture, Infusion
Hysteria:	Tincture*, Infusion*

Indigestion:	Tincture, Infusion
Jaundice:	Tincture*, Infusion
Kidney problems:	Tincture*, Powder
Measles:	Tincture, Infusion
Menstrual problems:	Tincture, Infusion
Nervous stomach:	Tincture, Infusion

External

Cramps:	Fomentation
Gas:	Fomentation
Swellings:	Fomentation

Chamomile is a valuable drink for insomnia, nervousness, to provide appetite and for weak stomachs. Six ounces of the infusion or one to two teaspoons of the tincture at a time is good for menstrual cramps, kidney, spleen or bladder problems. The tea is a good wash for sore eyes and open sores.

Chamomile is applied as a fomentation to sore muscles, swellings and painful joints.

CHAPARRAL *(Larrea divaricata)*

Part Used: leaves

Properties: Alterative, Antiobotic, Antiseptic, Parasiticide

Body Parts Affected: stomach, intestines, and blood

Preparation and Dosage:

Infusion:	Steep 5 to 15 minutes. 6 oz. three times daily
Tincture:	10 to 20 drops three times daily
Powder:	2 to 10 #0 capsules (10 to 60 grains) three times daily

Indicated Uses:

Internal

Acne:	Tincture, Infusion, Powder
Allergies:	Tincture*, Infusion*, Powder*
Arthritis:	Tincture, Infusion, Powder
Blood purifier:	Tincture, Infusion, Powder
Boils:	Tincture, Infusion, Powder
Bursitis:	Tincture, Infusion, Powder
Cancer:	Tincture, Infusion, Powder
Psoriasis:	Tincture, Infusion, Powder
Rheumatism:	Tincture, Infusion, Powder
Stomach cramps:	Tincture, Infusion
Tumors:	Tincture, Infusion, Powder

External

Arthritis:	Tincture, Fomentation, Liniment
Skin parasites:	Tincture, Fomentation, Salve

Chaparral is one of nature's best antibiotics used both internally and externally. It is good for treating bacterial, viral and parasitic infections. It is also an excellent addition to formulas in the treatment of kidney and bladder infections.

As a fomentation it is applied topically for skin diseases, herpes, scabies, eczema and arthritic pains. It contains an anti-tumor substance called NDGA (nordihydroguararetic acid) which has anti-cancer properties. It is very bitter and is usually mixed with other herbs or taken in tincture form. I do know of several people who drink it as a tea. Chaparral is a good addition to hair rinses.

CHICKWEED *(Stellaria media)*

Part Used: tops

Properties: Antipyretic, Demulcent; alterative

Body Parts Affected: blood, liver, lungs, kidneys and bladder

Preparation and Dosage:

Infusion:	Steep 5 to 15 minutes. 6 oz. three to four times daily, between meals
Decoction:	1 oz. to 1½ pints boiling water, simmered down to 1 pint. 3 oz. three to four times (or every two or three hours when needed)
Tincture:	½ tsp. as needed
Fluid Extract:	½ to 1 tsp. as needed
Powder:	5 to 10 #0 capsules (30 to 60 grains) three times daily

Indicated Uses:

Internal

Allergies:	Infusion*, Decoction*, Powder*
Anemia:	Infusion*, Decoction*, Powder*
Asthma:	Infusion*, Decoction*, Syrup*, Powder*
Bowel inflammations:	Infusion, Decoction, Powder
Bronchitis:	Infusion*, Decoction*, Powder*
Cleanser (lymphatics):	Infusion, Decoction, Powder
Constipation:	Decoction
Hay fever:	Infusion, Decoction, Powder
Hemorrhoids:	Infusion*, Decoction*, Powder*

Hoarseness:	Infusion, Decoction
Pleurisy:	Infusion*, Decoction*, Powder*, Syrup*

External

Boils:	Poultice
Itching:	Fomentation, Salve
Mouth sores:	Gargle
Ulcers:	Poultice

Chickweed can be used as a food or medicine. Nutritionally it is rich in B-complex vitamins, ascorbic acid, calcium, iron, sodium, zinc and molybdenum. Chickweed's best virtues are brought out when treating hot diseases like fevers and inflammations both internally and externally (fomentation).

It is excellent used in all cases of bronchitis, pleurisy, coughs, colds and hoarseness. It is good for all skin diseases applied as a fomentation. Add the tea to baths to soothe rashes and skin irritations. Drink the tea to build the blood. Make into a salve for dry, itchy skin.

CLEAVERS *(Galium aparine)*

Part Used: tops

Properties: Alterative, Astringent, Diuretic; antipyretic, laxative

Body Parts Affected: kidneys, bladder, blood and skin

Preparation and Dosage:

Infusion:	3 oz to 2 pints cold water; let stand three to four hours. 3 oz. (cold) three to four times daily; or 1½ oz. to 1 pint of warm water. Steep two hours. 1 cup three to four times daily
Tincture:	½ to 1 tsp. three to four times daily
Fluid Extract:	½ to 1 tsp. three to four times daily
Powder:	5 to 10 #0 capsules (30 to 60 grains) three to four times daily

Indicated Uses:

Internal

Blood purifier:	Infusion
Colds in the head:	Infusion
Edema:	Infusion, Fluid Extract
Kidney inflammation:	Infusion, Fluid Extract
Prostatitis:	Infusion*, Fluid Extract*
Skin diseases:	Infusion, Fluid Extract
Urinary obstructions:	Fluid Extract*, Infusion*

External

Burns and scalds:	Salve
Sunburn:	Fomentation, Salve
Tumors:	Salve*

Cleavers is excellent when used to help break fevers and when there is suppressed urine, inflammations of the kidneys and bladder and scalding urine during gonorrhea. It is a powerful diruetic and will rid the body of excess fluid. It will clean the blood and strengthen the liver. Combine with marshmallow root, uva ursi and buchu for urinary complaints.

CLOVES *(Caryophyllus aromaticus)*

Part Used: fruits

Properties: Antiseptic, Aromatic, Carminative, Stimulant; anodyne, antiemetic, aphrodisiac

Body Parts Affected: mouth, stomach, intestines, circulation and lungs

Preparation and Dosage:

Infusion:	Steep 5 to 15 minutes. 1 to 2 Tbsp. three times daily
Fluid Extract:	8 to 30 drops three times daily
Oil:	1 to 2 drops three times daily
Powder:	1 to 5 #0 capsules (2 to 10 grains) three times daily

Indicated Uses:

Internal

Bronchial expectorant:	Infusion*, Powder*
Cholera:	Infusion*, Powder*
Diarrhea:	Infusion*, Powder*
Dyspepsia:	Infusion, Powder
Fevers:	Infusion*
Flatulence:	Infusion, Powder
Nausea:	Infusion, Powder
Whooping cough:	Infusion*

External

Toothache:	Oil, applied externally

Clove oil will stop the pain of a toothache when applied directly to the cavity. A few drops of the oil in warm water will stop nausea and vomiting.

Cloves is very stimulating and warming to the system. It is a good addition to bitter formulas to cover the taste and improve digestion and circulation. It is especially good for those people with cold extremities.

As a carminative it is good for gas and intestinal spasms. Cloves promote sweating in colds, flu and fevers and is useful for treating whooping cough.

It is taken in small amounts and in frequent doses. Use one teaspoon of powdered root to one pint of boiling water, steep for 15 minutes in a covered pot. Strain and take two tablespoons as needed.

Chew whole cloves for bad breath and when garlic has been eaten.

COLTSFOOT *(Tussilago farfara)*

Part Used: leaf

Properties: Demulcent, Emollient, Expectorant

Body Parts Affected: lungs, stomach, intestines

Preparation and Dosage:

Infusion:	Steep 30 minutes. 6 oz. frequently
Tincture:	½ to 1 tsp. as needed
Fluid Extract:	½ to 1 tsp. as needed
Powder:	10 to 20 #0 capsules (60 to 120 grains) as needed

Indicated Uses:

Internal

Asthma:	Infusion*, Syrup*
Bronchitis:	Infusion*, Syrup*
Catarrh:	Infusion, Syrup
Colitis:	Infusion*
Coughs:	Infusion
Fevers:	Infusion*
Lung troubles:	Infusion
Stomach troubles:	Infusion

External

Piles:	Salve, Fomentation

Coltsfoot is an excellent remedy for catarrh, colds, whooping cough and other respiratory problems. Add coltsfoot to all spasmodic lung problem remedies. Coltsfoot is soothing to the stomach and intestines when there is inflammation and bleeding. As a cough syrup, combine it with horehound, ginger and licorice root.

COMFREY *(Symphytum officinale)*

Part Used: leaves and root

Properties: Demulcent, Expectorate, Mucilage, Vulnerary; alterative, astringent, nutritive

Body Parts Affected: bones and muscles, general effects on whole body

Preparation and Dosage:

Infusion (leaves);	Steep 30 minutes. 6 oz. three times daily
Decoction (root):	Simmer 30 minutes. 3 oz. frequently
Tincture:	½ to 1 tsp. three times daily
Fluid Extract:	½ to 2 tsp. three times daily
Powder:	5 to 10 #0 capsules (30 to 60 grains) three times daily

Indicated Uses:

Internal

Anemia:	Decoction*, Powder*, Syrup*
Arthritis:	Powder*, Decoction*
Asthma:	Powder, Decoction, Syrup
Bleeding internally:	Powder, Decoction, Infusion
Blood purifier:	Powder, Decoction, Syrup, Infusion
Bronchitis:	Powder, Decoction, Infusion, Syrup
Calcium deficiency:	Powder*, Decoction*, Syrup*
Colitis:	Decoction, Infusion, Powder
Coughs:	Decoction*, Infusion*
Diarrhea, dysentery:	Decoction
Emphysema:	Decoction, Syrup
Gall bladder inflammation	Decoction*, Powder*
Inflammations:	Infusion, Decoction, Syrup, Powder

External

Boils:	Poultice, Fomentation
Bruises:	Poultice, Fomentation
Burns:	Poultice, Fomentation, Salve
Psoriasis:	Salve, Fomentation
Sprains	Poultice or Fomentaton

Comfrey is a powerful remedy for coughs, catarrh, ulcerated bowels, stomach and lungs. It is one of the best remedies for internal bleeding anywhere in the body. Use a strong decoction for bleeding and to build new flesh during wasting diseases. It is excellent for dysentery and helps regulate blood sugar levels.

As a poultice, bruise the fresh leaves and apply to burns, wounds, open sores, gangrene and moist ulcers. The tea and decoction can be used as a fomentation for these also.

The dosage is 2 ounces of the decoction several times a day for internal hemorrhaging. Comfrey is a cell proliferator and will help heal broken bones, sprains and slow healing sores.

CORN SILK *(Zea mays)*

Part Used: leaves

Properties: Diuretic, Lithotriptic; demulcent

Body Parts Affected: kidneys, bladder and prostate

Preparation and Dosage:

Infusion:	Steep 5 to 15 minutes. 3 oz. as needed
Tincture:	5 to 20 drops three times daily
Fluid Extract:	¼ to ½ tsp. three times daily
Powder:	1 to 5 #0 capsules (5 to 30 grains) three times daily

Indicated Uses:

Internal

Bedwetting:	Infusion, Tincture
Chronic cystitis:	Infusion*
Inflammation of kidneys and bladder:	Infusion*
Kidney stones:	Infusion*
Prostatitis:	Infusion*, Fluid Extract, Tincture*
Uric acid (excess):	Infusion, Tincture
Urine retention:	Infusion, Tincture

Corn silk is used in irritated kidney and bladder conditions. It has the ability to remove gravel from the kidneys, bladder and prostate gland. It is good used in combination with other kidney herbs when the urinary tract needs opening up or when there is mucus in the urine. It is good for dropsy and edema when a weak heart is the cause. It has been a popular remedy for the aged when their urine is scanty and has heavy sediment. Corn silk is an excellent remedy for all inflammatory conditions of the urethra, bladder, prostate and kidneys.

CRAMPBARK *(Viburnum opulis)*

Part Used: bark

Properties: Antispasmodic; astringent, nervine

Body Parts Affected: nerves, heart and reproductive organs

Preparation and Dosage:

Infusion:	Steep 30 minutes. 3 oz. three to four times daily
Decoction:	1 oz. herb to 1 quart water. Simmer 30 minutes. 1 Tbsp. three to four times daily or as needed
Tincture:	½ to 1 tsp. three to four times daily

Fluid Extract:	½ to 2 tsp. three to four times daily
Powder:	5 to 10 #0 capsules (30 to 60 grains) three to four times daily

Indicated Uses:

Internal

Asthma:	Decoction*
Convulsions:	Tincture, Fluid Extract
Cramps:	Tincture, Fluid Extract, Decoction
Dysmenorrhea (painful menstruation)	Tincture*, Fluid Extract*, Powder*, Decoction*
Gas:	Tincture, Fluid Extract, Decoction
Hysteria:	Tincture, Fluid Extract
Menorrhagia (excessive uterine bleeding):	Tincture*, Fluid Extract*, Decoction*
Nervous conditions during pregnancy:	Tincture, Fluid Extract, Decoction
Neuralgia:	Tincture, Fluid Extract
Prevent miscarriage:	Tincture, Fluid Extract, Decoction
Spasms:	Tincture, Fluid Extract, Decoction

Cramp bark is used for menstural cramps, spasms of involuntary muscles, asthma, hysteria; especially when combined with angelica, black cohosh, ginger and chamomile. It is also good for heart palpitation and cramps during pregnancy.

CRANESBILL *(Geranium maculatum)*

Part Used: leaves, root

Properties: Astringent, Styptic; tonic

Body Parts Affected: stomach, intestines and kidneys

Preparation and Dosage:

Infusion (leaves):	Steep 5 to 15 minutes. 3 oz. when needed
Decoction (root):	Simmer 5 to 15 minutes. 1 Tbsp. to 1 cup three times daily
Tincture:	15 to 30 drops three times daily
Fluid Extract:	½ to 1 tsp. three times daily
Powder:	3 to 5 #0 capsules (20 to 30 grains) three times daily

Indicated Uses:

Internal

Bleeding piles:	Infusion, Decoction, Fluid Extract
Diarrhea:	Infusion, Decoction, Fluid Extract

Dysentery:	Infusion, Decoction, Fluid Extract
Hemorrhage of stomach and lungs:	Infusion, Decoction, Fluid Extract
Hematuria:	Infusion, Decoction, Fluid Extract
Leukorrhea:	Infusion, Decoction, Fluid Extract
Menorrhagia:	Infusion, Decoction, Fluid Extract
Night sweats:	Infusion, Decoction, Fluid Extract
Sore mouth:	Infusion, Decoction, Fluid Extract

Cranesbill (Geranium) is a powerful, non-irritating astringent which is used for weak, relaxed mucus membranes with copious discharges. It is of value in chronic diarrhea, dysentery, menorrhagia, blood in the urine and intestinal hemorrhaging. As a gargle, it is used for all mouth and throat diseases.

A decoction of the root used as a retention enema is excellent for bleeding hemorrhoids and anus swellings.

Externally, the powdered root can be applied to bleeding skin surfaces. Cover with a wet compress and it will stop the bleeding.

DAMIANA *(Turnera aphrodisiaca)*

Part Used: leaves

Properties: Emmenagogue, Tonic; aphrodisiac, cholagogue, diuretic

Body Parts Affected: reproductive organs, nerves, kidneys

Preparation and Dosage:

Infusion:	Steep 5 to 15 minutes. 1 to 2 cups, hot or cold, once daily
Tincture:	1 to 3 tsp. once daily
Fluid Extract:	15 to 30 drops, once daily
Powder:	5 to 20 #0 capsules (30 to 120 grains) once daily

Indicated Uses:

Internal

Acne caused by menstrual problems:	Fluid Extract, Powder
Aphrodisiac:	Fluid Extract, Powder
Hormone imbalance:	Fluid Extract*, Powder
Hot flashes (menopause):	Fluid Extract, Powder
Sexual stimulant:	Fluid Extract, Powder
Sexual neurasthenia (Nerve exhaustion):	Fluid Extract, Powder
Stimulant to central nervous system:	Fluid Extract, Powder

Suppressed
    menstruation: Fluid Extract, Powder
    Urinary irritations: Fluid Extract*, Powder*, Infusion*

Damiana is a sexual rejuvenator of the sexual organs. It has a tendency to overstimulate if used excessively. It mildly stimulates the flow of urine. It is a tonic to the nervous system in small, frequent doses.

DANDELION *(Taraxacum officinale)*

Part Used: leaf and root

Properties: Cholagogue, Diuretic, Hepatic, Lithotriptic, Stomachic; alterative, astringent, galactogogue

Body Parts Affected: liver, kidneys, gall bladder, stomach, pancreas, intestines and blood

Preparation and Dosage:

Infusion:	Steep 30 minutes. Three to four cups daily, hot or cold
Decoction:	Simmer root 30 minutes. 6 oz. frequently or three to four times daily, hot or cold
Tincture:	30 to 60 drops (½ to 1 tsp.) frequently
Powder (leaves)	10 to 20 #0 capsules (60 to 120 grains) frequently
Powder (root):	5 to 10 #0 capsules (30 to 60 grains) frequently

Indicated Uses:

Internal

Acne:	Tincture, Fluid Extract, Decoction
Anemia:	Decoction*, Powder*
Blood purifier:	Tincture, Fluid Extract, Powder, Decoction
Boils:	Tincture, Fluid Extract, Powder, Decoction
Bronchitis:	Powder*, Decoction*
Constipation:	Decoction
Cramps:	Tincture, Fluid Extract
Diabetes:	Infusion, Decoction
Gall stones:	Decoction*
Indigestion:	Infusion of leaves
Jaundice:	Infusion, Decoction
Kidney diseases:	Decoction
Kidney stones:	Decoction*
Low blood sugar:	Infusion, Decoction
Psoriasis:	Tincture, Fluid Extract, Infusion, Decoction
Skin diseases:	Tincture, Fluid Extract, Infusion, Decoction

Spleen, liver, pancreas, gall bladder obstructions:	Decoction

Dandelion is both a nutritive herb and one of nature's best medicines. Its main influence is upon the liver and it is an excellent blood purifier for conditions such as exzema, dropsy and diabetes. Because of its high content of mineral, it is used to treat anemia. It is good for enlargement of liver and for pancreas and spleen problems. Always use dandelion root when treating hepatitis and jaundice. It will increase the flow of urine and is good in kidney formulas. The roasted root is a coffee substitute.

DEVIL'S CLAW *(Harpagophytum procumbens)*

Part Used: root

Properties: Alterative; discutient, lithotriptic, stimulant

Body Parts Affected: liver, stomach, joints and kidneys

Preparation and Dosage:

Infusion:	Steep 30 minutes. 1 to 2 cups daily
Decoction:	Simmer 15 minutes. 6 oz. three times daily
Tincture:	30 to 60 drops three times daily
Fluid Extract:	½ to 1 tsp. three times daily
Powder:	2 to 3 #0 capsules (15 to 30 grains) three times daily

Indicated Uses:

Internal

Acid conditions:	Decoction, Powder, Fluid Extract
Arthritis:	Decoction, Powder, Fluid Extract
Blood purifier:	Decoction*, Powder*, Fluid Extract*
Gout:	Decoction, Powder, Fluid Extract
Rheumatism:	Decoction, Powder, Fluid Extract

Devil's claw is mainly used for gout, rheumatism and arthritis. It is a blood cleanser and will remove deposits in the joints and aid in elimination of uric acid from the body.

ECHINACEA *(Echinacea angustifolia)*
Part Used: Root
Properties: Alternative, Antiseptic, Lymphatic; parasiticide, sialagogue
Body Parts Affected: blood, lymph and kidneys

Preparation and Dosage:

Decoction:	Simmer 5 to 15 minutes. 1 Tbsp. three to six times daily
Tincture:	30 to 60 drops three to six times daily

| Fluid Extract: | ½ to 1 tsp. three to six times daily |
| Powder: | 2 to 5 #0 capsules (15 to 30 grains) three to six times daily |

Indicated Uses:

Internal

Acne:	Tincture, Fluid Extract, Powder
Bad breath:	Tincture, Fluid Extract, Powder
Bladder infections:	Tincture, Fluid Extract, Infusion, Decoction
Blood poisoning:	Tincture, Fluid Extract
Blood purifier:	Tincture, Fluid Extract
Boils:	Tincture, Fluid Extract, Powder
Fevers:	Tincture, Fluid Extract
Gangrene:	Tincture, Fluid Extract, Powder
Infections:	Tincture, Fluid Extract, Powder
Inflammation of mammary glands	Tincture, Fluid Extract
Intestinal antiseptic:	Tincture, Fluid Extract, Powder
Leukopenia (diminution of number of leukocytes in the blood):	Tincture, Fluid Extract, Powder
Lymphatic congestion:	Tincture, Fluid Extract, Powder
Skin diseases:	Tincture, Fluid Extract, Powder
Tonsilitis:	Tincture, Fluid Extract, Powder
Uremic poisoning (retention in the blood of toxins usually excreted by the kidneys):	Tincture, Fluid Extract, Powder
Venereal diseases:	Tincture, Fluid Extract, Powder

External

| Open wounds: | Fomentation, Tincture |
| Painful swellings: | Fomentation, Tincture |

Echinacea is one of the best blood cleansers and seems to be tolerated in large amounts. It is good for blood poisoning, carbuncles, all pus diseases, abscesses of the teeth, gangrene, all lymph swellings, snake and spider bites.

It is a valuable alternative to all antibiotics. It has a history of being used against syphilis and gonorrhea. Combine with myrrh to rid the body of pus or abscess formations. It acts as a digestive tonic.

ELDER *(Sambucus nigra)*

Part Used: flowers, bark, berries and root

Properties: Diaphoretic; alterative, laxative, stimulant

Body Parts Affected: blood, circulation, lungs, bowels and skin

Preparation and Dosage:

Infusion (flowers):	Steep 15 minutes. 6 oz. three times daily
Decoction (bark, berries, root):	Simmer 15 minutes. 1 cup at a time
Tincture (flowers):	15 to 30 drops three times daily
Fluid Extract (flowers):	½ to 1 tsp. three times daily
Powder (bark):	5 #0 capsules (30 grains) three times daily
Powder (berries/flowers):	5 to 10 #0 capsules (30 to 60 grains) three times daily
Powder (leaves):	10 #0 capsules (60 grains) three times daily

Indicated Uses:

Internal

Blood purifier:	Infusion
Bronchial and pulmonary afflictions:	Infusion*
Colds:	Infusion (mix with peppermint leaves)
Chills:	Infusion
Fevers:	Infusion
Influenza:	Infusion
Measles:	Infusion
Scarlet fever:	Infusion

Berries:

Colic:	Infusion
Diarrhea:	Infusion
Rheumatism:	Juice
Coughs:	Syrup
Colds:	Syrup

Seeds:

Powdered seeds are used for dropsy.

External (use the leaves or flowers)

Bruises:	Salve
Hemorrhoids:	Fomentation, Salve
Inflammations:	Salve, Fomentation
Sprains:	Salve, Fomentation
Wounds:	Salve, Fomentation

Michael Moore states, "the bark and root widely used in Europe, is not advisble in the West; our trees and bushes contain larger amounts of both hydrocyanic acid and sambuline, a nauseating alkaloid found mostly in the bark and root as well as the fresh plant."

In large doses, elder can act as a purgative and diuretic. Elder is used for urinary complaints, edema and rheumatic problems. The tea of the flowers is used as a diaphoretic to break fevers. Take a hot bath first, then combine elder flowers with equal parts peppermint and drink hot while in bed to promote sweating.

Elder flowers are used in salves for skin diseases.

ELECAMPANE *(Inula heminum)*

Part Used: root

Properties: Cholagogue, Diuretic, Expectorate, Stomachic; astringent, stimulant

Body Parts Affected: lungs, stomach and spleen

Preparation and Dosage:

Infusion:	Steep 15 to 30 minutes. 1 to 2 cups daily, hot or cold
Decoction:	Simmer 15 to 30 minutes. 1 Tbsp., as needed (see below) or 1 to 2 cups daily
Tincture:	30 to 60 drops (½ to 1 tsp.) one to two times daily
Fluid Extract:	½ to 1 tsp. one to two times daily
Powder:	3 to 10 #0 capsules (20 to 60 grains) one to two times daily. 5 is the average dose (30 grains)

Indicated Uses:

Internal

Asthma:	Tincture, Fluid Extract, Decoction, Syrup
Bronchitis:	Tincture, Fluid Extract, Decoction, Syrup
Cough:	Infusion, Decoction, Syrup
Digestive, respiratory, urinary tonic:	Tincture, Fluid Extract, Decoction, Syrup
Dyspepsia:	Tincture, Fluid Extract, Decoction, Syrup
Muscular weakness:	Fluid Extract*, Decoction*
Shortness of breath:	Fluid Extract, Infusion, Decoction, Syrup
Sluggish liver:	Decoction*, Syrup*
Tuberculosis:	Syrup*, Decoction*
Ulcers:	Infusion, Decoction, Syrup

Elecampane is useful in all respiratory problems. It is an excellent remedy for tuberculosis when combined with echinacea. It promotes expectoration. It is also good for whooping cough and weak digestion. The decoction taken in 1 tablespoon dosages will counteract stomach poisons and increase digestive power. The decoction or tincture is used for worms and as an external wash for skin diseases.

EPHEDRA *(Ephedra vulgaris)*
(Brigham tea, desert tea, Mormon tea, squaw tea)

Part Used: leaves

Properties: Expectorant; astringent, diaphoretic, stimulant

Body Parts Affected: circulation, lungs and heart

Preparation and Dosage:

Infusion:	Steep 5 to 15 minutes. 1 cup three to four times daily or as needed
Decoction:	Simmer 5 to 15 minutes. 1 cup three to four times daily or as needed
Tincture:	15 to 30 drops three times daily or as needed
Fluid Extract:	¼ to 1 tsp. three times daily or as needed
Powder:	5 to 10 #0 capsules (30 to 60 grains) three times daily or as needed

Indicated Uses:

Internal

Arthritis:	Tincture*, Fluid Extract*, Infusion*, Powder*
Asthma:	Tincture, Fluid Extract, Infusion
Fever:	Tincture, Fluid Extract, Infusion
Headaches:	Tincture, Fluid Extract, Infusion
Low blood sugar:	Tincture*, Fluid Extract*, Infusion*, Powder*
Rheumatism:	Tincture*, Fluid Extract*, Infusion*, Powder*
Sinus problems:	Tincture, Fluid Extract, Infusion
Skin eruptions:	Tincture*, Fluid Extract*, Infusion*, Powder*

External

Skin eruptions:	Fomentation

Ephedra tea is excellent for asthma, bronchitis, and other respiratory conditions. It is especially good for congestive sinus problems. It increases the blood pressure so it should not be used by persons who have high blood pressure. Weak or debilitated persons should only use it in formulas when it is in small amounts.

EYEBRIGHT *(Euphrasia officinalis)*

Part Used: above ground portion

Properties: Alterative; astringent, tonic

Body Parts Affected: eyes, liver and blood

Preparation and Dosage:

Infusion:	Steep 5 to 15 minutes. 6 oz. frequently
Tincture:	20 to 60 drops frequently
Fluid Extract:	1 tsp. frequently
Powder:	10 #0 capsules (60 grains) frequently

Indicated Uses:

Internal

Allergies:	Infusion, Fluid Extract
Cataracts:	Infusion, Fluid Extract
Diabetes:	Infusion*, Powder*, Fluid Extract*
Eye ailments (all):	Infusion, Fluid Extract
Hay fever:	Infusion*, Fluid Extract*, Powder*
Impure blood:	Infusion, Decoction, Fluid Extract, Powder
Indigestion:	Infusion, Decoction, Fluid Extract
Nose and throat congestion	Infusion, Fluid Extract
Upper respiratory problems:	Infusion, Fluid Extract, Powder

External

Cataracts:	Eyewash
Eye ailments (all):	Eyewash

Eyebright is cooling to the blood and will aid the liver to detoxify. This is the reason why it is said to help the eyes. Externally, it is used as an eyewash when combined with goldenseal or fennel for conjunctivitis, eye weakness, opthalmia and burning sore eyes.

FALSE UNICORN *(Chamailirium luteum)* (Helonias)

Part Used: root

Properties: Emmenagogue, Tonic; diuretic, emetic, parasiticide, stimulant

Body Parts Affected: uterus and kidneys

Preparation and Dosage:

Decoction:	Simmer 5 to 15 minutes. 6 oz three times daily
Tincture:	15 to 30 drops three times daily
Fluid Extract:	½ to 1 tsp. three times daily
Powder:	2 to 5 #0 capsules (15 to 30 grains) three times daily

Indicated Uses:

Internal

Amenorrhea:	Tincture*, Fluid Extract*, Decoction*, Powder*

Aphrodisiac:	Tincture, Fluid Extract, Powder
Diabetes:	Tincture*, Fluid Extract*, Powder*
Digestive tonic:	Tincture, Fluid Extract, Decoction, Powder
Dragging sensation in lower abdomen:	Tincture*, Fluid Extract*, Decoction*
Female hormone imbalances:	Decoction*, Powder*
Glandular tonic:	Decoction*, Fluid Extract*, Tincture*, Powder*
Infertility:	Tincture*, Fluid Extract*, Decoction*, Powder*
Intestinal weakness:	Tincture, Fluid Extract, Decoction, Powder
Irregular menstruation:	Tincture*, Fluid Extract*, Decoction*, Powder*
Leukorrhea:	Tincture*, Fluid Extract*, Decoction, Powder*
Menorrhagia:	Tincture*, Fluid Extract*, Powder*
Miscarriage (prevention):	Tincture, Fluid Extract, Decoction
Prolapsed uterus:	Decoction*, Fluid Extract*, Tincture*, Powder*
Spermatorrhea:	Tincture*, Fluid Extract*
Threatened abortion:	Tincture, Fluid Extract, Decoction
Urinary tract tonic:	Tincture*, Fluid Extract*, Decoction*, Powder
Uterine and ovarian problems:	Tincture*, Fluid Extract*, Powder*, Decoction*
Uterine displacement:	Tincture*, Fluid Extract*, Powder*, Decoction*

False unicorn is most commonly used for female infertility and impotence. It can be taken for several months. It also has been used for treating irregular menstruation and leukorrhea. It is usually combined with other herbs such as cramp bark or black haw, but it can be taken alone. During threatening situations, 15 drops of the tincture or ½ teaspoon of the fluid extract can be taken every hour. Do not confuse false unicorn with true unicorn.

FENNEL *(Foeniculum vulgare)*

Part Used: seed

Properties: Antispasmodic, Aromatic, Carminative; diuretic, expectorant, galactagogue, stimulant

Body Parts Affected: stomach, nerves, intestines and eyes

Preparation and Dosage:

Infusion:	Steep 5 to 15 minutes. 6 oz. three times daily

Fluid Extract:	5 to 60 drops three times daily
Oil:	1 to 5 drops three times daily
Powder:	3 is the average dose (15 grains)

Indicated Uses:

Internal

Colic:	Tincture, Fluid Extract, Infusion, Decoction
Coughs:	Decoction*, Syrup*
Cramps:	Tincture, Fluid Extract, Decoction
Emphysema:	Decoction*, Syrup*
Eyewash:	Infusion
Gas:	Tincture, Fluid Extract, Decoction
Hoarseness:	Decoction*, Syrup*
Indigestion:	Tincture, Fluid Extract, Decoction, Syrup, Powder
Jaundice:	Tincture*, Fluid Extract*, Decoction*
Rheumatism:	Tincture*, Fluid Extract*, Decoction*
Sinus congestion:	Tincture*, Fluid Extract*, Decoction*
Spasms:	Tincture, Fluid Extract

External

Eyewash:	Infusion

A few drops of the fluid extract or oil of fennel is good for flavoring foods and bitter medicines. It is used for treating gas, acid stomach, colic and cramps. It is excellent for children. In larger doses, Jethro Kloss used it to remove obstructions of the liver, spleen and gall bladder. Fennel will increase the flow of urine, menstrual blood and mother's milk, It can also be used as an eyewash.

FENUGREEK *(Trigonella foenumgraecum)*

Part Used: seed

Properties: Demulcent, Emollient, Expectorant; aphrodisiac, astringent, galactagogue, tonic

Body Parts Affected: lungs, stomach, intestines and reproductive organs.

Preparation and Dosage:

Infusion:	Steep 5 to 15 minutes. 1 cup during the day, hot or cold
Decoction:	Simmer 5 to 15 minutes. 6 oz. three times daily
Tincture:	30 to 60 drops three times daily
Fluid Extract:	½ to 1 tsp. three times daily
Powder:	2 to 10 #0 capsules (10 to 60 grains) three times daily

Indicated Uses:

Internal

Allergies:	Infusion*, Decoction*
Asthma:	Infusion, Decoction, Powder
Bronchitis:	Decoction
Coughs:	Infusion, Decoction, Syrup
Diabetes:	Powder*
Emphysema:	Infusion*, Decoction*, Powder*
Fever:	Infusion, Decoction
Hay fever:	Infusion*, Decoction*, Powder*
Heartburn:	Infusion, Decoction
Hoarseness:	Infusion, Decoction, Syrup
Migraine headaches:	Infusion
Mucus conditions (all):	Infusion, Decoction, Powder

External

Abscesses:	Poultice (seeds)
Boils:	Poultice (seeds)
Carbuncles:	Poultice (seeds)
Sore throat:	Gargle

Fenugreek is useful for all mucus conditions of the lungs. The decoction is useful for gas, stomach, ulcers, diabetes and gout. It is considered an aphrodisiac. Externally it can be used as a fomentation for boils, sores and dry skin problems. The tea is excellent for sore threats (drink and gargle) and for fevers.

FLAX *(Linum vsitatissimum)*

Part Used: seed

Properties: Demulcent, Emollient, Laxative, Mucilage

Body Parts Affected: lungs, throat, intestines and stomach

Preparation and Dosage:

Infusion:	Steep 5 to 15 minutes. 1 cup daily
Decoction:	2 oz. three times daily
Tincture:	15 to 40 drops three times daily or as needed
Fluid Extract:	15 to 30 drops three times daily or as needed
Powder:	10 to 20 #0 capsules (60 to 120 grains) once daily

Indicated Uses:

Internal

Asthma:	Decoction*
Bronchitis:	Decoction
Catarrh:	Decoction

Constipation:	Decoction, Soaked seeds
Coughs:	Decoction, Fluid Extract, Tincture
Diarrhea:	Decoction*
Enteritis:	Decoction
Flatulence:	Tincture, Fluid Extract, Decoction
Hemorrhoids:	Decoction*
Lung and chest disorders:	Tincture, Fluid Extract, Decoction
Pleurisy:	Decoction*

Flax seed has mucilagenous qualities which makes it good for all intestinal inflamations. A teaspoon of the powdered seed mixed in a cup of hot water or juice and taken three times a day will ease all ulcers and inflammations. The tea is good for coughs, asthma and pleurisy. Mixed in poultices it is one of the best remedies for sores, boils, carbuncles, inflammations and tumors. Combine with slippery elm bark for a very effective poultice for boils, pimples, oozing sores and burns. It is excellent added to diets which are low in fiber.

A good morning drink:

> 1 tablespoon of powdered flax seed
> 1 tablespoon of hulled sesame seed, powdered
> 1 tablespoon of unroasted carob powder
> 1 teaspoon of raw honey

Pour two cups of boiling water over ingredients and blend. Drink warm and it can take the place of hot chocolate. It is also a good drink for strengthening the teeth and bones. Drink this every day as a nutrient or to increase bowel movements. Several times people with bleeding, painful hemorrhoids have experienced easy bowel movements without pain when the tea or the above drink is taken every day.

FO-TI *(Polygonum multiflorum)*

Part Used: root

Properties: Stimulant, Tonic; astringent, diuretic

Body Parts Affected: liver, stomach, kidneys and reproductive organs

Preparation and Dosage:

Decoction:	Simmer 5 to 15 minutes. 2 oz. two to four times daily
Tincture:	15 to 30 drops three times daily
Fluid Extract:	5 to 20 drops three times daily
Powder:	2 to 3 #0 capsules (10 to 15 grains) three times daily

Indicated Uses:

Internal

Longevity:	Fluid Extract, Tincture, Powder
Tonic to endocrine glands:	Decoction, Powder

Fo-ti exerts a rejuvenating influence upon the endocrine glands which, in turn, strengthen the body. It acts as a tonic and nutritive herb. In large doses it is a safe aphrodisiac. Fo-ti is an excellent digestive tonic.

GARLIC *(Allium sativum)*

Part Used: bulb

Properties: Alterative, Antibiotic; antispasmodic, diaphoretic, expectorant, stimulant

Body Parts Affected: lungs, circulation, nerves and sinus

Preparation and Dosage:

Tincture:	30 to 60 drops (½ to 1 tsp.) three to four times daily
Juice:	10 to 30 drops three to four times daily
Oil:	2 to 3 drops or 1 tsp. (see below)
Syrup:	1 Tbsp. three to four times daily
Powder:	5 to 10 #0 capsules (30 to 60 grains) three to four times daily

Indicated Uses:

Internal

Arteriosclerosis:	Oil, Powder, Eat raw
Cancer:	Oil, Eat raw, Powder, Syrup
Contagious diseases:	Oil, Eat raw, Syrup, Powder
Coughs:	Syrup
Cramps:	Oil, Syrup
Diverticulitis:	Syrup, Powder, Eat raw
Emphysema:	Syrup*, Powder*
Gas:	Oil, Powder, Eat raw
Heart problems:	Powder, Eat raw, Oil
High blood pressure:	Powder*, Eat raw
Indigestion:	Eat raw, Oil, Powder
Liver congestion:	Eat raw, Powder
Parasites:	Eat raw, Powder, Oil
Rheumatism:	Eat raw, Powder, Oil
Sinus congestion:	Oil, Juice, Eat raw
Ulcers:	Syrup, Juice

External

Bowel problems and parasites:	Enemas

Ringworm:	Oil, Poultice
Skin parasites:	Oil, Poultice
Tumors:	Oil, Poultice
Warts:	Oil
Yeast infections:	Douche (using small amounts of tincture, juice, oil or powder)

Garlic has several outstanding characteristics. It is used for all lung and respiratory ailments. Use garlic as a tea or add it to syrups for coughs, colds, tuberculosis, fevers and blood diseases. It is good to use the tea as an enema for worms and bowel infections. Garlic is excellent for both high and low blood pressure, infections, stomach problems, indigestion and nervous headaches.

The best preparation is to use the fresh extract oil or eat the raw cloves.

Prepare the oil by peeling fresh garlic (4 to 8 ounces), mince it, and put into a wide-mouth jar and pour cold-pressed olive oil over it until all the garlic is covered. Close tightly and allow it to set for three to seven days. Shake it daily. Strain. Put in a dark bottle and store in a cool place. For fevers, intestinal infections, mucus of the stomach, colds and flu, take one teaspoon every hour in a little lemon juice or water. Put two to three drops in the ear for earaches twice daily. For skin problems, rub the oil directly into the skin. It is also good for aches, sprains and sore muscles.

See formula for Garlic Syrup.

GENTIAN *(Gentiana lutea)*

Part Used: root

Properties: Cholagogue, Stomachic, Tonic; anthelmintic

Body Parts Affected: stomach, liver, blood, spleen and circulation

Preparation and Dosage:

Decoction:	Simmer 5 to 15 minutes. ¼ to 1 tsp. three times daily to ½ to 1 cup daily
Tincture:	½ to 2 tsp. three times daily
Fluid Extract:	¼ to ½ tsp. three times daily
Powder:	2 to 4 #0 capsules (10 to 30 grains) three times daily

Indicated Uses:

Internal

Appetite (normalizes):	Tincture, Fluid Extract, Decoction
Chronic indigestion:	Tincture, Fluid Extract, Decoction
Dyspepsia:	Tincture, Fluid Extract, Decoction
Gas:	Tincture, Fluid Extract, Decoction
General debility (tonic):	Tincture, Fluid Extract, Decoction

Fevers:	Decoction
Gout:	Powder*, Decoction*
Intestinal inflammation:	Decoction*, Powder*
Liver congestion:	Tincture, Fluid Extract, Decoction
Jaundice:	Tincture*, Fluid Extract*, Decoction*
Stomach weakness:	Tincture, Fluid Extract, Decoction

Gentian's chief action is upon the liver and stomach. Gentian is a bitter tonic and as such finds its best field in atonic states of the intestinal tract and in slow digestion. It improves the appetite, increases digestion, augments circulation and is beneficial to the female organs. It is good for slow urination, colds, and gout. Because of its bitterness, combine it with aromatic herbs.

GINGER *(Zingiberis officinalis)*

Part Used: rhizome

Properties: Aromatic, Carminative, Diaphoretic, Stimulant; diuretic

Body Parts Affected: stomach, intestines, joints, muscles and circulation

Preparation and Dosage:

Infusion:	Steep 5 to 15 minutes. 1 fluid oz. at a time
Decoction:	Simmer 5 to 15 minutes. 2 oz. three times daily.
Tincture.	15 to 60 drops three times daily
Fluid Extract:	5 to 20 drops three times daily
Syrup:	½ to 1 tsp. three times daily
Powder:	2 to 4 #0 capsules (10 to 20 grains) three times daily, every two hours for nausea and vomiting

Indicated Uses:

Internal

Colds:	Infusion
Colon spasms:	Tincture, Infusion
Constipation:	Tincture*, Infusion*, Powder*
Contagious diseases:	Tincture*, Infusion*, Powder*
Coughs:	Tincture, Infusion
Cramps:	Tincture, Infusion
Indigestion:	Tincture, Infusion, Powder
Gas:	Tincture, Infusion, Powder
Headache:	Tincture, Infusion
Morning sickness:	Tincture, Infusion, Powder
Nausea:	Tincture, Infusion, Powder
Sinus congestion:	Tincture, Infusion, Powder
Stomach spasms:	Tincture, Infusion, Powder

External

Mumps:	Fomentation

Taken hot, ginger tea is good for suppressed menstruation and scanty urine. It is good to bring heat into the system and to stimulate digestion. The tincture is good for traveling sickness. Ginger prevents griping (use in laxative formulas) and treats bronchitis, gas, colds and flu. It will raise the body temperature when taken in frequent doses. (See ginger foot baths and fomentation.)

GINSENG *(Panax ginseng)*

Part Used: root

Properties: Alterative, Stimulant, Stomachic, Tonic

Body Parts Affected: heart and circulation, general effects on whole body.

Preparation and Dosage:

Decoction:	Simmer 15 to 60 minutes. Use about ¼ oz. of herb to 1 pint water. 4 oz. three times daily
Tincture:	20 to 60 drops three times daily
Fluid Extract:	½ to 2 tsp. three times daily
Powder:	2 to 5 #0 capsules (15 to 30 grains) three times daily

Indicated Uses:

Internal

Asthma:	Tincture, Fluid Extract*, Powder*
Endurance:	Tincture, Fluid Extract, Powder
Fevers:	Tincture, Fluid Extract, Decoction
Frigidity:	Tincture, Fluid Extract, Powder
Gas:	Tincture, Fluid Extract
Inflammation (intestines):	Tincture*, Fluid Extract*, Powder*
Longevity:	Tincture, Fluid Extract Powder
Prostate problems:	Tincture, Fluid Extract, Powder
Regulates hormones:	Tincture, Fluid Extract, Powder
Weak digestion:	Tincture, Fluid Extract, Powder

Ginseng is used as a general tonic affecting the whole body. It promotes appetite and is useful in digestive disturbances. The tea taken hot is effective for colds, chest troubles and coughs. It is used to normalize blood pressure, tone the heart, increase circulation and reduce cholesterol. It reduces blood sugar which makes it useful for diabetics. As a nutritive tonic it has been used to treat anemia.

Note: Do not use large amounts of ginseng on elderly or weak persons during high fevers, or when there is inflammation.

GOLDENSEAL *(Hydrastis canadensis)*

Part Used: rhizome

Properties: Alternative, Antibiotic, Antiseptic, Emmenagogue, Stomachic, Tonic; Laxative

Body Parts Affected: stomach, intestines, spleen, liver, eyes and all mucus membranes

Preparation and Dosage:

Infusion
(powdered root): Steep powder until cold. 1 to 2 tsp. three to six times daily
Decoction: Simmer 15 to 30 minutes. 1 to 2 tsp. three to six times daily
Tincture: 20 to 90 drops (⅓ to 1½ tsp.) three times daily
Fluid Extract: ¼ to 1½ tsp. three times daily
Powder: 2 to 5 #0 capsules (10 to 30 grains) three times daily. (5 is average dose)

Indicated Uses:

Internal

Alcoholism: Tincture*, Fluid Extract, Powder*, Infusion*
Allergies: Tincture, Fluid Extract, Powder, Infusion

Asthma: Powder*, Infusion*, Decoction*
Bad breath: Tincture, Fluid Extract, Powder, Infusion Decoction
Bladder diseases: Powder*, Infusion*, Decoction
Bronchitis: Powder*, Decoction*, Infusion*
Canker sores: Tincture, Fluid Extract, Infusion, Decoction
Chickenpox: Tincture, Fluid Extract, Infusion, Decoction
Colds: Tincture, Fluid Extract, Infusion, Decoction
Diabetes: Decoction*, Powder*
Eczema: Tincture, Fluid Extract, Infusion, Decoction
Gums (Bleeding,
infections): Tincture, Fluid Extract, Powder, Decoction
Hay fever: Infusion, Decoction, Powder, Tincture, Fluid Extract
Heart weakness: Decoction*, Infusion*, Powder*
Hemorrhoids: Tincture*, Fluid Extract*, Infusion*, Decoction*, Powder
Herpes: Tincture, Fluid Extract, Infusion, Decoction, Powder
Indigestion: Tincture, Fluid Extract, Infusion, Decoction, Powder

Infections:	Tincture, Fluid Extract, Infusion, Decoction Powder
Inflammations:	Tincture, Fluid Extract, Infusion, Decoction, Powder
Leukorrhea:	Tincture, Fluid Extract, Infusion, Decoction, Powder
Liver problems:	Decoction*, Infusion*, Powder*
Lymph congestion:	Decoction*, Infusion*, Powder*
Measles:	Tincture, Fluid Extract, Decoction, Powder, Infusion
Mammary and ovarian tumors:	Tinctures*, Fluid Extract*, Powder*
Morning sickness:	Tincture, Fluid Extract, Infusion, Powder, Decoction
Mouth (sores):	Infusion, Decoction, Tincture, Fluid Extract
Pyorrhea:	Mouthwash, Tincture, Fluid Extract, Infusion, Decoction
Tonsillitis:	Tincture, Fluid Extract, Decoction, Infusion
Ulcers:	Tincture*, Fluid Extract*, Powder*, Infusion*, Decoction

External

Burns:	Infusion, Decoction, Wash
Canker sores:	Gargle
Eye inflammations:	Infusion, Wash
Gums (bleeding, infections):	Gargle
Herpes (sores):	Fomentation, Tincture, Fluid Extract, Poultice
Leukorrhea:	Douche
Mouth sores:	Gargle
Ringworm:	Tincture, Fluid Extract, Fomentation, Wash
Skin inflammations:	Tincture, Fluid Extract, Poultice, Fomentation, Liniment, Wash
Tonsillitis:	Gargle
Wounds:	Tincture, Fluid Extract, Infusion, Decoction, Wash, Fomentation, Liniment

Goldenseal has been a popular remedy both externally and internally. As a fomentation, use externally on open sores, inflammations, eczema, ringworm, erysipelas or itchy skin afflictions.

Internally, it is a specific for all problems of the mucus membranes. It is excellent as a douche for vaginal infections, eyewash, antiseptic mouthwash for pyorrhea. Snuffed up the nose it is good for nasal catarrh. Small doses will relieve nausea during pregnancy. Use teaspoon doses of the tea combined with gotu kola as a brain tonic; used with cascara sagrada it is a bowel tonic. As a retention enema, it will reduce swollen hemorrhoids.

It is an excellent remedy used as a drink and gargle for tonsillitis and other throat problems. Use in all cases of catarrh of the intestines. Myrrh and goldenseal combined has great benefit in treating ulcers of the stomach.

For piles, hemorrhoids and prostate problems, combine two parts goldenseal and one part wild alum. Many times it is combined with other blood purifiers and toxic blood conditions.

Note: Do not use large amounts during pregnancy and hypoglycemia. Used over prolonged periods of time, it will reduce B vitamin absorption and destroy intestinal bacteria. Two to three #00 capsules daily is usually adequate for most conditions.

GOTU KOLA *(Centella Asiatica)*

Part Used: tops

Properties: Nervine, Tonic; alterative, antipyretic, diuretic

Body Parts Affected: brain, nerves, kidneys, bladder, heart and circulation

Preparation and Dosage:

Infusion:	Steep 5 to 15 minutes. 3 oz. three times daily
Tincture:	15 to 30 drops three times daily
Fluid Extract:	½ to 1 tsp. three times daily
Powder:	5 to 10 #0 capsules (30 to 60 grains) three times daily

Indicated Uses:

Internal

Brain food:	Tincture, Fluid Extract, Powder
Endurance:	Tincture, Fluid Extract, Powder
High blood pressure:	Tincture*, Fluid Extract*, Powder*
Longevity:	Tincture, Fluid Extract, Powder
Mental fatigue:	Tincture, Fluid Extract, Powder
Poor vitality:	Tincture, Fluid Extract, Powder
Senility:	Tincture, Fluid Extract, Powder

Gotu kola has remarkable rejuvenating properties similar to those of fo-ti and ginseng. It has been used in India as a diuretic as well as a blood purifier. It is valued for the treatment of depression, rheumatism, blood diseases and mental weaknesses. It neutralizes blood acids and will lower the temperature. It is known in India as a longevity herb. The usual dose is 3 ounces of the infusion three times daily.

GRAVEL ROOT OR QUEEN OF THE MEADOW
(Eupatorium purpureum)

Part Used: root

Properties: Diuretic, Lithotriptic; astringent, nervine, stimulant

Body Parts Affected: kidneys, bladder, nerves and joints

Preparation and Dosage:

Infusion (herb):	Steep 5 to 15 minutes. 1 to 2 cups daily
Decoction (Root):	Simmer 5 to 15 minutes. 1 to 2 oz. as needed up to 2 cups daily
Tincture:	30 to 60 drops (½ to 1 tsp.) three times daily
Fluid Extract:	½ to 1 tsp. three times daily
Powder:	5 #0 capsules (30 grains) three times daily

Indicated Uses:

Internal

Backache:	Tincture, Fluid Extract, Decoction
Bloody urine:	Tincture, Fluid Extract, Decoction
Bright's disease:	Tincture*, Fluid Extract*, Decoction*
Cystitis:	Tincture, Fluid Extract, Decoction
Endometritis:	Tincture, Fluid Extract, Decoction
Edema:	Tincture, Fluid Extract
Gonorrhea:	Tincture*, Fluid Extract*, Decoction*, Powder*
Gout:	Tincture, Fluid Extract, Decoction
Kidney and bladder disorders:	Tincture, Fluid Extract, Powder, Decoction
Prostate troubles:	Tincture, Fluid Extract, Decoction
Rheumatism:	Tincture*, Fluid Extract*, Decoction*, Powder*
Stones (kidney and bladder):	Decoction*, Fluid Extract*, Tincture*
Uterine inflammation:	Tincture*, Fluid Extract*, Decoction*
Uterine tonic:	Tincture*, Fluid Extract*, Decoction*
Weak pelvic organs:	Tincture, Fluid Extract, Decoction

Gravel root is used principally in the treatment of gravel or stones in the bladder, kidneys and urinary tract. It is also a nerve tonic. Gravel root is also good for uric acid deposits in the joints and for water retention.

It is also used for many female problems alone or in combination. A few of these conditons are endrometritis, leukorrhea, chronic uterine disease, labor pains, threatened abortions and dysmenorrhea.

HAWTHORN *(Crataegus oxycantha)*

Part Used: fruit

Properties: Tonic; antispasmodic, astringent, diuretic, sedative

Body Parts Affected: heart, circulation, nerves and kidneys

Preparation and Dosage:

Infusion (herb):	Steep 5 to 15 minutes. 1 cup two to three times daily

Decoction (berries):	Simmer 5 to 15 minutes. 6 oz. three times daily
Tincture:	15 to 30 drops (½ to 1 tsp.) three times daily
Fluid Extract:	10 to 15 drops three times daily
Powder:	10 #0 capsules (60 grains) three times daily

Indicated Uses:

Internal

Arteriosclerosis:	Tincture, Fluid Extract, Syrup
Arthritis:	Tincture, Fluid Extract, Syrup
Blood pressure (high or low):	Tincture*, Fluid Extract*, Syrup*
Cardiac dropsy:	Tincture, Fluid Extract
Heart tonic:	Tincture, Fluid Extract, Powder, Syrup
Nervous conditions:	Tincture*, Fluid Extract*, Powder*
Palpitation:	Tincture, Fluid Extract, Syrup
Tachycardia:	Tincture, Fluid Extract, Syrup
Vertigo:	Tincture, Fluid Extract

Hawthorn prevents hardening of the arteries and is excellent for feeble heart action, valvular insufficiency and irregular pulse. It is a cardiac tonic with antispasmodic properties and is valuable in angina pectoris. It is good for both high and low blood pressure, inflammation of the heart muscle and arteriosclerosis. A decoction of the berries is good for sore throats and acid conditions of the blood.

Extended use will lower the blood pressure. The tea is also good for nervous conditions and insomnia.

HOPS *(Humulus lupulus)*

Part Used: strobiles

Properties: Nervine, Stomachic; anodyne, antibiotic, carminative, cholagogue, tonic

Body Parts Affected: nerves, stomach, blood, liver and gall bladder

Preparation and Dosage:

Infusion:	Steep 5 to 15 minutes. 6 oz. three times daily, hot or cold
Tincture:	15 to 30 drops (½ to 1 tsp.) three times daily
Fluid Extract:	10 to 15 drops three times daily
Powder:	5 to 10 #0 capsules (30 to 60 grains) three times daily

Indicated Uses:

Internal:

Coughs:	Infusion*, Tincture*

Fever:	Infusion*, Tincture*
Headaches:	Infusion, Tincture
Indigestion:	Infusion, Tincture
Insomnia:	Infusion, Tincture
Jaundice:	Infusion*, Tincture*
Morning sickness:	Tincture, Infusion
Nerves (weak):	Tincture, Infusion
Stomach tonic:	Tincture, Infusion
Throat, bronchial tubes, chest ailments:	Infusion*
Toothache:	Tincture, Fluid Extract
Ulcers:	Tincture*, Infusion*

External

Boils:	Fomentation, Poultice
Bruises:	Fomentation, Poultice
Earaches:	Poultice
Inflammations:	Fomentation, Poultice
Rheumatic pains:	Fomentation*
Skin ailments:	Fomentation, Poultice
Ulcers:	Fomentation, Poultice

Hops is an excellent nervine and will produce sleep when insomnia is present. Three cups of the infusion daily will tone up the liver and digestive tract. Hops increases the flow of both the bile and urine. It is good to use for reduction of excessive sexual desires. The tea is good for nervous stomach, poor appetite, gas and intestinal cramps. The cold tea taken before meals will increase digestion. Hops as a poultice or fomentation is effective for boils, tumors, painful swellings and skin inflammations. Hops placed inside a pillow case will aid sleep.

HOREHOUND *(Marrubium vulgare)*

Part Used: tops

Properties: Diaphoretic, Expectorant; tonic

Body Parts Affected: lungs, chest and stomach

Preparation and Dosage:

Infusion:	Steep 20 minutes. 6 oz. at a time, frequently
Tincture:	20 to 60 drops three times daily
Fluid Extract:	½ to 1 tsp. three times daily
Syrup:	½ to 1 tsp. three times daily
Powder:	5 to 10 #0 capsules (30 to 60 grains) three times daily

Indicated Uses:

Internal

Asthma:	Infusion*, Syrup*

Coughs:	Infusion, Syrup
Colds:	Infusion
Dyspepsia:	Cold infusion, Fluid Extract
Fevers:	Infusion taken hot
Jaundice:	Cold infusion
Lung congestion:	Infusion, Syrup
Sore throats:	Infusion, Syrup

Horehound taken hot will increase perspiration. The infusion or tincture given cold is a bitter digestive tonic. In syrup it is a tonic and expectorant.

Horehound is effective for breaking up colds, bronchitis, bronchial catarrh, and it will expectorate mucus. It is very useful in chronic sore throats and pulmonary problems; use as a syrup for children.

HORSERADISH *(Cochleria amoracia)*

Part Used: root

Properties: Diaphoretic, Diuretic, Expectorant, Stomachic

Body Parts Affected: sinuses, stomach, gall bladder and urinary tract

Preparation and Dosage:

Decoction:	Simmer 5 to 15 minutes. 6 oz. one to two times daily, cold; or 2 to 3 Tbsp. warm three times daily

Indicated Uses:

Internal

Arthritis:	Fluid Extract*, Syrup*
Asthma:	Fluid Extract, Syrup
Circulation (stimulant):	Fluid Extract, Syrup, Infusion, Eat raw
Colds:	Infusion, Fluid Extract, Syrup
Coughs:	Syrup
Digestive stimulant:	Fluid Extract, Infusion, Syrup, Eat raw
Dropsy:	Infusion, Fluid Extract
Hoarseness:	Syrup
Liver problems:	Fluid Extract, Syrup, Eat raw
Lymphatic congestion:	Fluid Extract
Rheumatism:	Fluid Extract*, Infusion*
Sciatica:	Fluid Extract
Urine retention:	Fluid Extract, Syrup, Eat raw
Worms:	Fluid Extract, Syrup, Juice (½ tsp. in 1 cup water as needed)

External

Swellings of liver and spleen:	Poultice (mix with powdered mustard seed and slippery elm)

Horseradish is effective for promoting stomach secretions. A syrup of horseradish is excellent for sinus congestion and will promote digestion. It is good for dropsy and urine retention. Horseradish will stimulate the function of the pancreas. See horseradish syrup formula.

Note: Fresh horseradish left in contact with the skin will cause blistering. Avoid contact with the eyes.

HORSETAIL *(Equisetum arvense)*

Part Used: tops

Properties: Astringent, Diuretic, Lithotriptic; emmenagogue, galactagogue, nutritive, vulnerary

Body Parts Affected: kidneys, blood, heart and lungs

Preparation and Dosage:

Infusion:	Steep 45 minutes. A mouthful, four times daily, or 1 to 2 cups daily
Decoction:	Simmer 5 to 15 minutes. 2 oz. three to four times daily
Tincture:	5 to 30 drops three to four times daily
Fluid Extract:	5 drops three to four times daily
Powder:	5 to 10 #0 capsules (30 to 60 grains) three to four times daily

Indicated Uses:

Internal

Bedwetting:	Tincture, Fluid Extract, Infusion
Bleeding internallly:	Tincture, Fluid Extract, Infusion
Dropsy:	Tincture, Fluid Extract
Gravel:	Tincture, Fluid Extract, Infusion
Heart and lung tonic:	Tincture*, Fluid Extract*, Infusion, Powder*
Skin diseases:	Tincture*, Fluid Extract*, Infusion*
Spitting of blood:	Tincture*, Fluid Extract*, Infusion*

External

Bleeding wounds:	Fomentation
Ulcers:	Fomentation

The early settlers used horsetail as a diuretic in kidney and dropsical conditions. It is high in silica, so herbalists use it for skin and eye conditions. It is good for glandular swellings and pus discharges. It strengthens the heart and lungs and will remove gravel from the bladder and kidneys. It is specific for internal bleeding and urine retention. It is also used to clear fevers and release nervous tension.

Horsetail helps coagulate the blood and is useful during excessive bleeding and menstruation.

Note: Horsetail can be irritating to the kidneys when used for prolonged periods (e.g. daily for more than one month). It works best in small frequent doses.

HYSSOP *(Hyssopus officinalis)*

Part Used: leaves

Properties: Diaphoretic, Expectorant; cholagogue, stimulant, vulnerary

Body Parts Affected: lungs, sinuses and circulation

Preparation and Dosage:

Infusion:	Steep 5 to 15 minutes. 1 to 2 cups daily or frequently
Tincture:	½ to 1 tsp. frequently
Fluid Extract:	1 to 2 tsp. frequently
Powder:	10 #0 capsules frequently

Indicated Uses:

Internal

Asthma:	Infusion, Fluid Extract
Colds:	Infusion
Coughs:	Infusion
Fevers:	Infusion
Sluggish circulation:	Infusion
Weak digestion:	Infusion*

External

Muscular pains:	Fomentation
Cuts:	Poultice (use fresh green herb)

Hyssop has stimulating, expectorant qualities that make it excellent when trying to remove congestion from the lungs. Colds, coughs, asthma, sluggish circulation and weak digestion are treated with this herb.

The warm infusion mixed with equal parts of horehound is good for asthma and heavy mucus conditions. The infusion of hyssop alone is good for gas and to promote sweating when trying to break fevers.

Externally, a fomentation made from the leaves is used to relieve muscular rheumatism and bruises. A poultice made from the fresh green herb will help heal cuts.

IRISH MOSS *(Chondius crispus)*

Part Used: whole plant

Properties: Demulcent, Emollient, Nutritive

Body Parts Affected: lungs, kidneys and skin

Preparation and Dosage:

Infusion:	Steep 5 to 15 minutes. 2 oz. two to three times daily, up to 2 cups daily
Tincture:	30 to 60 drops (½ to 1 tsp.) two to three times daily
Fluid Extract:	½ to 1 tsp. two to three times daily
Powder:	4 to 6 #0 capsules (20 to 40 grains) two to three times daily

Indicated Uses:

Internal

Anemia:	Infusion*, Powder*
Coughs:	Infusion, Syrup
Goiter:	Infusion, Syrup
Kidney and bladder irritations:	Infusion*, Syrup*
Nutritional deficiencies:	Infusion*, Syrup*
Respiratory problems:	Infusion*, Syrup*
Thyroid problems:	Infusion
Ulcers of throat and stomach:	Infusion, Decoction, Syrup

External

Inflammations:	Poultice, Fomentation
Skin ailments:	Poultice

Irish moss is high in mucilage which makes it very soothing to the tissues. It is excellent for inflammations of the lungs, intestines and kidneys. Use it in hair rinses for dry hair and externally as a fomentation for dry and burning skin diseases.

Irish moss is one of the most nourishing of seasonings and can be used daily to supplement any diet. When making a decoction, sweeten it with licorice root, honey or an aromatic herb. Irish moss is also good for respiratory illnesses.

JUNIPER *(Juniperis communis)*

Part Used: fruit

Properties: Antispasmodic, Diuretic; anodyne, aromatic, astringent, carminative, lithotriptic, stimulant

Body Parts Affected: kidneys and stomach

Preparation and Dosage:

Infusion:	Steep 5 to 15 minutes. 3 oz. one to three times daily

Decoction:	Simmer 5 to 15 minutes. 1 to 2 cups daily
Tincture:	5 to 20 drops three times daily
Fluid Extract:	½ to 1 tsp. three times daily
Oil:	1 to 3 drops two times daily
Powder:	Up to 10 #0 capsules (up to 60 grains) daily

Indicated Uses:

Internal

Allergies:	Fluid Extract*, Infusion*, Decoction*, Powder*
Arthritis:	Fluid Extract*, Infusion*, Tincture*, Decoction*, Powder*
Bed wetting:	Oil, Tincture, Fluid Extract, Infusion
Bladder diseases:	Oil, Tincture, Fluid Extract, Infusion, Powder
Blood purifier:	Powder*, Fluid Extract*
Coughs:	Infusion, Decoction
Cystitis:	Oil, Fluid Extract, Tincture, Powder, Infusion
Diabetes:	Powder*, Infusion*, Decoction*
Gas:	Oil, Fluid Extract, Infusion, Decoction, Tincture
Hay fever:	Infusion*, Decoction*, Powder*
Intestinal putrification:	Infusion, Oil, Tincture, Fluid Extract, Powder
Leukorrhea:	Infusion, Powder, Oil
Lumbago:	Infusion*, Fluid Extract*, Powder*
Nephritis:	Infusion, Oil, Fluid Extract, Tincture, Decoction, Infusion

External

Leukorrhea:	Douche
Moist eczema:	Oil
Psoriasis:	Oil, Salve
Skin parasites:	Oil, Salve
Wounds:	Salve

Juniper berries are a stimulating diuretic, but in large doses it can be irritating. It is effective as a tea for urine retention, bladder problems, catarrh of the bladder, leukorrhea, gonorrhea, etc. Three drops of the oil can be taken three times a day on a teaspoon of honey for these ailments. It is a good douche for vaginal infections.

It is an excellent digestive tonic. The decoction or oil taken internally is good when there is putrification and gas in the stomach and intestines.

The berries, boiled and used as a spray will disinfect the rooms where sick people have been. Those who are nursing patients with serious illnesses such as scarlet fever, smallpox, typhus, cholera, etc. should chew a few juniper berries to protect themselves from pathogenic substances which may be inhaled.

Note: Juniper should not be used alone in large doses or with prolonged use during urinary tract or inflammatory problems.

KAVA KAVA *(Piper methysticum)*

Part Used: root

Properties: Anodyne, Antispectic, Antispasmodic, Diuretic; sedative, tonic

Body Parts Affected: nerves

Preparation and Dosage:

Infusion (ground root):	Steep 5 to 15 minutes. 2 oz. two times daily, up to 1 cup daily
Decoction	Simmer 5 to 15 minutes. 2 oz. two times daily, up to 1 cup daily
Tincture:	15 to 30 drops as needed
Fluid Extract:	¼ to ½ tsp. as needed
Powder:	3 to 7 #0 capsules (15 to 45 grains) as needed

Indicated Uses:

Internal

Insomnia:	Tincture, Fluid Extract, Infusion
Kidney infections:	Tincture, Fluid Extract, Infusion
Nervous conditions:	Tincture, Fluid Extract, Infusion, Powder
Neuralgia:	Tincture, Fluid Extract
Pain:	Tincture, Fluid Extract
Urinary antiseptic:	Tincture, Fluid Extract, Infusion

External

Analgesic:	Fomentation

Kava kava is an excellent herb for insomnia and nervousness. It will invoke sleep and relax the nervous system. It is used internally as a tincture or tea for pains associated with nerve or skin diseases and will relieve stress after injury.

Kava kava is an antiseptic which makes it good as a douche and valuable for urinary tract infections. When taken as a tea, it may be flavored with peppermint or some other aromatic. See "herpes" for further information.

Note: Regular use of large dosages will cause an accumulation of toxic substances in the liver.

KELP *(Fucus visiculosis)*

Part Used: whole plant

Properties: Demulcent, Nutritive; alterative, diuretic

Body Parts Affected: thyroid, nerves, brain, kidneys and bladder

Preparation and Dosage:

Infusion:	Steep 5 to 15 minutes. 1 to 2 cups daily
Tincture:	5 to 10 drops one to two times daily
Fluid Extract:	10 drops one to two times daily
Powder:	Sprinkle on food. 1 tsp. one to two times daily
Powder:	3 to 5 #0 capsules (10 to 30 grains) one to two times daily

Indicated Uses:

Internal

Anemia:	Powder*, Fluid Extract*
Colitis:	Powder*
Diabetes:	Powder*
Eczema:	Powder*, Fluid Extract*
Goiter:	Powder, Fluid Extract
Hot flashes (glandular food):	Powder, Fluid Extract
Obesity:	Powder, Fluid Extract
Psoriasis:	Powder*, Fluid Extract*
Thyroid problems (all):	Powder, Fluid Extract

Kelp is most helpful in the nourishment of the body due to its ability to stimulate metabolism. It is rich in iodine which the thyroid must have to properly function. Kelp absorbs wastes from the body fluids.

Studies at the Gastrointestinal Research Laboratories of McGill University in Montreal, found a factor called sodium alginate in kelp that binds with radioactive strontium-90 in the intestines and carries it out of the body. This factor aids in detoxification of the intestines.

Note: Excessive use of kelp can produce goiter-like symptoms due to the high content of iodine.

LADY'S SLIPPER *(Cypredium pubesceno)*

Part Used: root (fresh)

Properties: Antispasmodic, Nervine, Sedative

Body Parts Affected: nerves

Preparation and Dosage:

Infusion:	Steep 60 minutes. 1 Tbsp. every hour
Decoction:	Simmer 60 minutes. 1 Tbsp. in 6 oz. water three to four times daily
Tincture:	5 to 30 drops three times daily
Fluid Extract:	¼ tsp. three times daily
Powder:	2 to 10 #0 capsules (5 to 60 grains) three times daily

Indicated Uses:

Internal

Cholera:	Tincture, Fluid Extract
Epilepsy:	Tincture, Fluid Extract
Headache:	Tincture, Fluid Extract, Infusion, Decoction
Hepatitis:	Decoction*
Hysteria:	Tincture, Fluid Extract
Insomnia:	Tincture, Fluid Extract, Decoction
Irritability:	Tincture, Fluid Extract, Decoction, Powder
Nervous exhaustion:	Tincture, Fluid Extract, Decoction, Powder

Lady's slipper is an excellent nervine and acts as a tonic to exhausted nervous systems, improving circulation and nutrition. It is of value for such problems as cholera, hysteria, nervous headache, insomnia, fevers when nervousness is present, and nervous indigestion. This remedy can be mixed with small amounts of lobelia and ginger for the treatment of fevers and pneumonia. Combine with scullcap for hysteria and headaches. Combined with dandelion and chamomile, it is excellent for liver and digestive problems.

LEMON BALM *(Melissa officinalis)*

Part Used: tops

Properties: Diaphoretic, Sedative; antitryptic, antispasmodic

Body Parts Affected: nerves and circulation

Preparation and Dosage:

Infusion:	Steep 5 to 15 minutes 6 oz. as needed frequently
Tincture:	30 to 60 drops (½ to 1 tsp.) as needed
Fluid Extract:	½ to 2 tsp. as needed
Powder:	10 #0 capsules (60 grains) as needed

Indicated Uses:

Internal

Colds:	Infusion*
Fevers:	Infusion*
Flu:	Infusion*
Melancholy:	Tincture*, Fluid Extract*, Infusion*

The remedy is specific for children and infants when signs of fever, colds and flu approach. Prepare the tea and sweeten with honey and give hot to feverish children while they are covered with warm blankets. Combine with catnip tea for nervous fevers, or hyperactive children with digestive disturbances. Peppermint, spearmint and elder flowers are other herbs that combine well with lemon balm to treat fevers.

LICORICE *(Glycyrrhiza glabra)*

Part Used: root

Properties: Demulcent, Expectorant, Laxative; alterative

Body Parts Affected: lungs, stomach, intestines, spleen and liver

Preparation and Dosage:

Decoction:	Simmer 5 to 15 minutes. 1 Tbsp. as needed
Tincture:	30 to 60 drops (½ to 1 tsp.) two to three times daily
Fluid Extract:	½ to 1 tsp. two to three times daily
Syrup:	1 tsp. to 1 Tbsp. as needed
Powder:	Up to 10 #0 capsules (60 grains) daily

Indicated Uses:

Internal

Addison's disease:	Powder*, Fluid Extract*
Arthritis:	Powder*, Fluid Extract*
Asthma:	Powder*, Fluid Extract*
Bronchitis:	Powder*, Syrup*, Decoction*
Colds:	Decoction*
Constipation:	Decoction*, Powder*
Coughs:	Decoction*, Syrup*
Hoarseness:	Decoction*, Syrup*
Sore throat:	Decoction*, Syrup*
Ulcers:	Fluid Extract*, Decoction*, Syrup*

Licorice extract has been shown to have activities similar to those of cortisone and to a lesser extent, estrogen. It induces the adrenal cortex to produce larger amounts of cortisone and aldosterone. Glycyrrhizin, a component found in licorice, has a chemical structure similar to that of human steroid hormones. A derivative of glycyrrhizin, called carbenoxoline, has been successfully employed in ulcer therapy for the past two decades in Europe. Wild yam, ginseng and sarsparilla are herbs that also have hormone-like substances in them which combine well with licorice root.

Licorice root is added to bitter tonics to make them more palatable and to combinations of herbs to balance the formula. It is excellent for all kinds of stomach and intestinal ulcers. It is a specific for flu, colds and lung congestion and is added to cough syrups. It is a mild laxative and is effective for elderly people and children. For hoarseness and throat problems, combine with sage, ginger, horehound and coltsfoot. Combine licorice root powder with other herbs and make pills (see "Pills") for children's throat and lung problems.

Note: Large doses of licorice root are to be avoided with people who have high blood pressure or hyper adrenal function. Use smaller doses and combine other herbs with licorice in these situations. When licorice root is taken daily over an extended period of time, the dosage should

not exceed three grams per day. Larger doses may be taken for short periods of time, not to exceed 30 grams per week. The reason is because licorice root contains a substance similar to adrenal cortical hormones that may cause edema.

LOBELIA *(Lobelia inflata)*

Part Used: plant and seeds

Properties: Antispasmodic, Emetic, Nervine; expectorant

Body Parts Affected: nerves, lungs, stomach, muscles and circulation

Preparation and Dosage:

Infusion:	Steep 5 to 15 minutes. 1 Tbsp. as needed
Tincture:	10 to 30 drops as needed
Fluid Extract:	5 to 30 drops as needed
Powder:	1 to 2 #0 capsules (1 to 10 grains) as needed

Indicated Uses:

Internal

Allergies:	Powder*
Arthritis:	Tincture*, Fluid Extract*, Powder*
Asthma:	Tincture*, Fluid Extract*, Syrup*, Infusion*, Powder*
Bronchitis:	Infusion*, Decoction*, Syrup*, Tincture*, Fluid Extract*
Chicken pox:	Infusion*, Tincture*, Fluid Extract*
Contagious diseases:	Infusion*, Tincture*, Fluid Extract*, Powder*
Convulsions:	Tincture, Fluid Extract
Coughs:	Infusion*, Tincture*, Decoction*, Syrup*
Earache:	Tincture (drops in ear)
Ear infections:	Tincture (drops in ear)
Fevers (all kinds):	Tincture*, Infusion*, Decoction, Fluid Extract*, Powder*
Headache:	Tincture, Fluid Extract
Heart palpitation:	Tincture, Fluid Extract
Indigestion:	Tincture*, Fluid Extract*, Powder*, Infusion*, Decoction*
Jaundice:	Powder*, Infusion*, Decoction*, Syrup*
Pleurisy:	Infusion*, Decoction*
Pneumonia:	Infusion*, Decoction*
Poisoning (food):	Tincture (use as emetic)
St. Vitus dance:	Tincture, Fluid Extract
Teething:	Rub tincture or fluid extract on gums
Toothache:	Tincture (rub into gums)

External

Arthritis: Liniment*
Bites (snake, insect):   Poultice
Poison ivy: Tincture, Fluid Extract, Fomentation,
                                 Poultice
Ringworm: Tincture, Fluid Extract, Fomentation,
                                 Poultice
Tumors: Poultice

Lobelia is both a relaxant and a stimulant. Small doses of the tincture (5 to 10 drops) will act as a tonic and stimulant; larger doses will act as a sedative.

It is used internally for spasmodic lung and respiratory conditions (small doses, 15 drops of the tincture or one gelatin capsule) to relieve spasms and to act as an expectorant. It is a good herb to add to all cough medicines. Externally, lobelia is used as a wash for infected or itchy skin diseases. In large doses of the tincture (1 teaspoon to 1 tablespoon) it is an excellent emetic. Add lobelia to liniments for sore muscles, pains and rheumatism. Combine with lady's slipper for convulsions. As an expectorant, it is valuable in all respiratory treatments, especially the spasmodic type. Combined with scullcap and lady's slipper, it is good for lock jaw. Lobelia will relax the heart and lower rapid pulse taken in small doses.

Lobelia is suitable for fevers associated with phrenitis, meningitis, pneumonia, pleurisey, hepatitis, peritonitis, nephritis and periostitis. It is excellent for cramps, epilepsy, hysteria, chorea and convulsions.

LUNGWORT *(Pulmonaria officinalis)*

Part Used: leaves

Properties: Demulcent, Emollient, Expectorant, Mucilage; astringent, tonic, vulnerary

Body Parts Affected: lungs, bronchials, intestines, bowel and liver

Preparation and Dosage:

Infusion: Steep 5 to 15 minutes. 6 oz. at a time
Tincture: 15 to 30 drops three times daily
Fluid Extract: ½ to 1 tsp. three times daily
Powder: 10 #0 capsules (60 grains) three times daily

Indicated Uses:

Internal

Asthma: Tincture*, Fluid Extract*, Powder*, Infusion
Bronchial disorders: Infusion, Syrup
Colds: Infusion
Coughs: Infusion, Syrup*
Diarrhea: Infusion*, Powder*
Hay fever: Tincture, Fluid Extract
Hemorrhoids: Infusion*

Hoarseness:	Infusion, Syrup*
Influenza:	Infusion, Tincture, Fluid Extract, Syrup
Jaundice:	Infusion*, Syrup*
Pain in neck and between shoulders:	Tincture, Fluid Extract
Pleurisy:	Infusion*, Fluid Extract*, Tincture*
Pneumonia:	Infusion*, Fluid Extract*, Tincture*
Tuberculosis:	Infusion*, Fluid Extract*, Tincture*, Powder*, Syrup*
Ulcers:	Infusion*, Syrup*

External

Wounds:	Poultices, Fomentations

Lungwort exerts its actions mainly upon the respiratory system, especially when there is bleeding of the lungs. It is a reliable herb for coughs, asthma, colds, bronchial and catarrhal afflictions. It will heal weakened tissues and counteract inflammations. As a poultice, it is an excellent dressing for wounds and swellings. It is a good wash for infected sores.

When eaten fresh, lungwort nutritionally contains vitamin C, B-complex; minerals—iron, copper, silver, manganese, kerotin and nickel.

Lungwort has mild astringent properties and is used for diarrhea, hemorrhoids and mucus conditions of the throat.

MANDRAKE (AMERICAN) *(Podophyllum peltatum)*

Part Used: root

Properties: Cholagogue, Hepatic, Laxative; alterative, emetic, stimulant

Body Parts Affected: liver, gall bladder, intestines and skin

Preparation and Dosage:

Decoction:	Simmer 5 to 15 minutes. 1 Tbsp (cold) two times daily
Tincture:	1 to 10 drops two times daily
Fluid Extract:	¼ to ½ tsp. two times daily
Powder:	1 to 3 #0 capsules two times daily

Indicated Uses:

Internal

Constipation:	Tincture*, Fluid Extract*, Powder*
Fevers:	Tincture*, Decoction*, Fluid Extract*
Gall stones:	Tincture*, Fluid Extract*, Powder*
Jaundice:	Tincture*, Fluid Extract*, Powder*, Decoction*
Liver problems:	Tincture*, Fluid Extract*, Decoction*, Powder*

Pinworms:	Tincture*, Fluid Extract*, Decoction*, Powder*

Mandrake is a powerful glandular stimulant in small doses and is used to treat all skin diseases, lymphatic problems, obstructions of the liver and gall bladder, constipation, mercurial poisoning and digestive problems.

Externally, the tincture diluted in warm water (one tablespoon to two cups of water) is a wash for skin diseases. Cook down the tincture or evaporate the alcohol and paint on warts.

When taken internally, remember to take small doses. Mandrake is best combined with licorice root, ginger or some other carminative.

Note: Do not use during pregnancy or in large doses. Only moderate doses of this herb should be used. In large doses, it produces nausea and vomiting and even inflammation of the intestines and membranes of the stomach. Discontinue its use if any uncomfortable symptoms are noticed.

MARSHMALLOW *(Althea officinalis)*

Part Used: root, flowers and leaves

Properties: Demulcent, Diuretic, Emollient, Lithotriptic; alterative, nutritive, vulnerary

Body Parts Affected: intestines, kidneys and bladder

Preparation and Dosage:

Infusion (flowers/leaves):	Steep 5 to 15 minutes. 1 cup at a time, frequently
Decoction (root):	Simmer 5 to 15 minutes. 6 oz. three times daily
Tincture:	30 to 60 drops (½ to 1 tsp.) three times daily
Fluid Extract:	1 to 2 tsp. three times daily
Powder:	5 to 10 #0 capsules (30 to 60 grains) three times daily

Indicated Uses:

Internal

Allergies:	Decoction*, Powder*
Asthma:	Decoction*, Powder*
Bed wetting:	Tincture*, Fluid Extract*, Powder*, Decoction*
Bladder problems:	Tincture*, Fluid Extract*, Powder*, Decoction
Bleeding (urinary):	Powder*, Decoction*
Coughs:	Syrup, Decoction

Dysentery:	Infusion*, Decoction*
Emphysema:	Syrup*, Infusion*, Decoction*
Hoarseness:	Syrup, Decoction
Inflammations of intestines and respiratory tract:	Decoction, Syrup
Kidney stones:	Infusion*, Decoction*, Powder*, Tincture*, Fluid Extract*
Lactation:	Infusion*, Decoction*, Powder*, Tincture*, Fluid Extract*
Lung problems (all):	Fluid Extract, Infusion, Decoction
Throat inflammations:	Decoction, Syrup

External

Bee stings:	Poultice of leaves
Eye wash:	Infusion (use leaves)
Skin inflammations:	Poultice, Fomentation
Vaginal irritations:	Douche, Infusion, Decoction

Marshmallow is high in mucilage and is one of the best known remedies to lubricate the lungs, intestines and kidneys in cases of infections and inflammation. As a poultice it is excellent for inflamed parts such as gangrene, open wounds or burns. Internally, use for lung problems, diarrhea, dysentery and ulcers. It is excellent to add to douches for vaginal infections. The tea is good to bathe sore eyes. Use in combination with other diuretic herbs during kidney treatments to assist in the release of stones and gravel. It is high in minerals, especially calcium, and can be used in combination for its nutritive qualities.

MISTLETOE (AMERICAN) *(Viscum flavescens)*

Part Used: tops

Properties: Antispasmodic, Nervine; diuretic, emetic, emmenagogue, tonic

Body Parts Affected: nerves, heart, kidneys and bladder

Preparation and Dosage:

Infusion:	Steep 5 to 15 minutes. 1 cup during the day
Tincture:	30 to 60 drops (½ to 1 tsp.) two to three times daily
Fluid Extract:	¼ to 1 tsp. two to three times daily
Powder:	5 #0 capsules (30 grains) two to three times daily

Indicated Uses:

Internal

Blood flow to the brain:	Tincture, Fluid Extract

Chorea:	Tincture, Fluid Extract
Convulsions:	Tincture, Fluid Extract
Epilepsy:	Tincture, Fluid Extract
Hysteria:	Tincture, Fluid Extract
Nervous debility:	Tincture, Fluid Extract

American mistletoe shares with the European mistletoe the attributes to relieve tensions and minor spasms. The extract will increase uterine contractions and raise the blood pressure. It is a vasoconstrictor and should not be used with people that are prone to hypertension.

The dried plant has pronounced effects on the muscles of the uterus, stimulating contractions and lessening bleeding. It may be given early in labor to give tone to contractions and make them more regular as opposed to spasmodic.

Note: Viscum has been known to be toxic and should be carefully observed as to what effect it has in each indicated usage.

MISTLETOE (EUROPEAN) *(Viscum album)*

Part Used: tops

Properties: Stimulant, Tonic; diuretic

Body Parts Affected: heart, kidneys and circulation

Preparation and Dosage:

Infusion:	5 to 15 minutes. 3 oz. two to three times daily
Decoction:	Simmer 5 to 15 minutes. 1 Tbsp. three to four times daily
Tincture:	30 to 60 drops (½ to 1 tsp.) two to three times daily
Fluid Extract:	¼ to 1 tsp. two to three times daily
Powder:	2 to 5 #0 capsules (up to 30 grains) two to three times daily

Indicated Uses:

Internal

Arteriosclerosis:	Tincture*, Fluid Extract*, Decoction*
Cholesterol (high):	Tincture, Fluid Extract, Syrup
Digestion (poor):	Tincture, Fluid Extract, Decoction
Glandular stimulant:	Tincture, Fluid Extract, Decoction, Powder*
Heart tonic:	Tincture, Fluid Extract, Syrup
Weak pulse:	Tincture, Fluid Extract

External

Chilblains (frostbite):	Fomentation
Leg ulcers:	Fomentation

European mistletoe is used as a cardiac tonic and to stimulate circulation. At first it will raise the blood pressure, then lower it. The extract is a wonderful cure for prematurely aged arteries accompanied by high blood pressure. For arteriosclerosis, combine 1 cup of equal parts mistletoe, hawthorn berries and wild leeks. Cook them together in two pints of water for 15 minutes; strain and drink as a broth, one cup three times daily. Mistletoe extract combined with an equal amount of rauwolfia extract is beneficial in sudden heart palpitations, vascular spasms and difficult breathing during asthma attacks. Mistletoe is good for dizziness, vertigo and headaches.

Note: DO NOT EAT BERRIES. Use with care. In the American Materia Medica by Finley Ellingwood, M.D., mistletoe is reported to be used as an agent that affects the heart. Twenty to thirty drops of the fluid extract were used to treat hypertrophy of the heart with valvular insufficiency, drops, weak pulse and in later stages of disease when the heart was weak or irregular.

MOTHERWORT *(Leonurus cardiaca)*

Part Used: tops

Properties: Emmenagogue, Nervine, Tonic; antispasmodic, diaphoretic, laxative

Body Parts Affected: nerves, heart and uterus

Preparation and Dosage:

Infusion:	Steep 5 to 15 minutes. 6 oz. three to four times daily
Tincture:	30 to 60 drops (½ to 1 tsp.) three to four times daily
Fluid Extract:	½ to 1 tsp. three to four times daily
Powder:	5 to 10 #0 capsules (30 to 60 grains) three to four times daily

Indicated Uses:

Internal

Amenorrhea (absence of menstruation):	Infusion, Decoction, Tincture, Fluid Extract
Cramps:	Tincture, Fluid Extract, Infusion, Decoction
Disturbed sleep:	Tincture, Fluid Extract, Infusion, Decoction
Dysmenorrhea:	Tincture, Fluid Extract, Infusion, Decoction
Endocarditis:	Tincture, Fluid Extract, Infusion, Decotion
Fevers:	Tincture*, Fluid Extract*, Infusion*, Decoction
Fits:	Tincture, Fluid Extract, Infusion, Decoction
Heart tonic:	Tincture, Fluid Extract
Nervousness:	Tincture, Fluid Extract, Infusion, Decoction
Palpitation:	Tincture, Fluid Extract, Infusion, Decoction

Pericarditis:	Tincture, Fluid Extract, Infusion, Decoction
Pulmonary congestion:	Tincture, Fluid Extract, Infusion, Decotion
Spasms:	Tincture, Fluid Extract
Uterine pains:	Tincture, Fluid Extract, Infusion, Decoction

External

Stomach cramps:	Fomentation

Motherwort tea, taken warm, is an excellent remedy for suppressed menstruation and other female complaints. It is good for all nervous conditions, cramps, convulsions, sleeplessness and suppressed urine. Combined motherwort with cramp bark and squawvine for female cramping and suppressed menstrual flow and urine retention. A hot fomentation made from strong tea will relieve cramps and pain during menstruation. It is excellent for nervous conditions and acts as a heart tonic, especially when combined with hawthorn berries.

MUGWORT *(Artemisia vulgaris)*

Part Used: tops

Properties: Emmenagogue, Nervine, Stomachic; diaphoretic, diuretic

Body Parts Affected: nerves, circulation, stomach and uterus

Preparation and Dosage:

Infusion:	Steep 20 minutes, 1 tsp. as needed
Tincture:	30 to 60 (½ to 1 tsp.) as needed
Fluid Extract:	1 tsp. as needed
Powder:	Up to 10 #0 capsules (up to 60 grains) as needed

Indicated Uses:

Internal

Colds:	Infusion, Decoction
Epilepsy:	Tincture, Fluid Extract
Fevers:	Infusion, Decotion
Flu:	Infusion, Decoction
Insomnia:	Tincture, Fluid Extract, Infusion, Decoction
Menstrual cramps:	Tincture*, Fluid Extract, Infusion*, Decoction
Menstrual obstruction:	Infusion*, Decoction*, Powder*
Pains in the bowels and stomach:	Infusion, Decoction, Tincture, Fluid Extract
Stomach disorders:	Tincture, Fluid Extract, Infusion, Decoction

External

Abscesses:	Fomentation, Poultice
Bruises:	Fomentation, Poultice

| Carbuncles: | Fomentation, Poultice |
| Stomach pains: | Fomentation, Poultice |

Mugwort is excellent for female complaints such as suppressed menstruation and menstrual cramps. It is especially good when combined with cramp bark, marigold and black haw for these problems. Mugwort is good in kidney combinations when there are stones or gravel. For pains in the stomach and bowels, drink the tea in small frequent doses and apply a fomentation of the infusion over the painful area.

Mugwort may be applied externally as a poultice to boils, carbuncles and abscesses. Drink the tea for nervousness, shaking and insomnia.

MULLEIN *(Verbascum tapsus)*

Part Used: leaf

Properties: Demulcent, Expectorant; antispasmodic, astringent, diuretic, vulnerary

Body Parts Affected: lungs, glands and lymph

Preparation and Dosage:

Infusion:	Steep 5 to 15 minutes. 3 oz. frequently
Tincture:	30 to 60 drops (½ to 1 tsp.) frequently
Fluid Extract:	½ to 1 tsp. frequently
Oil:	2 to 3 drops two to three times daily
Powder:	Up to 10 #0 capsules (60 grains) frequently

Indicated Uses:

Internal:

Asthma:	Syrup*, Powder*, Infusion*
Bronchitis:	Syrup*, Powder*, Infusion*
Bruises:	Infusion
Constipation:	Infusion*, Syrup*
Coughs:	Infusion, Syrup
Diarrhea:	Infusion, Syrup
Glands, swollen (lymphatics):	Fluid Extract, Powder, Infusion
Hay fever:	Infusion*, Powder*, Fluid Extract*
Hemorrhage (bowels, lungs):	Infusion*
Sinus Congestion:	Infusion*, Tincture*, Fluid Extract*
Toothaches:	Oil rubbed on gums
Tumors:	Powder*, Fluid Extract*
Whooping cough:	Infusion, Syrup

External

| Diaper rashes: | Poultice, Fomentation |
| Eyes, inflammed: | Poultice, Fomentation |

Skin diseases:	Poultice, Fomentation
Tumors:	Poultice, Fomentation

The oil of mullein is considered one of the best remedies for ear infections. Put two to three drops of the warm oil in the ear overnight or two to three times daily. The dried leaves were smoked to relieve lung congestion by the Indians. Mullein tea is useful for coughs, colds and respiratory diseases. It is good for hemorrhoids, diarrhea, hemorrhages of the lungs and shortness of breath. It is used in kidney formulas to soothe inflammation. Mullein leaves are also used to treat lymphatic congestion.

MYRRH *(Commiphora nayrrha)*

Part Used: gum

Properties: Antiseptic, Emmenagogue; carminative, expectorant, stimulant

Body Parts Affected: stomach and lungs

Preparation and Dosage:

Infusion:	Steep 5 to 15 minutes. 3 oz. three to four times daily
Tincture:	30 to 60 drops (½ to 1 tsp.) three to four times daily
Powder:	2 to 6 #0 capsules (10 to 40 grains) three to four times daily

Indicated Uses:

Internal

Asthma:	Tincture*, Fluid Extract*, Powder*
Bad breath:	Tincture, Fluid Extract, Powder
Boils:	Tincture, Fluid Extract, Powder
Cankers:	Infusion, Tincture, Fluid Extract
Chronic catarrh:	Tincture, Fluid Extract, Powder
Colitis:	Decoction*, Powder*
Coughs:	Decoction*, Powder*
Digestive tonic:	Tincture, Fluid Extract, Powder, Decoction
Gums (bleeding):	Tincture, Fluid Extract, Infusion
Herpes:	Tincture, Fluid Extract*, Powder*
Indigestion:	Tincture, Fluid Extract, Powder, Infusion
Infections:	Tincture*, Fluid Extract*, Powder*, Infusion*, Decoction*
Leukorrhea:	Tincture, Fluid Extract, Powder, Infusion, Decoction
Mouth sores:	Tincture, Fluid Extract, Powder, Infusion
Skin disease:	Tincture*, Fluid Extract*, Powder*, Infusion*
Thrush:	Tincture, Fluid Extract
Ulcers:	Tincture*, Fluid Extract*, Powder*

External

Bad breath:	Gargle
Cankers:	Gargle
Cuts:	Wash, Infusion, Tincture, Fluid Extract
Gums (bleeding):	Gargle
Leukorrhea:	Douche, Infusion, Tincture, Fluid Extract
Mouth sores:	Gargle
Skin disease:	Fomentation
Thrush:	Gargle
Wounds:	Wash, Fomentation, Tincture, Fluid Extract

Myrrh gum is a powerful antiseptic. Goldenseal and myrrh in equal parts used in capsules or tea is a specific for intestinal ulcers, bad breath, catarrh of the intestines and all other mucus membrane conditions. The tincture added to water is an excellent mouth wash for spongy gums, pyorrhea and all throat diseases. Myrrh destroys putrification in the intestines and prevents blood absorption of toxins. It has been successful in treating chronic diarrhea, lung diseases and general body weaknesses. It is a good wash for wounds and skin diseases. Inject the tincture of myrrh in the sinuses for all sinus infections and inflammations. If the sinuses are too sensitive for the straight tincture, dilute it with water. The powder of myrrh can be applied to dry up moist skin conditions. Myrrh is best suited for all pus conditions both internally and externally as well as for mucus membrane problems.

Note: Do not take myrrh gum in large amounts or over a long period of time as it can be toxic.

NETTLES *(Urtica urens)*

Part Used: tops

Properties: Alterative, Nutritive; antiseptic, expectorant, hemostatic

Body Parts Affected: lungs, kidneys, bladder and blood

Preparation and Dosage:

Infusion:	Steep 5 to 15 minutes. 3 oz. frequently
Tincture:	5 to 15 drops frequently
Fluid Extract:	½ to 1 tsp. frequently
Powder:	3 to 10 #0 capsules (20 to 60 grains) frequently
Juice:	1 tsp. as needed

Indicated Uses:

Internal

Asthma:	Juice
Baldness:	Juice, Infusion
Calcium deficiency:	Infusion*, Powder*, Fluid Extract*,
Goiter:	Powdered seeds

Night sweats:	Infusion, Fluid Extract (take cold)
Nutritive:	Powder*, Infusion*
Stomach disorders:	Infusion, Fluid Extract
Urinary tract disorders:	Infusion*, Fluid Extract*

External

Baldness:	Hair rinse, Infusion

Nettles leaves pounded and used as a poultice is good for rheumatic pains. A poultice of nettles and slippery elm will stop bleeding when applied to the skin (use fresh leaves). The tea is good for diarrhea, dysentery, piles, hemorrhoids and gravel in the kidneys. The tea will expel phlegm from the lungs. The tea made from the root will help cure dropsy. The seeds are used in cough medicines. Use nettles as a hair rinse to restore natural color.

Use nettles with comfrey, mullein, horehound and lobelia for lung problems. It is a nutritive herb high in iron, silicon and potassium. It is good to use as a tea for anemia in children. Fresh leaves of nettles may be used in salads. Extract the fresh juice and take one teaspoon every hour to stop intestinal bleeding.

OAT *(Avena sativa)*

Part Used: stem and fruit

Properties: Nervine, Tonic; antispasmodic, stimulant

Body Parts Affected: nerves, uterus, stomach and lungs

Preparation and Dosage:

Infusion:	Steep 5 to 15 minutes. 6 oz. three times daily
Tincture:	30 to 60 drops three times daily
Fluid Extract:	1 tsp. three times daily
Powder:	Up to 10 #0 capsules (60 grains) three times daily

Indicated Uses:

Internal

Bedwetting:	Tincture, Fluid Extract, Infusion, Gruel
Calcium deficiency:	Infusion*, Gruel*
Epilepsy:	Tincture, Fluid Extract
Gout:	Tincture, Fluid Extract, Infusion, Gruel
Gravel (kidneys):	Tincture, Fluid Extract, Gruel
Heart Palpitation:	Tincture, Fluid Extract
Nerve stimulant:	Tincture, Fluid Extract
Nervous diseases:	Tincture, Fluid Extract, Infusion
Occipital headaches:	Tincture, Fluid Extract

Rheumatism:	Tincture, Fluid Extract, Infusion
Sexual neurasthenia:	Tincture, Fluid Extract
Skin diseases:	Tincture, Fluid Extract, Infusion, Gruel
Weak muscles from nerve exhaustion:	Tincture, Fluid Extract, Infusion

External

Skin inflammations:	Poultice, Fomentation

Oats are mainly used as a food for weak, debilitated digestion. It is good to use during gastroenteritis, dyspepsia and ulcers. The tincture and extract is a useful nerve tonic and uterine tonic. Use oat straw tea for kidney and chest ailments. The tea for children is good for bedwetting, colic and stomach problems. Add a gallon of the infusion of the straw to a warm bath for gout, rheumatic problems, lumbago and sore kidneys.

A tincture or extract can be made from fresh oats which should be picked when the milky substance is present in the grain. Its influence is directed to the brain and functions of the body. It is a specific for weak nerves and can be used as a nerve tonic to help recover from disease. It is important to remember that this remedy will help overcome most diseases caused by nervous disorders and exhaustion of all body parts. It is especially effective for ovarian and uterine disorders.

OREGON GRAPE ROOT *(Berberis aquifolium)*

Part Used: root

Properties: Alterative, Antiseptic, Cholagogue; laxative, tonic

Body Parts Affected: liver, stomach, intestines, blood and skin

Preparation and Dosage:

Infusion:	Simmer 10 minutes. 3 oz. three times daily
Decoction:	Steep 10 minutes. 3 oz. three times daily (before meals, made fresh daily)
Tincture:	30 to 60 drops (½ to 1 tsp.) three times daily
Fluid Extract:	½ to 1 tsp. three times daily
Powder:	2 to 5 capsules (15 to 30 grains) several times a day

Indicated Uses:

Internal

Blood purifier:	Tincture, Fluid Extract, Powder
Chronic constipation:	Tincture*, Fluid Extract*, Decoction
Chronic eczema:	Tincture, Fluid Extract
Creates appetite:	Tincture, Fluid Extract, Decoction
Gas:	Tincture, Fluid Extract
Improves absorption:	Tincture, Fluid Extract

Increases strength:	Tincture, Fluid Extract
Jaundice:	Tincture*, Fluid Extract*, Decoction*
Kidney and liver troubles:	Tincture*, Fluid Extract*, Decoction*, Powder*
Leukorrhea:	Tincture, Fluid Extract
Liver stimulant:	Tincture, Fluid Extract
Psoriasis:	Tincture, Fluid Extract
Rheumatism:	Tincture*, Fluid Extract*, Decoction*, Powder*
Skin diseases:	Tincture*, Fluid Extract*, Decoction*, Powder*

External

Leukorrhea:	Douche

Oregon grape root is an excellent blood purifier and is highly recommended in all chronic skin disease such as psoriasis, eczema, herpes and acne. The tincture is the most acceptable method of administering this botanical.

By stimulating the liver and gall bladder, it helps to overcome constipation. It has antiseptic qualities which influence the kidneys and can be used also as a douche. Oregon grape root is very similar to barberry in its action, but it has a stimulating effect on the thyroid gland.

PARSLEY *(Petroselinum sp.)*

Part Used: root, leaves, seeds

Properties: Diuretic; carminative, expectorant, nervine, tonic

Body Parts Affected: kidneys, bladder, stomach, liver and gall bladder

Preparation and Dosage:

Infusion (leaves):	Steep 5 to 15 minutes. 6 oz. two to three times daily
Decoction: (root/seed)	Simmer 5 to 15 minutes. 6 oz. two to three times daily
Tincture:	30 to 60 drops (½ to 1 tsp.) two to three times daily
Fluid Extract:	½ to 1 tsp. two to three times daily
Fresh juice:	2 oz. two times daily
Powder:	2 to 5 #0 capsules (10 to 30 grains) several times daily

Indicated Uses:

Internal

Anemia:	Fresh juice
Arthritis:	Tincture, Fluid Extract, Juice

Asthma:	Decoction*, Infusion*
Bad breath:	Eat raw, Juice, Infusion, Decoction
Bed wetting:	Tincture, Fluid Extract, Infusion, Decoction, Juice
Coughs:	Infusion*, Decoction*
Gall stones:	Infusion*, Decoction*
Gout:	Juice, Infusion, Decoction, Tincture, Fluid Extract
Hay fever:	Infusion*, Decoction
Kidney infections:	Tincture, Fluid Extract, Infusion, Decoction, Juice
Liver congestion:	Tincture, Fluid Extract, Infusion, Decoction, Juice, Eat raw
Low blood pressure:	Juice, Infusion, Eat raw
Lumbago:	Tincture*, Fluid Extract*, Infusion*, Decoction*, Juice
Prostate cleanser:	Tincture, Fluid Extract, Infusion, Decoction, Juice
Spleen (remove obstructions):	Juice, Decoction
Thyroid weakness:	Tincture, Fluid Extract, Infusion, Decoction, Powder, Juice
Water retention:	Tincture, Fluid Extract, Infusion, Decoction, Juice

External

Bites:	Poultice of fresh leaves

Parsley root or leaves is excellent for difficult urination, dropsy, jaundice, stones and obstructions of the liver and spleen. Combined with echinacea, plantain and marshmallow root it is a good remedy for kidney and bladder infections. The fresh juice of the leaves (2 ounces daily in apple juice) is an excellent blood tonic and remedy for anemia. Use the fresh leaves in salads. The root is excellent for jaundice. The seeds contain apiol, which is considered a safe and efficient emmenagogue and is used in amenorrhea and dysmenorrhea. Combine with buchu, cramp bark and black haw for female problems. The high chlorophyll content of the leaves makes this herb an excellent treatment for cancer. Drink the fresh juice daily.

Note: Parsley can be warming and should not be used if kidney inflammation exists.

PASSION FLOWER *(Passifloria incarnata)*

Part Used: plant and flower

Properties: Antispasmodic, Sedative; diaphoretic

Body Parts Affected: nerves and circulation

Preparation and Dosage:

Infusion:	Steep 5 to 15 minutes. 1 cup during the day
Tincture:	15 to 60 drops in water as needed
Fluid Extract:	10 to 20 drops as needed
Powder:	1 to 2 #0 capsules (3 to 10 grains) as needed

Indicated Uses:

Internal

Back tension:	Tincture, Fluid Extract, Infusion
Convulsion:	Tincture, Fluid Extract
Coughs:	Tincture, Fluid Extract, Infusion
Eye tension:	Tincture, Fluid Extract, Infusion
Fevers:	Infusion*
Headaches:	Tincture, Fluid Extract, Infusion
Hiccoughs:	Tincture, Fluid Extract, Infusion
High blood pressure:	Tincture, Fluid Extract
Insomnia:	Tincture, Fluid Extract, Infusion
Muscular twitching:	Tincture, Fluid Extract
Nervous tension:	Tincture, Fluid Extract, Infusion
Reduced pulse during high fevers:	Tincture*, Fluid Extract*, Infusion*
Spasms:	Tincture, Fluid Extract
Stimulates respiration:	Tincture, Fluid Extract, Infusion

External

Rheumatic pains:	Poultice

Passion flower is most commonly used for nervous conditions without pain, such as insomnia, restlessness, hysteria and nervous headaches. It tones the sympathetic nervous system. Passion flower is indicated in childhood nervous problems such as muscle twitching and irritability. In elderly people, it is good for sciatica and nerve debility.

PEACH *(Amygdalus persica)*

Part Used: bark and leaves

Properties: Laxative, Sedative, Stomachic; demulcent, mucilage

Body Parts Affected: stomach, liver, bladder, bowels and nerves

Preparation and Dosage:

Infusion (leaves):	Steep 5 to 15 minutes. 6 oz. three times daily
Decoction (bark):	Simmer 5 to 15 minutes. 1 tsp. to ½ cup at a time
Powder:	2 to 10 #0 capsules (15 to 60 grains) three times daily

Indicated Uses:

Internal

Bladder congestion:	Decoction of bark
Bronchitis:	Decoction of bark
Coughs:	Decoction of bark
Laxative:	Syrup made from the flowers*
Morning sickness:	Infusion of the leaves
Pain during colic:	Tincture of the flowers
Worms:	Infusion or syrup from the leaves
Vomiting:	Infusion, Fluid Extract

Peach tree leaves are laxative and have an excellent sedative effect upon the nervous system. The tea of the leaves is good for stomach problems, dyspepsia, jaundice and can be used to expel worms. It is excellent for bladder problems such as burning urine and urine retention. When the infusion of the leaves is taken hot in small doses, it is good for morning sickness during pregnancy. It has been added to lung remedies to help expectorate mucus.

Note: Avoid large doses in pregnant women as it can cause a purging of the bowels.

PENNYROYAL (AMERICAN) *(Mentha pulegium)*

Part Used: tops

Properties: Diaphoretic, Emmenagogue; carminative, stimulant

Body Parts Affected: circulation, uterus and lungs

Preparation and Dosage:

Infusion:	Steep 5 to 15 minutes. 6 oz. frequently
Tincture:	30 to 60 drops (½ to 1 tsp.) frequently
Fluid Extract:	¼ to 1 tsp. frequently
Oil:	1 to 2 drops frequently
Powder:	3 to 10 #0 capsules (20 to 60 grains) frequently

Indicated Uses:

Internal

Blood purifier:	Fluid Extract, Infusion
Colds:	Infusion
Colic:	Fluid Extract, Infusion
Congestion (lungs):	Infusion*
Convulsions:	Tincture, Fluid Extract
Cramps:	Tincture, Fluid Extract, Infusion
Fever:	Infusion
Headache:	Infusion, Fluid Extract

Itching:	Tincture, Fluid Extract, Infusion
Menstruation (delayed or scanty):	Tincture, Fluid Extract, Infusion
Nausea:	Infusion, Tincture, Fluid Extract
Regulates menstrual flow:	Tincture, Fluid Extract
Skin diseases:	Infusion*, Tincture*, Fluid Extract*
Spasms:	Tincture, Fluid Extract, Infusion

Pennyroyal is used to help break up fevers and for lung infections. The warm infusion used freely will promote perspiration and menstruation. Use hot foot baths of pennyroyal tea to bring on the menstrual flow. Pennyroyal is also good for nervousness, hysteria, cramps, colds and intestinal pains.

The tea is used for an external wash for skin eruptions, rashes and itching.

Note: Do not use pennyroyal when there is excessive menstrual flow. The tea has been used to induce abortions. Pregnant women should not use pennyroyal.

PEPPERMINT *(Mentha piperita)*

Part Used: leaves

Properties: Aromatic, Carminative, Diaphoretic, Stimulant; antispasmodic

Body Parts Affected: stomach, intestines, muscles and circulation

Preparation and Dosage:

Infusion:	Steep 5 to 15 minutes. 6 oz. three times daily
Tincture:	30 to 60 drops three times daily
Fluid Extract:	½ to 2 tsp. three times daily
Oil:	5 to 10 drops three times daily
Powder:	Up to 10 #0 capsules (up to 60 grains) three times daily

Indicated Uses:

Internal

Bronchitis:	Infusion*
Chills:	Oil, Infusion, Fluid Extract
Cholera:	Oil*, Infusion*, Fluid Extract*
Colds:	Infusion
Colic:	Oil, Infusion, Fluid Extract
Colitis:	Infusion*, Powder*
Coughs:	Infusion, Syrup, Oil
Diverticulitis:	Infusion*, Powder*
Dizziness:	Infusion, Oil, Fluid Extract
Fevers:	Infusion, Oil
Gas:	Infusion, Fluid Extract, Oil
Heartburn:	Infusion*, Powder*

Insomnia:	Infusion, Fluid Extract, Oil
Measles:	Oil, Infusion
Menstrual cramps:	Fluid Extract, Infusion, Oil
Migraine headaches:	Oil, Fluid Extract, Infusion
Morning sickness:	Infusion
Muscle spasms:	Fluid Extract, Infusion, Oil
Nausea:	Oil, Fluid Extract, Infusion
Nervous disorders:	Infusion*

External

Local anesthetic to local pains, inflammed joints:	Oil, Liniment
Skin itch:	Oil (2 drops added to two quarts of water and rubbed over affected area
Toothache:	Oil

Peppermint is one of the oldest household remedies. It is excellent for chills, colic, fevers, dizziness, gas, nausea, vomiting, diarrhea, dysentery and hysteria. Peppermint enemas are excellent for colon problems. Peppermint is good for spasms and convulsions in infants. When extremely cold and pale, use a strong peppermint tea. It may be used also for griping pain in the intestines. Do not boil the leaves as they contain extremely volatile medicinal properties.

Peppermint oil (5 to 10 drops poured into two quarts of hot water) breathed in through the mouth and nostrils will open up the sinuses. To do this, boil the water, add the oil, turn stove off, cover the head with a heavy blanket or towel and lean over the pot. Try to keep the steam from leaking out from under the blanket or towel. This is also good for facial steam baths.

PIPSISSEWA (PRINCE'S PINE) *(Chimaphila umbellata)*

Part Used: tops

Properties: Alterative, Diuretic; astringent, tonic

Body Parts Affected: urinary tract, liver, skin and circulation

Preparation and Dosage:

Infusion:	Steep 5 to 15 minutes. 3 oz. as needed
Tincture:	15 to 60 drops as needed
Fluid Extract:	½ to 1 tsp. as needed
Powder:	5 to 10 #0 capsules (30 to 90 grains) as needed

Indicated Uses:

Internal

Arthritis:	Tincture, Fluid Extract

Liver and kidney problems (combine with oregon grape root):	Tincture, Fluid Extract, Decoction, Powder
Rheumatism:	Tincture, Fluid Extract, Infusion
Skin diseases:	Tincture*, Fluid Extract*, Infusion*
Urinary infections:	Tincture, Fluid Extract
Urine retention:	Tincture, Fluid Extract

External:

Painful joints:	Fomentation, Poultice
Skin disease:	Fomentation

Pipsissewa is a good remedy for kidney and bladder problems. When combined with dandelion, goldenseal and yellow dock, it is good for all blood troubles and diseases of the urinary organs. Pipsissewa is excellent when used for burning urine, urethral and prostate irritation, catarrh of the bladder, relaxed bladder and for skin diseases. The tea, one cup three times daily, or tincture, 20 drops three times daily, are sufficient dosages for these conditions.

PLANTAIN *(Plantago major)*

Part Used: leaves and seeds

Properties: Diuretic, Emollient; alterative, antiseptic, astringent, deobstruent, expectorant, vulnerary

Body Parts Affected: kidneys, veins, intestines and skin (external application)

Preparation and Dosage:

Infusion (leaf):	Steep 5 to 15 minutes. 3 oz. three to four times daily
Decoction (seed):	Simmer 1 oz. seeds in 1½ pints water, reduce to 1 pint; sweeten with honey. 1 Tbsp. three to four times daily
Tincture:	2 to 60 drops three to four times daily
Fluid Extract:	½ to 1 tsp. three to four times daily
Powder:	Up to 10 #0 capsules (up to 60 grains) three to four times daily

Indicated Uses:

Internal

Diarrhea:	Infusion of leaves
Hemorrhoids:	Juice, Infusion of leaves*
Jaundice:	Infusion of leaves*, Powdered seeds
Liver obstructions:	Powdered seeds, Infusion of leaves*, Juice
Thrush:	Powdered seeds

External

Leukorrhea:	Douche with infusion of leaves
Thrush:	Gargle
Tumors:	Poultice of leaves
Ulcers:	Poultice of leaves
Wounds:	Poultice of leaves, Fomentation, Tincture

Plantain is used both internally and externally. It has soothing properties which makes it excellent for diarrhea, hemorrhoids, infections, ulcers and bronchitis. Plantain is excellent for acute neuralgia: take two to five drops of tincture every 20 minutes. Culpepper used the seeds for dropsy, epilepsy and yellow jaundice. Plantain is used for kidney and bladder infections. The seeds (similar to psyllium seeds) taken one teaspoon powdered in juice three times a day is an excellent bulk laxative. The seeds soaked overnight in water will produce a gel; bring it to a boil, turn off the heat and let steep for ten minutes. Press the gel through a strainer and use for ulcers, pains in the intestines and spitting up of blood.

İnject the tea (one cup) several times a day in the colon for hemorrhoids. Also use the tea as a douche for vaginal problems. Apply the freshly ground or chewed up leaves to snake and insect bites. Use the salve or fomentation on skin diseases such as eczema, boils and carbuncles. The fresh juice extract applied to the skin is good for itchy skin problems. Take a tablespoon of the fresh juice internally at the same time.

PLEURISY ROOT *(Asclepias tuberosa)*

Part Used: root

Properties: Diaphoretic, Expectorant; antispasmodic, carminative, diuretic, nervine, tonic

Body Parts Affected: lungs, kidneys and nerves

Preparation and Dosage:

Infusion:	Steep 30 minutes. 1 to 2 cups daily; for children 1 to 5 drops in hot water every one to two hours
Decoction	Simmer 5 to 15 minutes. 2 or 3 oz. as needed
Tincture:	30 to 60 drops every three hours
Fluid Extract:	½ to 1 tsp. three to four times daily
Powder:	3 to 5 #0 capsules (20 to 30 grains) three to four times daily

Indicated Uses:

Internal

Asthma:	Infusion, Decoction
Bronchitis:	Infusion, Decoction, Powder

Chicken pox:	Infusion, Decoction
Coughs:	Infusion, Decoction, Syrup
Fevers:	Infusion
Flu:	Infusion
Measles:	Infusion
Pleurisy:	Infusion*, Decoction*
Pneumonia:	Infusion*, Decoction*

Pleurisy root, when given as a hot decoction, is the ideal medicine for pleurisy and pneumonia. In severe cases it is excellent combined with equal parts of the infusion of scullcap given in small doses (2 ounces) every half hour while the patient is in bed and kept warm. The tincture of pleurisy root can be given in hot water for this also. It is an excellent sweating agent to break up colds, fevers, flu and all bronchial problems. It is especially good for stomach and bowel disorders of children exhibited by weakness, mucus discharges and gastric irritability with accompanying nervousness. A good enema for bowel complaints is to use a tablespoon to a quart of boiling water. Let it steep for 30 minutes and use warm.

The tea is good for asthma. A tincture of cayenne (5 to 15 drops) can be added to the tea to overcome chills.

POKE *(Phytolacca americana)*

Part Used: root, fruit

Properties: Alterative, Lymphatic; emetic, laxative

Body Parts Affected: blood, lymph and lungs

Preparation and Dosage:

Infusion (root):	Steep 10 minutes. 1 tsp. at a time, several times daily
Decoction (berries):	Simmer 10 minutes. 1 oz. three to four times daily
Tincture:	2 to 4 drops frequently
Fluid Extract:	½ to 1 tsp. (berries) three times daily; ¼ to ½ tsp. (root) three times daily
Powder:	1 to 2 #0 capsules (1 to 15 grains) three times daily

Indicated Uses:

Internal

Cirrhosis of liver:	Tincture*, Fluid Extract*, Powder
Eczema:	Tincture*, Fluid Extract*, Powder
Emetic (large doses):	Infusion, Decoction, Tincture, Fluid Extract
Enlargements of spleen and thyroid gland:	Tincture, Fluid Extract
Laxtive:	Tincture*, Fluid Extract*, Decoction*
Lymphatic congestion:	Tincture, Fluid Extract

Skin diseases:	Tincture, Fluid Extract
External	
Goiter:	Oil, Poultice, Salve
Skin diseases:	Poultice, Fomentation, Salve
Swollen breasts:	Fomentation, Oil, Poultice, Salve

Poke in large doses acts as an emetic and purgative, but is not recommended for these purposes. It is usually used in small doses as a blood and lymphatic cleanser and is combined with herbs such as red clover, yellow dock, echinacea and sassafras. It is good when used during rheumatism, tonsillitis, mumps, lymphatic swelling, breast tumors and laryngitis. In such cases, three parts of the decoction and one part vegetable glycerine taken in doses of one teaspoon three times daily is sufficient. Poke root is good for enlargement of the liver, spleen and thyroid glands.

Externally, it is added to salves for skin diseases such as scabies, eczema and infections. The decoction can also be used as a fomentation for these. It is a good poultice for breast tumors and caked breasts. Grind the root into a powder and mix with slippery elm and water and apply to the swellings. Keep this on all day and moisten when it becomes dry. This poultice should be changed every third day.

Note: Poke root contains toxic substances and it should not be used in excess of one gram a day. Toxic effects have been noticed while using poke root both internally and externally. Although it is an excellent herb, it should be used with caution.

PRICKLY ASH *(Xanthoxylum americanum)*

Part Used: bark

Properties: Stimulant; alterative, antispasmodic/astringent, emmenagogue, rubefacient

Body Parts Affected: blood, circulation and stomach

Preparation and Dosage:

Decoction:	Simmer 5 to 15 minutes. 1 to 2 oz. three to four times daily
Tincture:	5 to 20 drops three to four times daily
Fluid Extract:	½ to 1 tsp. three to four times daily
Powder:	2 to 5 #0 capsules (10 to 30 grains) three to four times daily

Indicated Uses:

Internal:

Asthma:	Powder*, Decoction*, Fluid Extract*
Cardiac stimulant:	Fluid Extract
Chronic rheumatism:	Fluid Extract*, Decoction*, Powder

Cold extremities:	Fluid Extract, Decoction
Colic:	Fluid Extract, Decoction,Powder
Dropsy:	Fluid Extract, Decoction
Flatulence:	Fluid Extract, Decoction, Powder
General stimulant:	Fluid Extract
Heart tonic:	Fluid Extract, Decoction
Indigestion:	Fluid Extract of the berries
Nerve stimulant:	Fluid Extract, Decoction, Powder
Skin diseases:	Fluid Extract*, Decoction*
Sluggish circulation:	Fluid Extract, Decoction

External

Wounds:	Use powdered bark as a poultice

Prickly ash bark is excellent when used to increase circulation and to produce warmth during chills. It is good for colds, rheumatism, poor digestion, weakness and arthritis. It is a good blood purifier for deposits in the joints. Add this herb to carminatives when there is colic, gas and weak digestion.

A decoction is excellent for cold extremities and acute ailments. When using as a diaphoretic, note that if excessive sweating manifests, cut the dosage down by 25% until the amount taken does not produce perspiration. The boiled fresh bark is a good wash for itchy skin. This herb is good to add to remedies when trying to break fevers. I have seen this herb bring on sweat when all else has failed.

PSYLLIUM *(Plantago psyllium)*

Part Used: seeds

Properties: Demulcent, Laxative

Body Parts Affected: bowels and intestines

Preparation and Dosage:

Infusion:	Steep 5 to 15 minutes. 2 to 4 tsp. after each meal; children, 1 tsp. after each meal
Powder·	1 trsp. in warm water or juice, three times daily
Powder:	6 to 8 #0 capsules (50 to 60 grains) three times daily

Indicated Uses:

Internal

Colitis:	Decoction, Powder, Soaked seeds or powder
Constipation:	Decoction, Soaked seeds or powder
Hemorrhoids:	Decoction, Soaked seeds or powder
Inflammed intestines:	Decoction, Soaked seeds or powder
Ulcers:	Decoction

Psyllium powder or the soaked seed will assist easy evacuation by increasing water content in the colon during colitis, ulcers and hemorrhoids. A teaspoon of the powder taken in warm water or juice three times a day will clean the intestine, removing putrefactive toxins. For children, the dose is one-half teaspoon.

Psyllium seed powder is added to poultices and unleavened bread which serves the purpose as a binder. Add a small amount while pouring water over the ingredients and stir until it becomes thick, similar to dough. Psyllium will draw out pus from boils, carbuncles and sores when used as a drawing agent in external application.

RASPBERRY *(Rubus idaeus)*

Part Used: leaf

Properties: Antispasmodic, Astringent; alterative, stimulant, tonic

Body Parts Affected: stomach, liver, blood, genitourinary system and muscles

Preparation and Dosage:

Infusion:	Steep 5 to 15 minutes. 6 oz. frequently
Tincture:	30 drops (½ to 1 tsp.) frequently
Fluid Extract:	1 to 2 tsp. frequently
Powder:	5 to 10 #0 capsules (30 to 60 grains) frequently

Indicated Uses:

Internal

Cankers:	Infusion, Tincture, Fluid Extract
Bowel tonic:	Cold infusion
Before childbirth:	Infusion, Tincture, Fluid Extract
Colds:	Infusion*
Coughs:	Infusion*, Syrup*
Diarrhea:	Infusion
Dysentery:	Infusion*, Tincture*, Fluid Extract*
Measles:	Infusion
Morning sickness:	Infusion
Mouth sores:	Infusion, Tincture, Fluid Extract
Ulcers:	Infusion*, Syrup*

External

Cankers:	Gargle
Eyewash:	Infusion
Leukorrhea:	Douche
Mouth sores:	Gargle
Wounds and burns:	Poultice of leaves mixed with slippery elm

Red raspberry is a mild, pleasant, stimulating, astringent tonic to the mucus membranes. It is splendid in the relief of urinary irritation, soothing the kidneys and the whole urinary tract. As a douche or an enema for dysentery, combine it with myrrh or goldenseal in equal parts. It will stop uterine hemorrhages.

Raspberry leaf tea is excellent to drink during pregnancy for relieving cramps and pain, morning sickness (good combined with peppermint), and an aid to ease in childbirth.

For relief of kidney infection, chronic dysentery and hemorrhages:

Tincture of witch hazel	25 drops
Tincture of goldenseal	12 drops
Tincture of raspberry	10 drops

Mix these together in two cups of water and take one tablespoon (adult dosage) as frequently as needed. This is also an excellent gargle for throat diseases.

RED CLOVER *(Trifolium pratense)*

Part Used: flowering tops

Properties: Alterative; nutritive, sedative, stimulant

Body Parts Affected: nerves, lungs, blood, liver and lymph

Preparation and Dosage:

Infusion:	Steep 30 minutes. 1 to 2 oz. frequently; or 4 to 6 cups daily
Tincture:	5 to 30 drops frequently
Fluid Extract:	1 tsp. frequently
Powder:	5 to 10 #0 capsules (30 to 60 grains) frequently

Indicated Uses:

Internal

Blood purifier:	Tincture, Fluid Extract, Infusion, Powder
Cancer:	Tincture*, Fluid Extract*, Infusion*, Powder*
Psoriasis:	Tincture, Fluid Extract, Infusion, Powder
Rheumatism:	Tincture*, Fluid Extract*, Infusion*, Powder*
Skin diseases:	Tincture, Fluid Extract, Infusion, Powder
Whooping cough:	Infusion

External

Cancerous growths:	Fomentation, Poultice

This herb is an excellent blood purifier when used alone or in combination with yellow dock, dandelion root, sassafras or other blood purifiers. It is a powerful remedy for cancerous growth. It is soothing to the nerves and is good for whooping cough and stomach problems. Red clover can be used in salves for all skin afflictions.

Use the tea as a gargle for all throat swellings and infections. Inject the tea into the bowel and uterus and retain for a few minutes for problems in those areas.

RHUBARB *(Rheum palmatum)*

Part Used: root

Properties: Astringent, Laxative, Stomachic; alterative, sialagogue

Body Parts Affected: stomach and intestines

Preparation and Dosage:

Decoction (root):	Simmer 5 to 15 minutes. 3 oz. three times daily
Tincture:	30 to 60 drops (½ to 1 tsp.) three times daily
Fluid Extract:	¼ tsp. three times daily
Powder:	1 to 2 #0 capsules (5 to 10 grains) (stomachic) three times daily
Powder:	3 to 5 #0 capsules (20 to 30 grains) (purgative) four times daily
Syrup:	1 tsp. as needed

Indicated Uses:

Internal

Constipation:	Tincture, Powder, Fluid Extract
Diarrhea:	Tincture, Powder, Fluid Extract
Dyspepsia:	Tincture, Powder, Syrup, Fluid Extract
Jaundice:	Tincture*, Powder*
Infantile digestion:	Tincture, Powder, Syrup, Fluid Extract
Worms:	Syrup*

Rhubarb is both laxative and astringent. Its dual properties make it a good herb for both diarrhea and constipation. It stimulates the walls of the colon and the secretory glands of the stomach and intestines. In small amounts, rhubarb is an excellent digestive tonic. Judge the amount on your own. 30 grains given every 2 or 3 hours has stopped diarrhea and hemorrhages in adults. Larger amounts will produce a laxative effect. If you do not desire a laxative effect, cut back on the dosage and it will act as a good tonic and blood cleanser. Finley Ellingwood, M.D. states in the American Materia Medica, "it is the laxative for debilitated patients, or for patients recovering from prostrating disease. Given to a nursing mother, like aloe, it relaxes the infant's bowels, and in some cases it is desirable to administer it to the mother for this purpose."

Rhubarb is used to treat chronic blood diseases. The dosage for a general digestive tonic and blood cleanser is one teaspoon of the tincture three times daily or one to three capsules three times daily.

Note: Do not use over prolonged periods as it tends to aggravate any tendency toward chronic constipation. Do not use during pregnancy.

ROSE *(Rosa spp.)*

Part Used: fruit, petals, buds

Properties: Nutritive, Stomachic; aperient, astringent

Body Parts Affected: heart, nerves and blood

Preparation and Dosage:

Infusion:	Steep 5 to 15 minutes. 1 cup at a time frequently
Decoction:	Simmer 5 to 15 minutres. 3 oz. three times daily
Powder:	5 to 10 #0 capsules (30 to 60 grains) frequently

Indicated Uses:

Internal

Circulation:	Tincture, Fluid Extract, Infusion
Colds:	Infusion
Intestinal putrification:	Syrup
Jaundice:	Syrup*, Infusion*
Sore throats:	Syrup
Ulcerated mouth:	Syrup
Vitamin C deficiency:	Infusion*, Syrup

The common red garden rose has long been a favorite medicine. It is a good vitamin C supplement and will ease cramps. The vitamin C content makes it a good remedy to combat colds and influenza. An infusion of the petals is used for headaches, dizziness and as a blood purifier. Use fresh rose hips for vitamin C, as the dried ones contain relatively little of this vitamin. Five to ten flowers or buds steeped in hot water for twenty minutes and taken as needed is a good treatment for diarrhea.

Euell Gibbons said, "There is hardly any other food that is comparable with rose hips in vitamin C content. We think of oranges as rich in this vitamin, but a single cup of pared rose hips may contain as much vitamin C as ten to twelve dozen oranges."

ROSEMARY *(Rosarinus officinalis)*

Part Used: leaves, flowers

Properties: Aromatic, Carminative, Diaphoretic, Stimulant; astringent

Body Parts Affected: stomach, intestines, liver, nerves and lungs

Preparation and Dosage:

Infusion:	Steep 5 to 15 minutes. 2 oz. three times daily
Tincture:	5 to 20 drops three times daily
Oil:	½ to 3 drops three times daily
Powder:	5 to 15 #0 capsules (30 to 60 grains) three times daily

Indicated Uses:

Internal

Colds:	Infusion
Digestive tonic:	Infusion, Fluid Extract
Gas:	Fluid Extract, Infusion
Migraine headaches:	Infusion, Oil
Nervousness:	Infusion
Prostate congestion:	Fluid Extract*, Infusion*, Powder*

External

Baldness:	Hair rinse with the infusion
Joint pains and sore muscles:	Liniment
Migraine headaches:	Rub diluted oil (1 part rosemary with 10 parts vegetable oil) on forehead and temples. Also use as a nasal vapor bath.

The tea is good for gas, colic, indigestion, nausea and fevers. It will promote liver function, the production of bile and improve circulation and digestion. It will raise the blood pressure. The oil added to liniments and salves is good for rheumatism, eczema, arthritis and wounds. The tea is a good hair rinse and makes a useful mouthwash for halitosis.

Note: Do not drink rosemary tea in excessive amounts. Three cups daily seems to be the limit in most cases.

RUE *(Ruta graveolens)*

Part Used: herb, leaves

Properties: Antispasmodic, Emmenagogue; rubefacient, stimulant

Body Parts Affected: nerves, tendons, circulation and uterus

Preparation and Dosage:

Infusion:	Steep 5 to 15 minutes. 2 oz. three times daily between meals
Tincture:	5 to 20 drops three times daily
Fluid Extract:	½ to 1 tsp. three times daily
Oil:	1 to 5 drops three times daily
Powder:	2 to 5 #0 capsules (10 to 30 grains) three times daily

Indicated Uses:

Internal

Bowel pains:	Infusion*, Fluid Extract*
Cramps:	Infusion, Fluid Extract
Dizziness:	Infusion
Headaches:	Infusion
Hysteria:	Infusion, Fluid Extract
Nervousness:	Infusion
Uterus congestion:	Infusion*

External

Headache:	Poultice (fresh leaves)
Sciatica:	Poultice (fresh leaves)

Rue is an excellent remedy for stomach problems, cramps in the bowel, nervousness, hysteria , spasms, dizziness and congestion in the female organs. The warm infusion is usually used for the above problems.

It is a good herb to add to cough medicines, especially when accompanied with poor digestion and gas.

Externally, the fresh, bruised herb is an irritant (rubefacient) used for sciatica. To relieve headache, a poultice is placed on the forehead. It is best to first rub a vegetable oil in the body part where the poultice is placed.

SAFFLOWER *(Carthamus tinctorious)*

Part Used: flowers

Properties: Diaphoretic; emmenagogue, laxative

Body Parts Affected: skin, kidneys and nerves

Preparation and Dosage:

Infusion:	Steep 5 to 15 minutes. 6 oz. two times daily
Tincture:	5 to 20 drops two times daily
Fluid Extract:	5 to 20 drops two times daily
Powder:	5 to 10 #0 capsules (30 to 60 grains) two times daily

Indicated Uses:

Internal

Arthritis:	Powder*, Infusion*, Fluid Extract*
Bronchitis:	Infusion*
Fevers:	Infusion
Gas:	Infusion, Fluid Extract
Heartburn:	Infusion*
Measles:	Infusion

Psoriasis: Infusion*, Fluid Extract*, Powder*
Uric acid: Fluid Extract*, Infusion*, Tincture*

The tea taken hot will produce perspiration and is used during colds, flu and fevers. It is very soothing to the nerves in cases of hysteria and associated with anemia.

When the flowers are stored for any length of time, oxygen combined with the volatile properties produces a sugarlike compound which induces the adrenal glands to produce more adrenalin and the pancreas to produce more insulin, although this herb is not a specific for pancreatic disease.

SAGE *(Salvia officinalis)*

Part Used: leaves

Properties: Antispasmodic, Astringent; anthelmintic, aromatic, vulnerary

Body Parts Affected: bowels, sinuses, bladder, mucus membranes and nerves

Preparation and Dosage:

Infusion (leaves):	Steep 5 to 15 minutes. 1 Tbsp. as needed or 1 to 2 cups daily, hot or cold
Tincture:	20 to 60 drops three to four times daily
Fluid Extract:	¼ to 1 tsp. three to four times daily
Powder:	2 to 5 #0 capsules (10 to 30 grains) three to four times daily

Indicated Uses:

Internal

Blood purifier:	Infusion
Bronchitis:	Infusion*
Dizziness:	Infusion
Gas:	Infusion
Headache:	Infusion
Head colds:	Infusion
Inflammed throat and tonsils:	Infusion
Lactation (to reduce):	Infusion (drink at body temperature)
Laryngitis:	Infusion, Oil
Liver complaints:	Infusion
Morning sickness:	Infusion
Mucus in respirtory tract:	Oil (1 to 3 drops), Infusion
Nausea:	Infusion
Nervous fevers:	Infusion
Night sweats:	Infusion
Tonsillitis:	Infusion
Weak digestion:	Infusion
Ulcers:	Infusion*, Syrup*

External

Inflammed throat and tonsils:	Gargle
Laryngitis:	Gargle
Rheumatic pains:	Oil, Liniment
Tonsillitis:	Gargle
Wounds:	Wash with the infusion

Sage tea is an excellent gargle when combined with freshly squeezed lemon juice and honey for all mouth diseases. Good for stomach troubles, diarrhea, gas, dysentery, colds and flu. It will expel worms in children and adults. Externally, it is a good wash for wounds that are slow to heal. It makes an excellent hair rinse to stimulate hair growth and it will remove dandruff. For fevers, clean the bowels with an enema and drink the hot tea while in bed.

Because of its astringent qualities, it is used alone for excessive night sweats and perspiration. The tea taken cold will cause the breast milk to cease during weaning. Sage can be combined with equal parts peppermint, rosemary and wood betony for an excellent headache remedy. Sage will decrease secretions of the lungs, sinuses, throat and mucus membranes.

SARSAPARILLA *(Smilax ornata)*

Part Used: root

Properties: Alterative, Carminative, Tonic; diaphoretic

Body Parts Affected: blood, skin, circulation and intestines

Preparation and Dosage:

Decoction:	Simmer 15 to 30 minutes. 3 oz. three times daily
Tincture:	5 to 15 drops three times daily
Fluid Extract:	2 to 4 tsp. three times daily
Powder:	5 to 10 #0 capsules (30 to 60 grains) three times daily

Indicated Uses:

Internal

Acne:	Fluid Extract, Tincture, Powder, Decoction
Blood purifier:	Fluid Extract, Tincture, Powder, Decoction
Boils:	Fluid Extract, Tincture, Powder, Decoction
Colds:	Decoction*
Fevers:	Decoction*
Heartburn:	Decoction*
Hot flashes:	Fluid Extract*, Tincture*, Powder*, Decoction
Rheumatism:	Fluid Extract, Tincture, Powder, Decoction
Uric acid (excessive):	Fluid Extract*, Decoction*, Powder*

External

Ringworm:	Fomentation
Sores and wounds:	Wash with the decoction

Sarsaparilla is useful for skin eruptions, ringworm, rheumatism, arthritis and gout. It contains a hormone like substance which makes it good in glandular formulas. The tea will increase the flow of urine, break up gas, and taken hot it is a good diaphoretic for fevers. It is also a good eyewash. It is one of the best herbs to use for infants infected with venereal disease. Combine sarsaparilla with yellow dock and sassafras for a spring tonic. Pustules and sores may be washed with a tea made from the root.

SASSAFRAS *(Sassafras officinale)*

Part Used: root bark

Properties: Alterative, Aromatic, Carminative, Diaphoretic; diuretic, stimulant

Body Parts Affected: blood, skin, circulation and intestines

Preparation and Dosage:

Decoction:	Simmer 5 to 15 minutes. 3 oz. three to four times daily
Tincture:	15 to 30 drops three to four times daily
Fluid Extract:	¼ to 1 tsp. three to four times daily
Powder:	5 to 10 #0 capsules (30 to 60 grains) three to four times daily

Indicated Uses:

Internal

Acne:	Decoction*, Fluid Extract*
Blood purifier:	Decoction*, Fluid Extract*
Boils:	Decoction*, Fluid Extract*
Colic:	Fluid Extract, Decoction
Cramps:	Fluid Extract*, Decoction*
Rheumatism:	Decoction*, Fluid Extract*, Powder*
Stomach cramps:	Decoction, Fluid Extract

External

Disinfectant:	Oil
Rheumatic pains:	Oil, Liniment

Sassafras is a spring tonic. It will thin the blood after a heavy winter. It stimulates and cleans the liver of toxins. Given during painful mentstruation, it will relieve the suffering and is effective in afterpains from childbirth. Sassafras is usually combined with other alterative herbs when used to purify the blood.

The oil of sassafras will relieve toothaches and used externally, it is good for rheumatic pains.

Note: People with anemia or thin blood should not use sassafras. The oil is toxic and should not be taken internally.

SAW PALMETTO *(Serenoa serrulata)*

Part Used: fruit

Properties: Diuretic, Tonic; antiseptic, sedative

Body Parts Affected: lungs, throat, reproductive organs and kidneys

Preparation and Dosage:

Infusion:	Steep 5 to 15 minutes. 6 oz. two to three times daily
Tincture:	15 to 60 drops two to three times daily
Fluid Extract:	10 drops two to three times daily
Powder:	2 to 4 #0 capsules (10 to 20 grains) two to three times daily

Indicated Uses:

Internal

Asthma:	Fluid Extract*, Powder*, Decoction*
Bronchitis:	Decoction*, Powder*
Colds:	Decoction*
Dysmenorrhea:	Fluid Extract*, Powder*, Decoction*
Enlarged prostate:	Fluid Extract, Tincture, Decoction
Frigidity:	Fluid Extract, Decoction, Tincture
Impotence in young men:	Tincture, Fluid Extract, Powder
Nerve tonic:	Tincture, Fluid Extract, Powder, Decoction
Ovarian enlargement:	Tincture, Fluid Extract, Powder
Sexual neurasthenia:	Tincture (combine with tincture of oats "avena sativa"), Fluid Extract
Sinus and respiratory problems:	Decoction, Tincture, Fluid Extract, Powder
Sterility:	Tincture, Fluid Extract, Powder

Saw palmetto berries improve the digestion and increase weight and strength. This herb is a useful agent in all throat diseases, colds, bronchitis, whooping cough and head and nose congestion. It is a sexual stimulant and valuable in treating diseases of the reproductive organs, ovaries, prostate and testes. When recovering from diseases of the glands, it is an especially good tonic and will speed recovery.

SCULLCAP *(Scutellaria spp.)*

Part Used: tops

Properties: Antispasmodic, Nervine; antipyretic

Body Parts Affected: nerves and stomach

Preparation and Dosage:

Infusion:	Steep 15 to 30 minutes. 3 oz. four to five times daily
Tincture:	10 to 40 drops three to four times daily
Fluid Extract:	¼ tsp. three to four times daily
Powder:	3 to 5 capsules (15 to 30 grains) two or three or more times daily

Indicated Uses:

Internal

Alcoholism:	Infusion*, Powder*
Convulsions:	Tincture, Fluid Extract
Coughs:	Infusion*, Tincture*, Fluid Extract*
Epilepsy:	Tincture, Fluid Extract
Hysteria:	Tincture, Fluid Extract
Indigestion:	Tincture, Fluid Extract, Infusion
Insanity:	Tincture, Fluid Extract, Powder
Insomnia:	Tincture, Fluid Extract, Infusion
Nervous tension:	Tincture, Fluid Extract, Infusion
Nervous headache:	Tincture, Fluid Extract, Infusion

Scullcap is an excellent herb for almost any nervous system malfunction, mild or chronic, from insomnia to hysteria. It has been used as an aid in weaning individuals from barbiturate addictions and excessive use of valium. In combination with American ginseng (¼ ounce), scullcap (½ ounce), taken in small frequent doses, it is a good treatment for alcoholism. Make the decoction of ginseng root, then an infusion of scullcap and combine the two.

Scullcap has been used as a substitute for quinine for pains of ovarian or uterine origin. Combined with pennyroyal and crampbark, the tea is good for excessive sexual desires. Its action is through the cerebrospinal centers, calming the heart and hysterical excitement. The hot tea is good to break fevers when nervousness is present. Scullcap is a sedative and nerve tonic. It should be used as fresh as possible, since much of its activity is lost with prolonged storage.

SENNA *(Cassia acutipolia)*

Part Used: leaves, pods

Properties: Laxative, Vermifuge; diuretic

Body Parts Affected: intestines

Preparation and Dosage:

Infusion:	Steep 30 minutes. 2 oz. three times daily

Tincture:	30 to 40 drops two to three times daily
Fluid Extract:	½ tsp. two to three times daily
Powder	2 to 10 #0 capsules (10 to 60 grains) two to three times daily

Indicated Uses:

Internal

Jaundice:	Infusion*, Powder*
Laxative:	Fluid Extract, Infusion, Powder
Parasites:	Infusion*, Powder*
Purgative:	Fluid Extract, Infusion

Senna is an effective laxative and should be modified by combining it with an aromatic herb such as ginger, anise, fennel or coriander to avoid griping (cramping). The pods are milder than the leaves. Use 6 to 12 pods for adults and 3 to 6 pods for children. Make an infusion and drink cold. Use an ounce of senna to one pint of water; add 10% of an aromatic herb. Steep for 20 minutes. Drink the infusion cold. It seems to gripe less when taken cool.

Note: Senna should not be used when there is inflammation anywhere in the intestinal tract, piles, prolapsed intestines or rectum and it should not be used during pregnancy.

SHEPHERD'S PURSE *(Capsella bursa-pastorial)*

Part Used: tops

Properties: Astringent, Diuretic; stimulant

Body Parts Affected: kidneys, bladder and blood

Preparation and Dosage:

Infusion:	Steep 30 minutes. 6 oz. one to two times daily
Tincture:	20 to 60 drops one to two times daily
Fluid Extract:	¼ to ½ tsp. one to two times daily
Powder:	2 to 10 #0 capsules (15 to 60 grains) one to two times daily

Indicated Uses:

Internal

Bowels (bleeding):	Tincture, Fluid Extract, Infusion
Blood in urine (hematuria):	Tincture, Fluid Extract, Infusion
Chronic menorrhagia:	Tincture*, Fluid Extract*, Infusion*
Dysentery:	Tincture, Fluid Extract, Infusion
Gastric hemorrhage:	Tincture, Fluid Extract, Infusion
Hemorrhoids:	Tincture, Fluid Extract, Infusion

Lungs (bleeding):	Tincture*, Fluid Extract*, Infusion
Uterine bleeding:	Tincture, Fluid Extract, Infusion

External

Rheumatic joint pains:	Poultice
Wounds:	Salve

Shepherd's purse is an excellent astringent which will stop bleeding of the lungs, colon, kidneys and bladder; the tops should be used fresh for this purpose. It is good for excessive menstrual bleeding and bedwetting. This herb is excellent for intermittent fevers, piles and hemorrhoids. I have seen it stop diarrhea when nothing else would.

Culpepper says, "The juice being dropped into the ears, heals the pains, noise and muttering. A good ointment may be made of it for all wounds, especially wounds on the head."

SLIPPERY ELM *(Ulmus fulva)*

Part Used: inner bark

Properties: Demulcent, Emollient, Nutritive; astringent

Body Parts Affected: general effects on the whole body

Preparation and Dosage:

Infusion (powder):	Slowly pour 1 pint of boiling water over 1 oz. powdered bark, stirring constantly. Simmer 5 to 15 minutes. 6 oz. three to four times daily
Decoction (whole bark):	Simmer 5 to 15 minutes. 3 oz. three to four times daily
Tincture:	15 to 30 drops three to four times daily
Fluid Extract:	½ to 1 tsp. three to four times daily
Gruel:	Mix 1 tsp. powder with sufficient cold water to make a thin and very smooth paste. Stirring steadily, pour 1 pint of boiling water onto the paste. Flavor with honey, lemon rind, cinnamon, cloves, nutmeg or other spices. ½ to 1 pint (warm) one to three times daily
Syrup:	1 Tbsp. as needed
Powder:	5 to 10 #0 capsules (30 to 60 grains) three to four times daily

Indicated Uses:

Internal

Bladder inflammation:	Decoction*
Bronchitis:	Decoction, Syrup

Colitis:	Decoction, Gruel
Constipation:	Decoction*, Syrup*, Gruel
Cramps (ovarian):	Decoction*, Syrup*
Coughs:	Syrup, Decoction
Cystitis:	Decoction*
Diarrhea:	Gruel
Diverticulitis:	Decoction*
Dysentery:	Decoction*
Eczema:	Decoction*, Powder*
Flu:	Decoction*
Gas:	Decoction, Syrup
Hemorrhage:	Decoction*, Powder*, Syrup*
Hemorrhoids:	Decoction*, Gruel
Hoarseness:	Syrup
Lung congestion:	Syrup, Decoction
Stomach problems:	Decoction, Gruel
Tonsillitis:	Syrup*, Decoction, Throat lozenges
Ulcers:	Decoction, Gruel

External

Burns:	Poultice
Colitis:	Enema
Constipation:	Enema
Diverticulitis:	Enema
Dysentery:	Enema
Gangrenous wounds:	Poultice (combine with wormwood and charcoal)
Hemorrhoids:	Enema
Leukorrhea:	Douche
Open sores:	Poultice
Rheumatic and gouty afflictions:	Poultice of bran, apple cider vinegar and slippery elm. Mix into a paste and apply
Wounds:	Poultice

Slippery elm used as a gruel is nourishing for children and the elderly with weak stomachs, ulcers and those recovering from diseases. It will relieve constipation and diarrhea. Slippery elm tea is good for coughs and bronchitis when added to cough medicines.

Slippery elm is also used to bind the materials of suppositories, boluses, lozenges and unleavened breads together.

Externally, use it as a poultice applied to sores, wounds, burns, open sores and infected skin problem areas. It is a good addition to douches and enemas when there is inflammation and burning. If used as a douche or enema, it will need to be diluted with water so it will not plug the apparatus as it is a mucilaginous herb.

SPEARMINT *(Mentha viridus)*

Part Used: leaves

Properties: Aromatic, Carminative, Diaphoretic, Stimulant; antispasmodic, diuretic

Body Parts Affected: stomach, intestines, muscles and circulation

Preparation and Dosage:

Infusion:	Steep 5 to 15 minutes. 6 oz. three to four times daily
Tincture:	½ to 1 tsp. three to four times daily
Fluid Extract:	¼ to ½ tsp. three to four times daily
Powder:	5 to 10 #0 capsules (30 to 60 grains) three to four times daily

Indicated Uses:

Internal

Colds:·	Infusion*
Cramps:	Infusion, Oil*
Fevers:	Infusion
Flu:	Infusion*
Gas:	Infusion, Gas
Indigestion:	Infusion, Oil
Spasms:	Infusion*, Oil*

Spearmint is non-toxic and is soothing to the stomach with mild diuretic and diaphoretic properties. Its main uses are during colds, flu, indigestion, gas, cramps and slight spasms. Use spearmint in bitter herb combinations to give flavor. Spearmint with horehound or elder flowers is used to break fevers in children. This herb is excellent when used as an enema for restlessness. It is also good when used to stop vomiting. When combined with pleurisy root and scullcap, it is a good remedy for pleurisy and pneumonia. Do not boil the herb as the medicinal volatile oil will be steamed off.

SQUAW VINE *(Mitchella repens)*

Part Used: whole plant

Properties: Emmenagogue; astringent, diuretic

Body Parts Affected: uterus, bladder and colon

Preparation and Dosage:

Infusion:	Steep 5 to 15 minutes. 3 oz. three to four times daily
Tincture:	15 to 60 drops three to four times daily
Fluid Extract:	½ to 1 tsp. three to four times daily
Powder:	5 to 10 #0 capsules (30 to 60 grains) three to four times daily

Indicated Uses:

Internal

Childbirth (for cramping and pains before and during labor):	Tincture, Fluid Extract, Decoction
Congestion and pelvic organs:	Tincture, Fluid Extract, Decoction
Gravel and urinary irritation:	Tincture, Fluid Extract, Decoction
Leukorrhea:	Tincture, Fluid Extract, Decoction
Painful menstruation:	Tincture, Fluid Extract, Decoction
Uterine and ovarian pains:	Tincture, Fluid Extract, Decoction

The American Indian women used squaw vine as a tea or infusion all during pregnancy to assure the proper development of the child and render the delivery safe and easy, and to help develop proper lactation. It is a uterine tonic and will relieve congestion of the uterus and ovaries. It is excellent for absent or painful mentstruation. The berries, crushed and added to a tincture of myrrh, allowed to steep for three days and strained iş a good fomentation for sore nipples. It is good combined with raspberry leaf when used during pregnancy.

Squaw vine combined with witch hazel leaves makes an excellent injection for leukorrhea, dystenery and bleeding piles. This herb is a good diuretic and can be used for gravel, kidney and bladder complaints.

ST. JOHN'S WORT *(Hypericum perforatum)*

Part Used: tops

Properties: Astringent; alterative, aromatic, diuretic, nervine, sedative

Body Parts Affected: stomach, bladder, blood, liver and nerves

Preparation and Dosage:

Infusion:	Steep 5 to 15 minutes. 1 oz. as needed, up to 1 cup during the day
Tincture:	10 to 20 drops as needed
Fluid Extract:	½ to 1 tsp. as needed
Powder:	5 to 10 #0 capsules (30 to 60 grains) as needed

Indicated Uses:

Internal

Afterbirth pains:	Tincture, Fluid Extract
Bedwetting:	Tincture, Fluid Extract
Blood purifier:	Tincture, Fluid Extract

Coughs:	Infusion*
Hysteria:	Tincture, Fluid Extract
Irregular menstruation:	Infusion*, Tincture, Fluid Extract, Powder*
Lung problems (expectorant):	Infusion
Muscular bruises and pains:	Tincture, Fluid Extract
Spine (tenderness and pains):	Tincture, Fluid Extract
Uterine disorders:	Infusion*, Tincture, Fluid Extract, Powder*

External

Breast tumors:	Oil, Salve, Fomentation
Bruises:	Oil, Salve, Fomentation
Enlarged glands:	Oil, Salve, Fomentation
Swellings:	Oil, Salve, Fomentation

The tea is a good blood purifier and is used for boils, uterine pain, suppressed urine, diarrhea, dysentery and jaundice. A small amount of aloe powder added to the tea will strongly influence the liver. The tea can be taken for uterine cramping, insomnia, bedwetting and other nervous conditions.

The extracted oil makes a good external application for burns, wounds, bruises and other sensitive skin problems. Steep the flowers in olive oil for two weeks, strain and apply topically for swollen breasts, hard tumors, wounds, ulcers and burns.

STONEROOT *(Collinsonia canadensis)*

Part Used: root

Properties: Astringent; diuretic, hepatic

Body Parts Affected: veins, liver and colon

Preparation and Dosage:

Decoction:	Simmer 5 to 15 minutes. 1 Tbsp. three times daily; or up to 1 cup during the day
Tincture:	30 to 60 drops three times daily
Fluid Extract:	¼ to 1 tsp. three times daily
Powder:	2 #0 capsules (5 grains) three times daily

Indicated Uses:

Internal

Bladder stones:	Tincture, Fluid Extract, Decoction
Diarrhea:	Tincture, Fluid Extract, Decoction
Digestive tonic:	Tincture, Fluid Extract, Decoction
Dysentery:	Tincture, Fluid Extract, Decoction
Heart tonic:	Tincture, Fluid Extract, Decoction, Powder

Hemorrhoids:	Tincture, Fluid Extract, Decoction, Powder
Increases appetite:	Tincture, Fluid Extract, Decoction, Powder
Laryngitis:	Tincture, Fluid Extract, Decoction
Varicose veins:	Tincture, Fluid Extract, Decoction, Powder
Weak veins and arterioles:	Tincture, Fluid Extract, Decoction, Powder

External

Hemorrhoids:	Tincture, Salve

Stoneroot is a good astringent and a specific tonic to relax the walls of the veins and arterioles which makes it a remedy for varicose veins in both the legs and rectum. It is especially good for piles and hemorrhoids. The tincture taken one teaspoon three times daily or two capsules three times daily is a sufficient amount. It is one of the best remedies to take for pain after surgical operations of the rectum for piles, ulcers or fistula.

The continued use of collinsonia will strengthen the heart with corresponding improvements in the general circulation. It is especially good for the heart when it has been overstrained by fever or sickness.

The decoction is a good diuretic and is used for water retention and gravel in the kidneys and bladder. The fresh leaves are a good poultice for wounds and sores.

TANSY *(Tanacetum vulgare)*

Part Used: herb, seed, root

Properties: Anthelmintic; emmenagogue, stimulant, tonic

Body Parts Affected: intestines

Preparation and Dosage:

Infusion (herb):	Steep 30 minutes. 1 tsp. three to four times daily
Decoction (seed, root):	Simmer 5 to 15 minutes. 3 oz. two to three times daily
Tincture:	½ to 1 tsp. two to three times daily
Fluid Extract:	½ to 2 tsp. two to three times daily
Syrup (root):	1 tsp. two to three times daily
Powder:	5 to 10 #0 capsules (30 to 60 grains) two to three times daily

Indicated Uses:

Internal

Fever:	Infusion*
Hysteria:	Infusion, Tincture, Fluid Extract
Nervousness:	Tincture, Fluid Extract, Infusion
Worms:	Syrup*, Infusion*

External

Arthritic pains:	Fomentation
Skin diseases:	Poultice (use the green leaves)

Tansy is used for expelling worms in both children and adults. The infusion is usually used for this taken in teaspoonfuls morning, midday and evening. I have seen worms expelled beautifully in children by making one cup of the infusion and pouring it over one-half cup of raisins. Let the raisins swell up with the liquid. Then give three teaspoon dosages of the mixture daily.

It is valuable in treating hysteria and kidney weaknesses. During menstruation when there is uneasiness accompanied with nervous tension and fever, the infusion and fluid extract is excellent.

A poultice made of the fresh, bruised green leaves is good for skin eruptions and swellings. A hot fomentation is good for arthritic pains.

THYME *(Thymus vulgaris)*

Part Used: tops

Properties: Antiseptic, Carminative, Diuretic; antispasmodic, expectorant, parasiticide

Body Parts Affected: intestines, lungs, throat, stomach and skin

Preparation and Dosage:

Infusion:	Steep 30 minutes. 1 oz. frequently, up to 2 cups a day
Tincture:	30 to 60 drops (½ to 1 tsp.) two to three times daily
Fluid Extract:	1 tsp. two to three times daily
Powder:	5 to 10 #0capsules (30 to 60 grains) two to three times daily

Indicated Uses:

Internal

Bronchial problems:	Infusion*
Diarrhea:	Infusion
Gastritis:	Infusion*
Laryngitis:	Infusion
Whooping cough:	Infusion

External

Mouth sores:	Mouthwash (infusion)
Crabs:	Fomentation, Poultice, Oil (add 4 drops oil to 4 oz. vegetable oil and rub on skin)
Lice:	Fomentation, Poultice, Oil (add 4 drops oil to 4 oz. vegetable oil and rub on skin)

Scabies:	Fomentation, Poultice, Oil (add 4 drops oil to 4 oz. vegetable oil and rub on skin)

As a tincture, extract of infusion, thyme is good for all throat and bronchial problems, especially bronchitis, laryngitis and whooping cough. It is good for all stomach and intestinal problems such as diarrhea, gastritis, lack of appetite, gas and colic. An infusion of the leaves will relieve headaches.

Externally, the tincture or oil diluted with vegetable oil (1 part thyme to 10 parts oil) is a useful antiseptic for ringworm, athlete's foot, scabies, crabs and lice.

A salve made of thyme, myrrh and goldenseal is good for herpes and other skin problems. For itchy skin problems, add 15 drops of the oil to a hot bath and soak for 45 minutes. Wash all wounds with this marvelous antiseptic.

TORMENTIL ROOT *(Potentilla tormentilla)*

Part Used: root

Properties: Astringent, Hemostatic, Styptic; anticatarrhal

Body Parts Affected: bowel and intestinal tract

Preparation and Dosage:

Decoction:	Simmer 5 to 15 minutes. 3 oz. three times daily
Tincture:	15 to 30 drops three times daily or 5 to 10 drops in water every hour
Fluid Extract:	½ to 1 tsp. three times daily
Powder:	5 to 10 #0 capsules (30 to 60 grains) three times daily

Indicated Uses:

Internal

Diarrhea:	Fluid Extract, Tincture, Decoction, Powder
Gonorrhea:	Fluid Extract*, Tincture*, Decoction*, Powder*
Leukorrhea:	Fluid Extract, Tincture, Decoction, Powder
Mild hemorrhage (lungs):	Fluid Extract, Decoction
Mouthwash:	Gargle
Prolapsed uterus:	Fluid Extract, Tincture, Decoction, Powder
Spleen obstruction:	Fluid Extract, Tincture, Decoction, Powder
Stomach bleeding:	Fluid Extract, Tincture, Decoction, Powder
Varicose veins:	Fluid Extract, Tincture, Powder

External

Leukorrhea:	Douche
Varicose veins:	Fomentation
Wounds:	Fomentation

The decoction or tincture is used for diarrhea, enteritis, stomach inflammations, mouthwashes and douches. The root is an excellent astringent and is used for dysentery, diarrhea and jaundice. Drink three ounces three times daily or an ounce every two hours. The tincture is taken five to ten drops in water every hour. Four ounces of the decoction injected into the bowel is good for bleeding, prostate enlargement, hemorrhoids and prolapsed anus (retain as long as possible). Gargle with the diluted decoction or fifteen drops of the tincture in a cup of water for tonsillitis, laryngitis and canker sores.

UVA URSI *(Arctostaphylos uva ursi)*

Part Used: leaves

Properties: Astringent, Diuretic; alterative, tonic

Body Parts Affected: kidneys and urinary tract

Preparation and Dosage:

Infusion:	Steep 30 minutes. 3 oz. as needed, up to 3 cups a day
Tincture:	10 to 20 drops, three or more times daily
Fluid Extract·	½ to 1 tsp. three times daily
Powder:	3 to 10 #0 capsules (20 to 60 grains) three times daily

Indicated Uses:

Internal

Bedwetting:	Tincture, Fluid Extract, Infusion
Bladder diseases:	Tincture, Fluid Extract, Infusion
Bronchitis:	Infusion*
Cystitis:	Tincture, Fluid Extract, Infusion
Diabetes:	Tincture*, Fluid Extract*, Infusion*
Dysentery:	Tincture, Fluid Extract, Infusion
Hemorrhoids.	Tincture, Fluid Extract, Infusion
Kidney congestion:	Tincture, Fluid Extract, Infusion
Leukorrhea:	Tincture, Fluid Extract, Infusion
Liver problems:	Tincture*, Fluid Extract*, Infusion*, Powder*
Lumbago:	Tincture, Fluid Extract, Infusion
Piles:	Tincture, Fluid Extract, Infusion

External

Dysentery:	Retention enema, Infusion
Hemorrhoids	Retention enema, Salve
Leukorrhea:	Douche
Piles:	Retention enema, Salve

Uva ursi is a specific for nephritis, cystitis, urethritis or kidney and bladder stones. For these purposes it should be combined with other diuretics, but always add marshmallow root or some other mucilaginous diuretic. Uva ursi leaves are astringent and tonic and are particularlly good for chronic diarrhea, dystentery and profuse menstruation, piles and diabetes. It has a direct sedative and tonic effect to the bladder walls, imparting tone and decreasing excessive discharges.

The leaves (one cup) put in a stocking and added to a hot tub of water makes a good bath for after childbirth, inflammations, hemorrhoids and skin infections. It is good for gonorrhea. Use as a douche (infusion) for vaginal infections and other problems in the pelvic region.

Note: Uva ursi should not be used in large quantities during pregnancy because it is a vasoconstrictor to the uterus (cuts down circulation to the uterus.)

VALERIAN *(Valeriana officinalis)*

Part Used: root

Properties: Antispasmodic, Nervine; carminative, stimulant

Body Parts Affected: nerves

Preparation and Dosage:

Decoction:	Simmer 5 to 15 minutes. 3 oz. three times daily
Tincture:	½ to 1 tsp. three times daily
Fluid Extract:	½ tsp. three times daily
Oil:	5 drops three times daily
Powder:	2 to 3 #0 capsules (10 to 15 grains) three times daily

Indicated Uses:

Internal

Afterpain (afterbirth):	Tincture, Fluid Extract, Powder
Calms the brain/ nervous system:	Tincture, Fluid Extract
Colds:	Powder*, Decoction*
Colic:	Tincture, Fluid Extract, Decoction
Convulsions:	Tincture, Fluid Extract
Fever:	Decoction*
Gas:	Tincture, Fluid Extract, Decoction*
Hangover:	Tincture, Fluid Extract
Hysteria:	Tincture, Fluid Extract
Insomnia:	Tincture, Fluid Extract, Powder
Measles:	Tincture, Fluid Extract, Powder*, Decoction*
Nerve weakness:	Tincture, Fluid Extract, Powder
Pain:	Tincture, Fluid Extract
Palsy:	Tincture, Fluid Extract

Paralysis:	Tincture, Fluid Extract, Powder
Spasms:	Tincture, Fluid Extract, Decoction*
Stomach pains:	Tincture, Fluid Extract
Ulcers:	Tincture, Fluid Extract*, Powder*, Decoction*

Valerian is a strong sedative and nerve tonic. It is especially active when under emotional stress and pain. The tea or tincture will lessen menstrual cramps, muscle pains, intestinal cramps and bronchial spasms. It is useful in colic, low fevers, colds and gravel in the bladder.

At first valerian may seem to be a stimulant because the essential oil of valerian must be broken down by body enzymes to valeramic acid (the calming principle) before the sedative effect can be felt. Large dosages can bring on depression. The dosage of the tincture is usually ½ to 1 teaspoon.

VERVAIN *(Verbena officinalis)*

Part Used: tops

Properties: Antipyretic, Antispasmodic, Diaphoretic; astringent, expectorant, galactagogue, vulnerary

Body Parts Affected: circulation, lungs and intestines

Preparation and Dosage:

Infusion:	Steep 5 to 15 minues. 3 oz. frequently
Tincture:	10 to 20 drops frequently
Fluid Extract:	½ to 1 tsp. frequently
Powder:	3 #0 capsules (15 grains) frequently

Indicated Uses:

Internal

Colds:	Infusion
Convulsions:	Tincture, Fluid Extract, Infusion
Coughs:	Infusion
Fevers:	Infusion
Headaches:	Infusion, Tincture, Fluid Extract
Measles:	Infusion*
Nerve weakness:	Tincture, Fluid Extract, Infusion
Pain in the bowels:	Infusion
Pleurisy:	Infusion*

External

Rheumatism, neuralgia, sciatica:	Make a poultice out of flax seed meal and use a strong infusion of vervain instead of water to moisten it.
Swellings of the spleen:	Poultice (mix with wheat flour or bran)

Vervain is one of the palliatives for the onset of colds, flu, coughs and upper respiratory inflammations. It will promote sweating to allay fevers. Combine with boneset for fevers and take ½ to 1 hot cup every hour. The tea will settle a nervous stomach and is good for insomnia. It is good for pneumonia, asthma and all other congestive chest diseases. The tea can also be applied to sores to increase healing. Drink the warm tea for pain or cramps in the stomach and bowels.

Large amounts of vervain will act as an emetic. It is bitter and can be made more palatable if combined with lemon grass or peppermint and honey. Start with one teaspoonful when treating children and increase if needed; one tablespoon to 1 cup with adults.

WHITE OAK BARK *(Quercus alba)*

Part Used: bark

Properties: Astringent; antiseptic, diuretic

Body Parts Affected: skin, gastro-intestinal tract and kidneys

Preparation and Dosage:

Decoction:	Simmer 5 to 10 minutes. 3 oz. as needed
Tincture:	15 to 30 drops as needed
Fluid Extract:	½ to 1 tsp. as needed
Powder:	3 to 10 #0 capsules (15 to 60 grains) as needed

Indicated Uses:

Internal

Bladder weakness:	Decoction*, Tincture, Fluid Extract, Powder*
Canker:	Tincture, Fluid Extract, Decoction
Diarrhea:	Tincture, Fluid Extract, Decoction Powder
Hemorrhage (intestines, bowels, lungs, kidneys):	Tincture, Powder, Fluid Extract, Decoction
Hemorrhoids:	Tincture, Fluid Extract, Powder, Decoction
Herpes:	Tincture*, Fluid Extract*, Powder*, Decoction
Leukorrhea:	Tincture, Fluid Extract, Powder, Decoction
Nose bleeds:	Snort teaspoon of decoction up nostrils
Uterus, prolapsed:	Decoction, Tincture, Fluid Extract, Powder
Varicose veins:	Tincture, Fluid Extract, Powder, Decoction

External

Canker:	Gargle
Diarrhea:	Enema
Fever blisters:	Fomentation, Salve

Goiter:	Fomentation, Poultice
Gums (soft):	Gargle
Hemorrhage (intestines, bowel, lungs, kidneys):	Retention enema
Hemorrhoids:	Salve, Retention enema
Herpes:	Fomentation, Salve, Poultice
Leukorrhea:	Douche
Mouth Ulcers:	Gargle
Pyorrhea:	Gargle
Ringworm:	Fomentation, Salve, Poultice
Skin diseases:	Fomentation, Salve, Poultice
Sores (antiseptic):	Salve, Fomentation
Thrush:	Gargle
Tonsillitis:	Gargle
Ulcers:	Fomentation, Poultice of ground bark
Varicose veins:	Fomentation, Poultice, Salve

White oak bark is a most excellent astringent. The decoction is good as an injection for vaginal infections, piles or hemorrhoids. The tea is taken for bleeding of the stomach, lungs and rectum. It will stop spitting up of blood. It will increase the flow of urine and help remove gallstones and kidney stones.

Externally, the tea is good for bathing scabs, sores, poison oak, and insect bites. Soak a towel in the tea and tie over the weak vessels and broken capillaries. It is excellent for varicose veins (both internally and externally as a poultice). Use the fomentation and apply overnight to swollen glands, tumors, mumps, goiter and lymphatic swellings.

Drink the tea for blood urine, chronic diarrhea, mucus discharges and hemorrhages. It will clean the stomach. Oak bark is an antiseptic and is a good skin wash for wounds. Applied to the gums it will strengthen them (correct the diet first).

WHITE WILLOW *(Salix alba)*

Part Used: bark

Properties: Anodyne, Antispasmodic, Tonic; astringent, diaphoretic, diuretic, febrifuge

Body Parts Affected: stomach, kidneys, bowel, intestines and head

Preparation and Dosage:

Infusion:	Steep 5 to 15 minutes. 1 cup during the day
Decoction (bark):	Simmer 5 to 15 minutes. 1 cup during the day
Tincture:	15 to 60 drops as needed
Fluid Extract:	¼ to 1 tsp. as needed
Powder:	6 to 10 #0 capsules (30 to 50 grains) as needed

Indicated Uses:

Internal

Alleviate pain:	Powder, Tincture, Fluid Extract
Dyspepsia:	Powder, Tincture, Fluid Extract, Decoction
Dysentery:	Powder*, Decoction*, Fluid Extract*
Enlarged prostate:	Powder, Tincture, Fluid Extract
Headache:	Tincture, Fluid Extract, Powder
Internal bleeding:	Tincture, Fluid Extract, Powder, Decoction
Kidney infections:	Tincture*, Fluid Extract*, Powder*, Decoction*
Mouth (sores):	Tincture, Fluid Extract, Decoction
Spermatorrhea:	Powder, Tincture, Fluid Extract
Tonsillitis:	Tincture, Fluid Extract, Decoction
Urine retention:	Tincture, Fluid Extract, Decoction

External

Mouth (sores):	Gargle
Tonsillitis:	Gargle

White willow has the ability to alleviate pain and reduce fevers. White willow is our natural alternative to aspirin. The principle active ingredient in white willow is salicin. Its uses are many: headaches, fevers, neuralgia and pains in the joints. The glucoside salicin is excreted in the urine as salicylic acid and related compounds which renders the tea useful for kidney, urethra and bladder irritabilities and acts as an analgesic to those tissues. Willow bark is a strong antiseptic and is a good poultice and fomentation for infected wounds, ulcerations, eczema and all other skin inflammations. A decoction is an excellent gargle for throat and tonsil infections.

Taken internally it is good for gout, rheumatism and arthritic pains. The tea is also a good eyewash and a snuff to stop nose bleeds and other surface bleeding.

WILD CHERRY BARK *(Prunus serotina)*

Part Used: dried inner bark

Properties: Sedative, Stomachic; astringent, stimulant tonic

Body Parts Affected: lungs, stomach and nerves

Preparation and Dosage:

Infusion:	Steep 5 to 15 minutes. 6 oz. three to four times daily between meals
Decoction:	Simmer 5 to 15 minutes. 2 oz. three times daily
Tincture:	30 to 60 drops three times daily
Fluid Extract:	½ to 1 tsp. three times daily
Syrup:	½ to 2 tsp. three times daily
Powder:	5 #0 capsules three times daily

Indicated Uses:

Internal

Asthma:	Syrup, Decoction
Colds:	Decoction*
Flu:	Decoction*
Dyspepsia:	Syrup, Tincture, Fluid Extract, Decoction
Nervous stomach:	Syrup*, Decoction*
Tuberculosis:	Syrup*, Decoction*
Whooping cough:	Syrup*, Decotion*

Wild cherry bark is a tonic to the digestive tract and respiratory tract. It is a common remedy in the treatment of chronic coughs, especially those accompanied by excessive mucus. It is a popular remedy for heart palpitations when this condition is caused by a stomach disorder. It is a tonic for the stomach and improves digestion by stimulating the gastric glands. It is good for treating dyspepsia. It soothes nerve irritations of both the stomach and lungs and loosens mucus in the throat and chest.

WILD YAM (Dioscorea villosa)

Part Used: root

Properties: Cholagogue; antispasmodic, diaphoretic

Body Parts Affected: muscles, joints, uterus, liver and gall bladder

Preparation and Dosage:

Decoction:	Simmer 5 to 15 minutes. 2 to 3 oz. in water three to four times daily, up to 2 cups per day
Tincture:	10 to 40 drops three to four times daily
Fluid Extract:	1 tsp. three to four times daily
Powder:	5 to 10 #0 capsules (30 to 60 grains) three to four times daily

Indicated Uses:

Internal

Cramps:	Tincture, Fluid Extract, Decoction
Gas (excellent):	Tincture, Fluid Extract, Decoction, Powder
Griping pains in bowels and stomach:	Tincture, Fluid Extract, Decoction
Hepatitis:	Tincture*, Fluid Extract*, Decoction*, Powder*
Hiccoughs:	Tincture, Fluid Extract, Decoction
Morning sickness:	Tincture, Fluid Extract, Decoction, Powder
Nausea:	Tincture, Fluid Extract, Decoction
Neuralgic dysmenorrhea:	Tincture, Fluid Extract, Decoction

Ovarian neuralgia:	Tincture, Fluid Extract, Decoction
Pain while passing gallstones	Tincture, Fluid Extract, Decoction*
Spasmodic asthma:	Tincture, Fluid Extract
Ulcers:	Tincture*, Fluid Extract*, Decoction*, Powder*

Wild yam has steroid-like substances that are used in the process of making birth control pills. This is why wild yam is present in many gland balancing formulas. Wild yam is a valuable antispasmodic and is used for abdominal cramps, bowel spasms and menstrual cramps.

Wild yam provides excellent benefits to the function of the gall bladder and liver. It will counteract nausea (use in 2 ounce dosage with honey added).

It is combined with other blood cleaners and will aid in removing wastes from the system, relieving stiff and sore joints. To prevent miscarriage, Kloss says, "Combine with powdered ginger to prevent miscarriage. One teaspoon of wild yam to ½ teaspoon of dried ginger." I suggest adding one teaspoon of red raspberry to this combination and steep in one pint of water for twenty minutes, strain and take a mouthful every half hour when threatened by this problem.

For arthritis and pain take the following in a cup of warm water three times daily.

Tincture of burdock root	20 drops
Tincture of black cohosh	15 drops
Tincture of motherwort	15 drops
Tincture of wild yam	30 drops

Note: *When given for afterbirth pains, it is better to use ten drops of the tincture in cold water. The hot decoction causes too great of relaxation to the uterus and could permit hemorrhage.*

WITCH HAZEL *(Haemamelis virginiana)*

Part Used: bark, leaves

Properties: Astringent, Hemostatic, Tonic; sedative

Body Parts Affected: skin, stomach and intestines

Preparation and Dosage:

Infusion (leaves):	Steep 10 to 15 minutes. 6 oz. as needed
Decoction (bark):	Simmer 10 to 15 minutes. 3 oz. as needed, up to 2 cups daily
Tincture (bark):	15 to 60 drops as needed
Fluid Extract (bark):	½ tsp. as needed
Powder (bark):	5 to 10 #0 capsules (30 to 60 grains) as needed

Indicated Uses:

Internal

Diarrhea:	Tincture, Fluid Extract, Decoction, Powder
Diptheria:	Tincture, Fluid Extract, Decoction, Powder
Hemorrhoids:	Tincture, Fluid Extract, Decoction, Powder
Leukorrhea:	Tincture, Fluid Extract
Prolapsed bowel and uterus:	Tincture, Fluid Extract, Powder, Decoction
Stop bleeding from lungs, uterus and other internal organs:	Tincture, Fluid Extract, Decoction
Varicose veins:	Tincture, Fluid Extract, Decoction, Powder

External

Burns:	Fomentation
Bruises:	Fomentation
Diptheria:	Gargle
Insect bites:	Fomentation, Tincture, Fluid Extract
Leukorrhea:	Retention douche
Sore breasts:	Fomentation, Salve
Sore muscles:	Fomentation, Liniment
Tonsillitis:	Gargle
Varicose veins:	Fomentation

The tea or fluid extract is one of nature's best remedies for stopping excessive menstruation, hemorrhages from the lungs, stomach, uterus and bowels. It can be used as an injection for bleeding piles and vaginal discharges and infections. Also take a tablespoon of the tea several times internally daily for these conditions. Use the tincture diluted in water for gargles and mouthwashes for infections and as a maintenance procedure.

As a fomentation or poultice, it is good for bed sores, wounds, sore and inflammed eyes and oozing skin diseases. Use this herb when making boluses and suppositories. There is hardly an inflamed condition internally or externally that will not respond to this remedy.

WOOD BETONY (Betonica officinalis)

Part Used: tops

Properties: Nervine; alterative, aromatic, hepatic, parasiticide

Body Parts Affected: nerves and liver

Preparation and Dosage:

Infusion:	Steep 5 to 15 minutes. 3 oz. three to four times daily
Tincture:	30 to 60 drops (½ to 1 tsp.) three to four times daily

| Fluid Extract: | ½ to 1 tsp. three times daily |
| Powder: | 5 to 10 #0 capsules (30 to 60 grains) three to four times daily |

Indicated Uses:

Internal

Bronchitis:	Infusion*
Colds, coughs:	Mix the powder with honey and take in ¼ teaspoon dosages whenever needed
Convulsions:	Tincture, Fluid Extract, Infusion
Cramps:	Powder*, Infusion*, Fluid Extract
Dizziness:	Infusion
Dyspepsia:	Infusion
Headache:	Infusion
Jaundice:	Infusion
Menstrual cramps:	Infusion*, Fluid Extract*
Nerve disorders:	Infusion*, Fluid Extract*, Powder*
Nervousness:	Infusion, Tincture, Fluid Extract
Palsy:	Infusion*, Powder*
Worms:	Infusion

External

Old sores and ulcers:	Poultice of the green herb
Splinters:	Poultice of the green herb
Wounds:	Poultice of the green herb

Betony is an excellent remedy for most head problems such as pain in the head, headaches and nerve twitching of the face. It is used in combination with other herbs for treating rheumatism and other diseases which stem from impurities of the blood. The infusion and powder has been used to treat jaundice, gout, convulsions and colds. Betony is frequently combined with other nervines and antispasmodics to treat nerve diseases and to calm the nerves when stress is present from other diseases. It is good for palsy, insanity, neuralgia, colds and cramps.

The infusion taken three to four times daily in three ounce dosages will kill worms and open up obstructions of the liver and gall bladder. The fresh, green herb, bruised and used as a poultice will draw out splinters and help heal open wounds.

WORMWOOD *(Artemisia absinthium)*

Part Used: tops, leaves

Properties: Anthelmintic; antiseptic, aromatic, diaphoretic, tonic

Body Parts Affected: liver, gall bladder, stomach, intestines, uterus and joints

Preparation and Dosage:

Internal

Infusion:	Steep 5 to 15 minutes. 3 oz. as needed, up to 2 cups daily
Tincture:	10 to 30 drops three to four times daily
Fluid Extract:	15 to 60 drops three to four times daily
Powder:	2 to 4 #0 capsules (15 to 20 grains) three to four times daily

Indicated Uses:

Internal

Diarrhea:	Infusion*, Powder*
Fevers:	Infusion
Gas:	Infusion, Powder, Fluid Extract
Indigestion:	Infusion
Jaundice:	Infusion*
Weak digestion:	Infusion, Fluid Extract
Worms:	Infusion

External

Boils:	Fomentation
Rheumatism:	Fomentation, Liniment
Swelling:	Fomentation, Liniment

Wormwood is an intensely bitter herb and will stimulate sweating and improve digestion. It is an excellent stomach tonic. The hot tea stimulates the uterus and will help bring on suppressed menstruation. The tea will expel roundworms and pinworms. It is an excellent remedy for bilious and liver troubles. Add wormwood to liniments for excellent results in rheumatism, swellings and sprains.

Wormwood is good for all digestive problems when the liver and gall bladder are involved. It will relieve pain during labor also.

Externally, the tea as a fomentation is used for insect bites, bruises and injuries. As a folk medicine, its reputation lies in its use for gastritis, stomach ulcers, dysentery, tuberculosis, liver and spleen conditions, kidney and bladder problems. Bleeding of the bowel can be treated by an injection of the tea and retained for 5 minutes several times daily as needed.

YARROW *(Achillea millefolium)*

Part Used: flower and leaves

Properties: Astringent, Diaphoretic, Hemostatic; stimulant

Body Parts Affected: circulation

Preparation and Dosage:

Infusion:	Steep 5 to 15 minutes. 6 oz. three to four times daily

Tincture:	5 to 20 drops three to four times daily
Fluid Extract:	½ to 1 tsp. three to four times daily
Oil:	5 to 20 drops three to four times daily
Powder:	5 to 10 #0 capsules (30 to 60 grains) three to four times daily

Indicated Uses:

Internal

Bleeding piles:	Infusion
Blood purifier:	Infusion, Tincture, Fluid Extract
Blood in urine:	Infusion, Fluid Extract, Tincture, Powder*
Colds:	Infusion
Deficient urinary function:	Infusion, Fluid Extract, Tincture
Epdidymitis:	Infusion, Tincture, Fluid Extract
Hemorrhage (lungs):	Infusion*, Powder*
Hemorrhoids:	Infusion, Tincture, Fluid Extract
Jaundice:	Powder*, Infusion*, Tincture*, Fluid Extract*
Leukorrhea, menorrhagia, amenorrhea:	Tincture, Fluid Extract, Infusion*
Measles:	Infusion
Piles:	Tincture, Fluid Extract, Infusion
Skin diseases:	Infusion
Tonic to urinary organs:	Infusion, Tincture, Fluid Extract, Powder*
Uremic poisoning:	Infusion, Tincture, Fluid Extract

External

Bleeding piles:	Retention enema
Hemorrhoids:	Retention enema
Piles:	Retention enema

Yarrow tea is excellent for shrinking hemorrhoids, hemorrhages and bleeding of the lungs. It can be taken in tincture form with excellent results. For piles, vaginal secretions and hemorrhage, use as a douche or enema. Inject into the colon after each bowel movement (two ounces) if there is swelling or bleeding. If there is much pain, inject a warm tea (112 to 115 degrees Farenheit) and it will soothe and alleviate the pain. It is excellent for diarrhea when taken internally for infants. It will expel gas from the stomach. It is an excellent fever remedy in conditions such as measles, colds, flu and skin eruptions. It is a good antiseptic because of its tannin and essential oils. Add yarrow to salves and boluses.

YELLOW DOCK (Rumex crispus)

Part Used: root

Properties: Alterative, Astringent; cholagogue, laxative, nutritive

Body Parts Affected: blood, skin, spleen, liver and gall bladder

Preparation and Dosage:

Decoction:	Simmer 5 to 15 minutes. 1 Tbsp. in 6 oz. water, three times daily
Tincture:	5 to 30 drops three times daily
Fluid Extract:	½ to 1 tsp. three times daily
Syrup:	1 tsp. three t four times daily
Powder:	5 to 10 #0 capsules (30 to 60 grains) three times daily

Indicated Uses:

Internal

Acne:	Infusion, Powder*, Tincture, Fluid Extract
Anemia:	Powder*, Infusion*, Syrup*
Blood purifier:	Infusion, Tincture, Fluid Extract, Powder
Boils:	Infusion, Tincture, Fluid Extract, Powder
Cancer:	Infusion*, Tincture*, Fluid Extract*, Powder*
Jaundice:	Tincture, Fluid Extract, Powder*, Infusion*
Leukorrhea:	Tincture, Fluid Extract, Powder*, Infusion*
Piles:	Infusion, Tincture, Fluid Extract
Psoriasis:	Infusion, Tincture, Fluid Extract, Powder*
Skin diseases:	Infusion, Tincture, Fluid Extract, Powder*
Tonic to stomach:	Infusion, Tincture, Fluid Extract, Powder

External

Boils:	Fomentation, Salve
Leukorrhea:	Retention douche
Piles:	Retention enema
Psoriasis:	Wash, Fomentation
Tumors:	Fomentation

Yellow dock is an astringent blood purifier. It will tone up the entire system and is good for diseases such as skin infections, tumors, liver and gall bladder problems, ulcers and skin itch. It acts as a laxative because it stimulates the flow of bile. It makes an excellent salve for itchy skin diseases and swellings of glands or otherwise.

Yellow dock is high in iron and is used in the treatment of anemia and will nourish the spleen. Use in formulas when treating jaundice and hepatitis. Combine in teas and salve with echinacea, burdock root and sarsparilla.

Externally, it is applied to bleeding piles and wounds. When there is running of the ears, ulcertated eyelids, scurvy, blood or lymph problems, drink three cups of the tea daily.

YERBA SANTA *(Eriodictyon californisum)*

Part Used: leaves

Properties: Expectorant; astringent, stimulant

Body Parts Affected: lungs and stomach

Preparation and Dosage:

Infusion:	Steep 30 minutes. 2 to 3 oz. three times daily
Tincture:	10 to 30 drops, three to four times daily
Fluid Extract:	½ to 1 tsp. three to four times daily
Powder:	2 to 10 #0 capsules (15 to 60 grains) three to four times daily

Indicated Uses:

Internal

Asthma:	Smoke the leaves, Infusion*, Powder*
Bronchitis:	Infusion*, Powder*
Colds:	Infusion
Dry coughs:	Infusion, Syrup
Fevers:	Infusion
Headache:	Infusion
Tuberculosis:	Infusion*, Syrup*

External

Insect bites:	Fomentation
Mouthwash:	Gargle

Yerba santa is a specific for all forms of bronchial congestion. At times bronchial and lung congestion is caused by digestive problems where excess mucus builds up in the intestinal tract. Yerba santa will stimulate the digestive juices, improving digestion, thus correcting the lung congestion. Thus, yerba santa is an excellent remedy for all respiratory problems to help remove mucus. It is a good remedy for dysentery and diarrhea also.

Yerba santa dilates the bronchial tubes which makes it excellent for asthma and hay fever. The leaves can be smoked for mild bronchial spasms.

HERBS USED FOR SPECIFIC PARTS OF THE BODY

Herbs have certain effects on specific body parts because of the healing properties they possess. This chart will help you identify the proper herbs when treating particular systems or parts of the body.

Body Parts Affected	Herbs
Adrenal glands	Licorice
Bladder	Buchu, celery, chickweed, cleavers, corn silk, gotu kola, gravel root, kelp, marshmallow, mistletoe (American), nettles, parsley, peach, sage, shepherd's purse, squaw vine, St. John's wort
Blood	Alfalfa, barberry, black walnut, blessed thistle, buckthorn, burdock, calendula, chaparral, chickweek, cleavers, dandelion, devil's claw, elder, eyebright, gentian, hops, horsetail, nettles, oregon grape root, poke, prickly ash, raspberry, red clover, rose, sarsparilla, sassafras, shepherd's purse, St. John's wort, yellow dock
Bones	Comfrey
Bowels	Bistort, elder, lungwort, peach, psyllium, sage, tormentil root, white willow
Circulatory system	Angelica, bayberry, boneset, bugleweed, cayenne, cloves, elder, ephedra, garlic, gentian, ginger, ginseng, gotu kola, hawthorn, hyssop, lemon balm, lobelia, mistletoe (European), mugwort, passion flower, pennyroyal, peppermint, pipsissewa, prickly ash, rue, sarsparilla, sassafras, spearmint, vervain, yarrow
Colon	Aloe vera, cascara sagrada, squaw vine, stoneroot
Digestive tract	Barberry
Eyes	Eyebright, fennel, goldenseal
Gall bladder	Buckthorn, cascara sagrada, dandelion, hops, horseradish, mandrake, parsley, wild yam, wormwood, yellow dock
Gastrointestinal tract	White oak bark

General effects	Comfrey, ginseng, slippery elm
Genito-urinary tract	Raspberry
Head	White willow
Heart	Angelica, black cohosh, blessed thistle, bugleweed, cayenne, cramp bark, ephedra, ginseng, gotu kola, hawthorn, horsetail, mistletoe (American and European), motherwort, rose
Intestinal tract	Agar-agar, agrimony, angelica, bayberry, blackberry, black haw, black walnut, boneset, buckthorn, catnip, chaparral, cloves, coltsfoot, cranesbill, dandelion, fennel, fenugreek, flax, ginger, goldenseal, licorice, lungwort, mandrake, marshmallow, oregon grape root, peppermint, plantain, psyllium, rhubarb, rosemary, sarsparilla, sassafras, senna, spearmint, tansy, thyme, tormentil root, vervain, white willow, witch hazel, wormwood
Joints	Blue cohosh, devil's claw, ginger, gravel root, wild yam, wormwood
Kidneys	Buchu, burdock, cayenne, celery, chamomile, chickweed, cleavers, corn silk, cranesbill, damiana, dandelion, devil's claw, echinacea, false unicorn, fo-ti, gotu kola, gravel root, hawthorn, horsetail, juniper, kelp, marshmallow, mistletoe (American and European), nettles, parsley, plantain, pleurisy root, safflower, saw palmetto, shepherd's purse, uva ursi, white oak bark,white willow
Liver:	Agrimony, barberry, boneset, buckthorn, burdock, cascara sagrada, chamomile, chickweed, dandelion, devil's claw, eyebright, fo-ti, gentian, goldenseal, hops, licorice, lungwort, mandrake, oregon grape root, parsley, peach, pipsissewa, raspberry, red clover, rosemary, St. John's wort, stoneroot, wild yam, wood betony, wormwood, yellow dock
Lungs	Angelica, beth root, bistort, black cohosh, bugleweed, chickweed, cloves, coltsfoot, elder, elecampane, ephedra, fenugreek, flax, garlic, horehound, horsetail, hyssop, irish moss, licorice, lobelia, lungwort, mullein, myrrh, nettles, oat, pennyroyal, pleurisy root, poke, red clover, rosemary, saw palmetto, thyme, vervain, wild cherry bark, yerba santa

Lymphatic system	Echinacea, mullein, poke, red clover
Mammary glands	Blessed thistle
Mouth	Cloves
Mucus membranes	Goldenseal, sage
Muscles:	Comfrey, ginger, lobelia, peppermint, raspberry, spearmint, wild yam
Nervous system	Black cohosh, black haw, black walnut, blue cohosh, catnip, celery, chamomile, cramp bark, damiana, fennel, gotu kola, gravel root, hawthorn, hops, kava kava, kelp, lady's slipper, lemon balm, lobelia, mistletoe (American), motherwort, mugwort, oat, passion flower, peach, pleurisy root, red clover, rose, rosemary, rue, safflower, sage, scullcap, St. John's wort, valerian, wild cherry bark, wood betony
Pancreas	Cascara sagrada, dandelion
Prostate	Corn silk
Reproductive system	Cramp bark, damiana, fenugreek, fo-ti, saw palmetto
Sinuses	Garlic, horseradish, hyssop, sage
Skin	Aloe vera, calendula, cleavers, elder, irish moss, mandrake, oregon grape root, pipsissewa, plantain, safflower, sarsparilla, sassafras, thyme, white oak bark, witch hazel, yellow dock
Spleen	Barberry, chamomile, elecampane, gentian, goldenseal, licorice, yellow dock
Stomach	Agrimony, alfalfa, aloe vera, angelica, bayberry, bistort, blackberry, black haw, blessed thistle, boneset, cascara sagrada, cayenne, chamomile, chaparral, cloves, coltsfoot, cranesbill, dandelion, devil's claw, elecampane, fennel, fenugreek, flax, fo-ti, gentian, ginger, goldenseal, hops, horehound, horseradish, juniper, licorice, lobelia, mugwort, myrrh, oat, oregon grape root, parsley, peach, peppermint, prickly ash, raspberry, rhubarb, rosemary, scullcap, spearmint, St. John's wort, thyme, white willow, wild cherry bark, witch hazel, wormwood, yerba santa

Tendons	Rue
Throat	Flax, saw palmetto, thyme
Thyroid	Kelp
Urinary tract	Blue cohosh, horseradish, pipsissewa, uva ursi
Uterus	Beth root, black cohosh, black haw, blessed thistle, blue cohosh, false unicorn, motherwort, mugwort, oat, pennyroyal, rue, squaw vine, wild yam, wormwood
Veins	Plantain, stoneroot

HERBAL FORMULATIONS

When using herbs, the herbalist generally combines several herbs rather than using a single herb. Some single herbs are very strong and need to be buffered by a demulcent or carminative herb to make it easier for weak stomachs to digest. A single herb doesn't always have all the healing qualities you need to cover the symptoms being treated, so other herbs are added to your combination. By mixing several herbs, a variety of symptoms can be treated at one time.

There are situations when single herbs can be used. The first is during treatment of a chronic ailment; oftentimes acute symptoms or new symptoms such as nervousness, tension, stomach upset and so forth manifest. Usually these can be treated with one herb taken several times a day. Continue any treatment previously being used, but supplement it with the appropriate single herb. A second example of using a single herb is during sweating therapy. A hot bath is given, then a hot diaphoretic herb tea is given. You can use more than one herb, but usually one is enough. Sometimes a little stimulation is needed or there may be stomach upset. Ginger tea would cover both these symptoms. So, single herbs are used mainly as instruments in treating less problematic conditions or added to an already existing treatment to help control the disease.

When studying the properties of herbs, you will notice that they have primary and secondary properties. The primary property is the herb's strongest healing activity and is used to treat the major symptoms of the disease. There are also secondary symptoms that usually accompany the illness which are treated by the secondary properties of the herbs chosen. Here is a chart which tells you the primary and secondary properties. This will help you decide which properties are needed to treat the specific symptoms. It is important to remember to use the primary properties to treat the most aggravating symptoms.

	ALTERATIVE	ANODYNE	ANTHELMINTIC	ANTACID	ANTIBIOTIC	ANTICATARRHAL	ANTIEMETIC	ANTIPYRETIC	ANTISEPTIC	ANTISPASMODIC	APERIENT	APHRODISIAC	AROMATIC	ASTRINGENT	CARDIAC	CARMINATIVE	CATHARTIC	CHOLAGOGUE	CONDIMENT	DEMULCENT	DEOBSTRUENT	DIAPHORETIC	DISCUTIENT	DIURETIC
AGAR-AGAR																				●				
AGRIMONY														•										•
ALFALFA	●								•															
ALOE VERA																				●				
ANISE																●								
ANGELICA	•															●						●		
BARBERRY	•								●		•													
BAYBERRY														●										
BETH ROOT									●					●										
BISTORT									•					●										
BLACKBERRY														●										•
BLACK COHOSH	•									●														•
BLACK HAW										●														
BLACK WALNUT	•								●					●										
BLESSED THISTLE	•																							
BLUE COHOSH										●														•
BONESET								•														●		
BUCHU									●													•		●
BUCKTHORN																								
BUGLEWEED														●										
BURDOCK, ROOT	●																					•	●	●
BURDOCK, LEAVES																								
BURDOCK, SEEDS	●																							•
CALENDULA									•					●								•		
CARAWAY													●			●								
CARDAMON													●			●								
CASCARA SAGRADA											•													
CATNIP																●						●		
CAYENNE									•				•			●								
CELERY																●								●
CINNAMON													●			●								
CHAMOMILE																	•					•		
CHAPARRAL	●				●				●															
CHICKWEED	•						●													●				

Herb	EMOLLIENT	EXPECTORANT	FEBRIFUGE	GALACTAGOGUE	HEMOSTATIC	HEPATIC	LAXATIVE	LITHOTRIPTIC	LYMPHATIC	MUCILAGE	NERVINE	NUTRITIVE	OPTHALMIC	OXYTOCIC	PARASITICIDE	PURGATIVE	RUBEFACIENT	SEDATIVE	SIALAGOGUE	STIMULANT	STOMACHIC	STYPTIC	TONIC	VERMICIDE	VERMIFUGE	VULNERARY
AGAR-AGAR							●					•														
AGRIMONY						●														●			•			
ALFALFA												●														
ALOE VERA	●					●																				●
ANISE																				●						
ANGELICA		•																		●			•			
BARBERRY						●														●			•			
BAYBERRY																					•					
BETH ROOT																							•			
BISTORT																						●				
BLACKBERRY						●															●		•			
BLACK COHOSH																										
BLACK HAW											●												●			
BLACK WALNUT																									●	
BLESSED THISTLE				●															•	●	●					
BLUE COHOSH														●												
BONESET							•													●						
BUCHU																										
BUCKTHORN		•			●	●																				
BUGLEWEED																		●					•			
BURDOCK, ROOT																										
BURDOCK, LEAVES																							●			
BURDOCK, SEEDS																										
CALENDULA																										●
CARAWAY																				●						
CARDAMON																				●						
CASCARA SAGRADA					●	●																				
CATNIP											•							●								
CAYENNE																				●						
CELERY											●									•					•	
CINNAMON																				●						
CHAMOMILE											●							●					•			
CHAPARRAL															●											
CHICKWEED																										

	ALTERATIVE	ANODYNE	ANTHELMINTIC	ANTACID	ANTIBIOTIC	ANTICATARRHAL	ANTIEMETIC	ANTIPYRETIC	ANTISEPTIC	ANTISPASMODIC	APERIENT	APHRODISIAC	AROMATIC	ASTRINGENT	CARDIAC	CARMINATIVE	CATHARTIC	CHOLAGOGUE	CONDIMENT	DEMULCENT	DEOBSTRUENT	DIAPHORETIC	DISCUTIENT	DIURETIC	EMETIC	EMMENAGOGUE
CLEAVERS	●								•					●										●		
CLOVES		•					•		●			•	●			●										
COLTSFOOT																				●						
COMFREY	•													•						●						
CORIANDER	•															●								●		
CORN SILK																				•				●		
CRAMPBARK										●				•												
CRANESBILL														●												
CUMIN										•						●										
DAMIANA												•						•						•		●
DANDELION	•													•				●						●		
DEVIL'S CLAW	●																						•			
ECHINACEA	●								●																	
ELDER	•																					●				
ELECAMPANE														•				●						●		
EPHEDRA														•							•					
EYEBRIGHT	●													•												
FALSE UNICORN																								•	•	●
FENNEL										●		●				●								•		
FENUGREEK												•		•						●						
FLAX																				●						
FO-TI														•										•		
GARLIC	●				●				•													•				
GENTIAN			•															●								•
GINGER													●			●						●		•		
GINSENG	●																									
GOLDENSEAL	●				●				●																	●
GOTU KOLA	•							•																•		
GRAVEL ROOT														•										●		
HAWTHORN										•				•										•		
HOPS			•		•											●		•								
HOREHOUND																						●				
HORSERADISH																						●		●		
HORSETAIL														●										●		•
HYSSOP																			•			●				

Herb	EMOLLIENT	EXPECTORANT	FEBRIFUGE	GALACTAGOGUE	HEMOSTATIC	HEPATIC	•LAXATIVE	LITHOTRIPTIC	LYMPHATIC	MUCILAGE	NERVINE	NUTRITIVE	OPTHALMIC	OXYTOCIC	PARASITICIDE	PURGATIVE	RUBEFACIENT	SEDATIVE	SIALAGOGUE	STIMULANT	STOMACHIC	STYPTIC	TONIC	VERMICIDE	VERMIFUGE	VULNERARY
CLEAVERS																										
CLOVES																				●						
COLTSFOOT	●	●																								
COMFREY		●								●		•														●
CORIANDER																										
CORN SILK								●																		
CRAMPBARK											•															
CRANESBILL																						●	•			
CUMIN																				●						
DAMIANA																							●			
DANDELION				•		●	●													●						
DEVIL'S CLAW							•													•						
ECHINACEA									●					•				•								
ELDER							•													•						
ELECAMPANE		●																		•	●					
EPHEDRA		●																		•						
EYEBRIGHT																							•			
FALSE UNICORN														•						•			●			
FENNEL		•		•																•						
FENUGREEK	●	●		•																			•			
FLAX	●						●			●																
FO-TI																				●			●			
GARLIC		•																		•						
GENTIAN																					●		●			
GINGER																				●						
GINSENG																				●	●		●			
GOLDENSEAL						•															●		●			
GOTU KOLA											●												●			
GRAVEL ROOT								●			•									•						
HAWTHORN																		•					●			
HOPS											●										•		•			
HOREHOUND		●																					•			
HORSERADISH		●																			●					
HORSETAIL			•					●				•														•
HYSSOP		●																		•						•

	ALTERATIVE	ANODYNE	ANTHELMINTIC	ANTACID	ANTIBIOTIC	ANTICATARRHAL	ANTIEMETIC	ANTIPYRETIC	ANTISEPTIC	ANTISPASMODIC	APERIENT	APHRODISIAC	AROMATIC	ASTRINGENT	CARDIAC	CARMINATIVE	CATHARTIC	CHOLAGOGUE	CONDIMENT	DEMULCENT	DEOBSTRUENT	DIAPHORETIC	DISCUTIENT	DIURETIC	EMETIC
IRISH MOSS																				●					
JUNIPER		•								●		•	•			•								●	
KAVA KAVA			●						●	●														●	
KELP	•																			●				•	
LADY'S SLIPPER										●															
LEMON BALM								•		•												●			
LICORICE	•																			●					
LOBELIA										●															●
LUNGWORT														•						●					
MANDRAKE (AMERICAN)	•																	●							•
MARSHMALLOW	•																			●				●	
MISTLETOE (AMERICAN)										●													•	•	
MISTLETOE (EUROPEAN)																								•	
MOTHERWORT										•													•		
MUGWORT																							•	•	
MULLEIN										•				•						●				•	
MYRRH									●							•									
NETTLES	●									•															
OAT										•															
OREGON GRAPE ROOT	●									●								●							
PARSLEY																•								●	
PASSION FLOWER										●													•		
PEACH																					•				
PENNYROYAL																•						●			
PEPPERMINT								•					●			●						●			
PIPSISSEWA	●													•										●	
PLANTAIN	•								•					•									•	●	
PLEURISY ROOT										•						•						●		•	
POKE	●																								●
PRICKLY ASH	•									•						•									
PSYLLIUM																				●					
RASPBERRY	•									●				●											
RED CLOVER	●																								
RHUBARB	•													●											

	EMOLLIENT	EXPECTORANT	FEBRIFUGE	GALACTAGOGUE	HEMOSTATIC	HEPATIC	LAXATIVE	LITHOTRIPTIC	LYMPHATIC	MUCILAGE	NERVINE	NUTRITIVE	OPTHALMIC	OXYTOCIC	PARASITICIDE	PURGATIVE	RUBEFACIENT	SEDATIVE	SIALAGOGUE	STIMULANT	STOMACHIC	STYPTIC	TONIC	VERMICIDE	VERMIFUGE	VULNERARY
IRISH MOSS	●											●														
JUNIPER								•												•						
KAVA KAVA																		•					•			
KELP												●														
LADY'S SLIPPER											●							●								
LEMON BALM																		●								
LICORICE		●					●																			
LOBELIA		•									●															
LUNGWORT	●	●								●													•			•
MANDRAKE (AMERICAN)						●	●													•						
MARSHMALLOW	●							●				•														●
MISTLETOE (AMERICAN)											●											•				
MISTLETOE (EUROPEAN)																				●			●			
MOTHERWORT							•				●												●			
MUGWORT											●										●					
MULLEIN		●																								•
MYRRH	•																			•						
NETTLES	•			•								●														
OAT											●									•			●			
OREGON GRAPE ROOT							•																•			
PARSLEY		•									•												•			
PASSION FLOWER																		●								
PEACH							●				•							●			●					
PENNYROYAL																		•								
PEPPERMINT																		●								
PIPSISSEWA																							•			
PLAINTAIN	●	•																								•
PLEURISY ROOT		●									•												•			
POKE							•		●																	
PRICKLY ASH															•					●						
PSYLLIUM							●																			
RASPBERRY																				•			•			
RED CLOVER											•								•	•						
RHUBARB							●													•	●					

	ALTERATIVE	ANODYNE	ANTHELMINTIC	ANTACID	ANTIBIOTIC	ANTICATARRHAL	ANTIEMETIC	ANTIPYRETIC	ANTISEPTIC	ANTISPASMODIC	APERIENT	APHRODISIAC	AROMATIC	ASTRINGENT	CARDIAC	CARMINATIVE	CATHARTIC	CHOLAGOGUE	CONDIMENT	DEMULCENT	DEOBSTRUENT	DIAPHORETIC	DISCUTIENT	DIURETIC	EMETIC
ROSE											●			●											
ROSEMARY												●	·			●						●			
RUE										●															
SAFFLOWER																						●			
SAGE			·							●			·	●											
SASSPARILLA	●															●						·			
SASSAFRAS	●												●			●						●		·	
SAW PALMETTO									·															●	
SCULLCAP									·	●															
SENNA																								·	
SHEPHERD'S PURSE														●										●	
SLIPPERY ELM														·						●					
SPEARMINT										·			●			●						●		·	
SQUAW VINE														·										·	
ST. JOHN'S WORT	·												·	●										·	
STONEROOT														●										·	
TANSY			●																						
THYME										●	·					●								●	
TORMENTIL ROOT							·							●											
UVA URSI	·													●										●	
VALERIAN										●						·									
VERVAIN							●			●				·								●			
WHITE OAK BARK									·					●											·
WHITE WILLOW		●							●					·										·	·
WILD CHERRY BARK														·											
WILD YAM										·								●				·			
WITCH HAZEL														●											
WOOD BETONY	·											·													
WORMWOOD			●						·			·												·	
YARROW														●								●			
YELLOW DOCK	●													●				·							
YERBA SANTA														·											

	EMOLLIENT	EXPECTORANT	FEBRIFUGE	GALACTAGOGUE	HEMOSTATIC	HEPATIC	LAXATIVE	LITHOTRIPTIC	LYMPHATIC	MUCILAGE	NERVINE	NUTRITIVE	OPTHALMIC	OXYTOCIC	PARASITICIDE	PURGATIVE	RUBEFACIENT	SEDATIVE	SIALAGOGUE	STIMULANT	STOMACHIC	STYPTIC	TONIC	VERMICIDE	VERMIFUGE	VULNERARY
ROSE												●									●					
ROSEMARY																				●						
RUE																	●			●						
SAFFLOWER					●																					
SAGE																										●
SASSPARILLA																							●			
SASSAFRAS																				●						
SAW PALMETTO																		●					●			
SCULLCAP											●															
SENNA							●																		●	
SHEPHERD'S PURSE																				●						
SLIPPERY ELM	●											●														
SPEARMINT																				●						
SQUAW VINE																										
ST. JOHN'S WORT											●							●								
STONEROOT						●																				
TANSY																				●			●			
THYME		●													●											
TORMENTIL ROOT				●																		●				
UVA URSI																							●			
VALERIAN											●									●						
VERVAIN		●	●																							●
WHITE OAK BARK																										
WHITE WILLOW			●																				●			
WILD CHERRY BARK																		●		●	●		●			
WILD YAM																										
WITCH HAZEL				●														●					●			
WOOD BETONY						●					●				●											
WORMWOOD																								●		
YARROW				●																●						
YELLOW DOCK							●					●														
YERBA SANTA	●																			●						

There are two formula types to consider: One for acute ailments and one for chronic. We will first consider the formulas for treating acute diseases.

7 to 8 parts (70%-80%)	— Primary herbs
1 part (10%)	— Carminative (aromatic) - secondary
1 part (10%)	— Optional demulcent - secondary or
1 part (10%	— Optional stimulant, laxative or anti-spasmatic - secondary

The largest part of your formula is the primary herb or herbs. Generally, one to three herbs are chosen for this part. As was mentioned, herbs have several properties. Your main objective is to cover all the symptoms with the primary herbs and then choose the secondary herbs which have properties in common with the primary herbs to help support them by strengthening their properties. For example, a specific carminative is chosen because it has secondary properties that are in common with the properties of the primary herbs. You might be treating a kidney infection and your primary herb is uva ursi. Uva ursi is an antiseptic diuretic. In choosing your carminative, ginger would be a good choice because it not only has carminative qualities, but it is also a diuretic. Sometimes there may be additional symptoms that are not covered by the primary herbs. If this happens, make sure the secondary herbs are chosen with properties that will cover those symptoms. When one becomes experienced enough, there will not be any problem in finding primary herbs to cover all the symptoms present. Occasionally, when the primary herb or herbs are supported by one of the secondary herbs, and you want to choose another secondary herb that supports it indirectly, like choosing one that is a good blood cleanser or liver and kidney stimulant, this can be done.

The secondary herbs that you choose are determined by the symptoms present. That is why demulcent, stimulant, laxative, and anti-spasmodic herbs are optional. If the circulation is slow and sluggish, you will add a stimulant to the formula to help break up blockages. If there are spasms or tension in the body caused by the illness, an antispasmodic herb will be added. If the person is constipated, a laxative can be added. Laxatives are optional because they are usually taken alone, used for a short period of time.

If inflammations, ulcers, intestinal bleeding, and irritations are part of the symptom complex, demulcents are used in the formula. If there is no sign of the latter, then demulcents may still be kept in the formula as a small percentage, or deleted. Bitter herbs sometimes need a demulcent herb to make it easier on individuals with sensitive digestion. If the bitter herb must be tasted in order to produce a certain effect on the digestive glands and to aid intestinal secretions or as a tonic to the stomach, a demulcent is not necessary.

When using demulcents in formulas, sometimes more of this quality is needed. This is true especially when treating inflammations and ulcers. It is good to remember that roots have more of the demulcent property than leaves and if two parts demulcent is indicated, certain leafy herbs will not have enough, so roots would be a better choice.

Herbs have multiple properties. Let us say we are building a formula that calls for one part aromatic and one part antispasmodic. Some herbs have both these properties. Ginger and cumin are examples. Using either of these herbs will cover two properties in your formula. Instead of using 10% of the herb, you would use 20% because 10% of each property is needed.

The carminative or aromatic herb which is 10% of the weight of your formula is a constant. This is the only secondary herb that usually remains in the formula. It acts as a stimulant to the circulation, causes some inner heat, and aids assimilation of the formula.

Here are some guidelines you can follow in building a formula for acute diseases and chronic diseases.

a. Write out the symptoms and arrange them in order from the most primary, aggravating symptom down to the most minute symptoms.

b. Begin matching the healing properties of herbs to the primary and secondary symptoms. The chart in this chapter will assist you in doing this. Usually one to three herbs are chosen (70 to 80% by weight of the formula) to cover these symptoms. The percentage and weight of these primary herbs are determined by the symptoms. Instead of having all primary herbs equal parts, you may need more of one property than another. A larger percentage of that herb should be used.

c. Make sure all primary and most secondary symptoms are covered by the properties of your primary herbs.

d. Choose your secondary herbs so that they have properties in common with the primary ones. Secondary herbs that have other properties besides having one or more in common with the primary herbs can also be used. The body will benefit from these also.

e. In choosing secondary herbs you might find that all the properties of the primary herbs are already backed up and supported by other secondary herbs. In this case just pick a good secondary herb which will support the overall problem. A good blood cleanser is an example.

f. If emetic herbs are used in formulas, they should be buffered by sweeter herbs so no vomiting is induced. Licorice, fennel, anise are a few sweeteners.

g. When making formulas for douches, gargles, or for an external use, there is no set formula. Usually equal parts of the herbs are used and less if the herb is harsh or irritating (rubefacients)

h. Use a standard weight as one part. Ex: 1 part = 1 ounce; then 7 to 8 parts would equal 7 or 8 ounces; or 1 part = ¼ ounce, then 7-8 parts is about 2 ounces.

An example of a formula to treat a cold would be

	SYMPTOMS	PROPERTIES
Primary —	Cough	Antispasmodic
	Lung Congestion	Expectorant
Secondary —	Burning urine	demulcent, diuretic

Primary Herbs (7 parts or 70%)

3 parts or 30% — mullein-expectorant, demulcent; antispasmodic, astringent
2 parts or 20% — marshmallow-demulcent, lithotriptic, emollient, diuretic; alterative
2 parts or 20% — lobelia-nervine, antispasmodic, emetic; expectorant

Secondary Herbs (3 parts to 30%)

1 part or 10% — angelica-stimulant, carminative; expectorant, tonic, alterative
1 part or 10% — mistletoe (American)-antispasmodic, nervine; diuretic, emmenagogue, emetic
1 part or 10% — licorice root-expectorant, demulcent, laxative; alterative

Mullein was chosen because of its expectorant and demulcent primary properties. The demulcent property will soothe the kidneys and the expectorant property will help remove mucus from the lungs. It also has a secondary antispasmodic property to counteract the cough. Mistletoe with its primary antispasmodic nervine properties would be specific for cough, and it has diuretic secondary properties to influence the kidneys.

Marshmallow is an excellent diuretic with demulcent properties which will soothe the lungs and kidneys and counteract the burning urine. It is also lithotriptic which will aid in removing gravel in the kidneys. Lobelia is a powerful antispasmodic, nervine which was chosen to sedate the cough. It has a secondary property (expectorant) that will help remove excess mucus from the lungs.

All the primary and secondary symptoms are covered by the properties of the primary herbs.

The secondary herbs support the primary. Angelica acts as a stimulant and carminative, and supports the primary herb mullein with its expectorant property. Mistletoe supports the antispasmodic, nervine properties in lobelia and mullein. It also has diuretic properties which supports marshmallow root.

Licorice root is chosen not only for its demulcent, expectorant properties which support the primary herbs, but whenever an emetic is added to a formula, and you do not want to cause vomiting, it should be buffered. By this I mean balanced with a sweet herb like licorice root, fennel, anise seed, or cinnamon.

Another example of a formula for treating a cold which is an acute ailment:

	Symptoms	Properties
Primary —	chills	stimulant, diaphoretic
	fever	diaphoretic
7 to 8 parts (70-80%)	primary herb	boneset
1 part (10%)	carminative	ginger-secondary
1 part (10%)	demulcent	licorice root-secondary

When treating chills, a stimulant herb is needed to produce inner heat and increase circulation. To help break a fever, diaphoretic herbs are used to produce sweating.

Boneset is the primary herb. It was chosen because of its stimulating diaphoretic properties. Ginger was chosen to support the primary herb. It is also a stimulant, diaphoretic. Licorice root was chosen for its demulcent properties and to sweeten the taste of the formula. This is an example when the secondary herb, ginger, supports the primary herb, but licorice root does not. This is because the primary symptoms are already supported by ginger so licorice root can be chosen to benefit the body by its other properties. Licorice root is a good demulcent and a good herb to treat colds, flu, and fevers. It is sweet so it will make this formula taste better. Also, it is an alterative (blood cleanser) so actually, it is supporting the primary herb in an indirect way.

We will now discuss how to build an herbal formula for chronic diseases. Here is a basic formula to follow

  7 parts or 70% — primary herbs
  1 part or 10% — blood cleanser
  1 part or 10% — stimulant or carminative
  ½ part or 5% — stomachic (stomach tonic)
  ½ part or 5% — nervine

The treatment of a chronic disease should be one of a systemic approach. The whole body has been weakened by the illness. This is why diet and other therapies such as manipulations, massage, hydrotherapy, etc. are always used along with herbal therapy. It is important never to use an extreme in any therapy. The body should not be pushed in any one direction too fast. An example would be if a person was eating a junk food diet, you wouldn't advise a raw food diet immediately. The body would detoxify too rapidly and only become weaker. That is why we discussed ten therapies, and said that at any time a therapy may need to be changed to another therapy. If the body gets weak, you tone it up; if it gets sluggish, we use stimulation therapy. The energy level is always changing. This is important to remember while using a formula during chronic diseases. You might be using a formula to detoxify an individual and they begin getting weak. The formula may need to be changed to a more toning formula.

Basically the same rules are followed in building a formula for a chronic disease as in building one for an acute. The primary herbs (usually 1 to 3 herbs, more if needed) are chosen to treat the most specific (primary) symptoms. Then the secondary herbs are chosen to support the primary ones. Every property of the primary herb which is being used to treat a symptom should be supported at least once by a secondary herb. This means that a primary herb may have four properties covering four symptoms. Each secondary herb does not have to have all of its properties in common with the primary herb. It can have one or two in common with it as long as the properties of the other secondary herbs cover the properties that remain.

Ten percent of the formula is a blood cleanser (alterative). This is added to the formula to influence the healing activity of the whole body. If the blood is clean, the whole body will be effected. An herb is chosen that has one, two or more properties in common with the primary herbs.

Ten percent of the formula is a stimulant or carminative. If the body needs inner heat, a carminative is chosen. If body heat is normal, just add a stimulant. A stimulant helps raise the activity of the body, break through blockage, and increase circulation. A stimulant is also chosen to have one or more properties in common with the primary herbs.

Five percent of the formula is a stomachic (digestive tonic). The digestion is the first line of defense. A tonic will increase absorption of nutrients and the herb in the formula. The whole body benefits from good digestion. It is chosen to have one or more properties in common with the primary herbs.

Five percent of the formula is a nervine. The nerve energy is usually low during chronic diseass. It takes nerve power to digest, eliminate toxins, and every other function of the body. A nervine, like the blood cleanser, is chosen to aid the whole system. It should also have properties in common with the primary herbs.

Follow the same rules for building formulas for both acute and chronic diseases.

	Symptoms	Properties Needed
Primary	lung congestion (asthma)	expectorant
Secondary	skin eruptions	alterative
	burning urine	demulcent, diuretic

Your formula can look something like this:

Primary Herbs (7 parts or 70%)

3 parts or 25% — comfrey-expecorant, mucilage, demulcent; alterative
2 parts or 25% — elecampane-expectorant, diuretic, cholagogue, stomachic; astringent
2 parts or 20% — plantain-emollient, diuretic; expectorant, deobstruent, astringent, antiseptic, alterative

Secondary Herbs

1 part or 10% — pipsissewa-alterative, diuretic; astringent, tonic
1 part or 10% — angelica-stimulant, carminative, diaphoretic, emmenagogue; expectorant alterative, tonic
½ part or 5% — dandelion-stomachic, lithotriptic, hepatic, diuretic, cholagogue; astringent, alterative
½ part or 3% — lobelia-nervine, emetic, antispasmodic; expectorant

70% of your formula is the primary herbs which cover all the symptoms of the disease. The primary herbs can also be divided up into different percentages. Usually the herbs that have properties which treat the primary symptoms should be in large amounts. Comfrey and elecampane are 25% each because of their expectorant properties. Comfrey root is an expectorant which will help remove the lung congestion and the asthma symptoms. It also has major properties as a mucilage and demulcent which will treat the burning urine by soothing the kidneys. Comfrey root also has a secondary property as an alterative (blood cleanser) to help treat the skin eruptions. In treating skin problems, the blood must be cleansed because the skin is being used as an eliminatory organ.

Elecampane was chosen because it also has expectorant properties to treat the major symptoms but it also has a primary property as a diuretic which will improve kidney functions. It is also a good stomach tonic (stomachic) and will aid gall bladder activity (cholagogue).

Plantain has primary properties as a diuretic and emollient which will aid the kidneys and secondary properties like expectorant and alterative for the lungs and skin problems.

As a blood cleanser (alterative) pipsissewa was chosen because it has a primary property as a diuretic which supports the diuretic properties in the primary herbs to treat the kidney ailment.

Angelica was chosen as the stimulant because it has corresponding secondary properties such as expectorant, alterative with the primary herbs. So it acts as a good stimulant and supporting herb to the primary herbs.

Dandelion is an excellent stomachic, plus supporting diuretic, alterative properties.

Lobelia is good nervine, plus expectorant. Its antispasmodic property will aid in relaxing the lungs and other body parts.

Another example:

	SYMTOMS	PROPERTIES
Primary	blood in the urine (chronic, reoccuring)	diuretic, demulcent, astringent or hemostatic
Secondary	indigestion headaches (usually caused by indigestion)	stomachic

PRIMARY HERBS

25%-30%	— horsetail-astringent, diuretic, lithotriptic; galactagogue, nutritive
25%	— marshmallow-demulcent, diuretic, emollient; nutritive
20%	— dandelion-stomachic, lithotriptic, hepatic, diuretic, cholagogue, astringent, alterative

Secondary Herbs

10%	—Cleavers (Blood cleaner)-Alterative, astringent, diuretic; antipyretic laxative
10%	— cinnamon-stimulant, astringent, aromatic
10%	— elecampane-stomachic, expectorant, diuretic; astringent
10%	— lady's slipper-nervine, sedative, antispasmodic

Horsetail was chosen because of its astringent, diuretic, and lithotriptic properties. Its lithotriptic property will help remove any blockages in the kidneys, and the astringency will stop the bleeding. It has a secondary property as being an antipyretic. This is good and helps cool down any inflammations in the urinary tract. Marshmallow root was chosen because of its demulcent, diuretic qualities to soothe the kidneys and remove pain and inflammations.

Dandelion is an excellent stomachic to treat the indigestion, has diuretic and lithotriptic properties, and is a secondary astringent.

Cleavers was chosen as a blood purifier because it backs up the primary astringent, diuretic properties.

Cinnamon is both a stimulant and astringent. It will help the taste of the formula and aid in stopping the bleeding.

As a stomachic, elecampane was picked. It has diuretic plus astringent properties aiding the primary herbs.

The nervine is lady's slipper. Because all the primary properties were supported already by other secondary herbs, lady's slipper was chosen as a good nervine (tonic). Here is an example of not supporting the primary herbs directly by having properties in common with them, but indirectly with its sedative, antispasmodic properties. In treating a problem like this, there is sometimes tension both mentally and physically. So indirectly, by influencing the nerves, the whole body benefits. This is only done when the primary properties are well supported by the other herbs. Then try to choose an herb that seems to support the overall symptom complex of the disease.

In treating chronic diseases when the individual begins to improve, healing crises may manifest. In these cases continue on with your main formula and choose a single herb or put another formula together to treat the acute symptoms. When the symptoms are gone, stop the use of the added formula. This may have to be done several times. I have seen several healing crises take place in an individual within just a one or two month period. Tinctures are very convenient to treat unexpected symptoms. They absorb fast and the sick individual does not have to worry about making teas.

These formula formats are excellent to follow. However, not all of the formulas in the chapter "Comprehensive Therapies For Common Ailments" follow these suggested formats. This is due to the fact that once an individual becomes skilled in knowing the properties of herbs, slight changes can be made to suit specific cases.

DIET AND CLEANSING

One of the main reasons why therapies fail, whether herbal therapy or otherwise, is because the correct use of foods is not properly incorporated into the program. This difficulty is easily overcome if one understands the true meaning and use of a cleansing diet, proper food combining and a transition diet. A change from a traditional diet to a vegetarian or raw food diet is a progressive regime.

The bloodstream should receive vitamins, minerals, amino acids, fatty acids, simple sugars and water from the intestines; not poisons. When proteins are digested properly, their end products, amino acids, pass from the intestines to the blood. If proteins are improperly combined with other types of food, putrefactive bacteria ferment them into skatol, intol, phenol, hydrogen sulfide and other poisons.

When starches and sugars are properly prepared for assimilation by good digestion, their final stage is simple sugars called monosaccharides which the body uses without difficulty. But when starches undergo putrification from staying in the intestines too long, or when mixed with incompatible substances, they are broken down into acetic acid, alcohol and carbon dioxide. These by-products of putrification are absorbed into the bloodstream and affect muscle tissues, joints, organs, glandular ducts and genetically weak areas, causing tumors, pains, arthritis, gout, etc.

The main objective of dietary therapy is to learn how to adapt to stressful situations and purify your body, particularly the intestinal tract, so larger amounts of nutrients can be absorbed .The cleaner you are internally, the more you absorb, the less you need to eat. The more congested you are the less you absorb, the more you must consume. In a pure body, more energy can manifest while eating small amounts of food.

If an individual has the will, constitution, spiritual attitude and climate, he or she can evolve to a diet of raw fruits, sprouts, leafy green vegetables and small amounts of seeds and nuts. With this mentioned diet, I have overcome early signs of arthritis, thirty-three allergies, and achieved a weight loss of 85 pounds. It usually takes from one to three years for transition to an all raw food diet. This is very difficult if not impossible to do when living in a cold climate.

Elimination is an important process since the removal of waste products and toxins is an essential part of maintaining health. Whether changing to a lighter vegetarian diet or undertaking a fast, a purification diet will remove most of the surface waste and prepare the body for a better diet and other purification regimes.

During the cleanse, a variety of symptoms may manifest. Mucus discharge from the nose, lungs, kidneys and bowels can result. Vomiting, skin rashes, headaches and neuralgia may also occur. These are signs that the cleansing is taking place. Many people get enthusiastic about a pure body but give up when they get a little sick when the body releases poisons. It must be understood that it is better to rid the body of these obstructions and experience some acute symptoms now than let them remain within the body and cause a chronic disease later. If one takes the proper measures and uses enemas, exercise, takes warm baths, etc. these will aid the body in elimination and some of the adverse symptoms will not have to be experienced. Herbs can be used to counteract any possible symptoms that manifest. Refer to the sections on "Herbs for Specific Diseases" and "Diseases and Their Remedies" to determine the proper remedy. During the acute symptoms, herb teas, tinctures, etc. are usually taken every two hours.

If flatulence persists after a few days, this may sugggest that the diet is not quite correct, or improper food combinations are being used. Other problems could be a weakness in digestion and absorption or an imbalance in colon bacteria. Obviously, a cleaned out digestive system that does a good job of absorbing nutrients should not have fermentation producing gases.

PURIFICATION DIET FOR INNER CLEANLINESS

The purpose of this diet is to purify and cleanse the body. It may be used for a period of six to fourteen days, or longer if needed. Usually an individual that has been eating a diet with meat and refined, processed foods should start with a six day cleanse. A person who has been on cleansing diets before or is eating a vegetarian diet can use this cleansing diet longer. If adverse symptoms persist over a three to six day period, it usually means the body is very toxic and that shorter cleaning periods can be used with a progressive change in diet between cleanses. A good regime is to use a three day cleanse at the end of every month while improving your diet between cleanses.

Juices will help neutralize toxins in the body and aid their elimination through the kidneys and liver. Drink one or two cups of freshly squeezed fruit or vegetgable juice between meals. They should be taken one-half hour before or one hour after meals. It is good to dilute the juices with 25% distilled water or drink no more than four to eight ounces of the juice at one time. Chew your juices until most of the flavor is gone before swallowing. This is especially true if symptoms of diabetes or hypoglycemia are present.

If the juices cause gas or bloating, cut down the amount taken or delete them entirely. Vegetable broths or distilled or purified water can be substituted. Use enemas if gas and bloating is still a problem.

Liquid chlorophyll (the juice of green plants) is one of the best blood purifiers and nutritional supplements. Drink two ounces twice daily during this cleanse. It should be taken on an empty stomach one-half hour before or one hour after meals. If nausea or stomach upset is experienced, mix the chlorophyll juice with apple, orange or pineapple juice.

Enemas or colonics (see chapter on enemas) can be used during this cleansing diet, either in the morning, evening or whenever needed. When gas pains, nausea, bloating or a burning feeling is felt in the stomach or bowels, an enema is indicated. Add four ounces of liquid chlorophyll to two quarts of water, or use specific herb teas for enemas.

Herbs can be taken during this cleanse, such as blood purifiers and laxatives. It is important to use the herbs or juices specific for the problem being treated. If it is just a general clean-up, the diet with juices, broth and liquid chlorophyll suggestions are all that is needed.

Some of the symptoms that manifest during the cleanse, like nausea, headaches, burning feet, fatigue, etc. can be overcome by the use of foot baths, whole baths and cool baths. Directions on when and how to use them are given in the chapter on hydrotherapy. When there is body odor or minor skin problems, soak in a warm tub of water for twenty to sixty minutes with one to four pounds of epsom salts added. This bath will help draw out the poisons from the blood and take the stress off the liver and kidneys. Brush the skin after it is dried, with a natural bristle brush or loofa to activate the lympth flow and circulation. These can be purchased at your local health food stores.

During the diet we are about to discuss, try to rest as much as possible or do light exercises if you feel well enough. Skip a meal if the recommended foods are too much for you to eat. Everyone is a little different in the amount of solids and liquids they can handle. If a meal is skipped, substitute one or two cups of freshly squeezed juice in its place.

BREAKFAST

One-half hour before eating breakfast mix one heaping teaspoon of psyllium seed powder in eight ounces of orange, pineapple or apple juice. Drink this immediately or it will thicken. Psyllium seed powder may cause bloating. If this becomes uncomfortable, use an enema or herbal laxatives (cascara sagrada, turkey rhubarb or a cold infusion of senna tea mixed with a little ginger) for a few days until most of the surface waste clears from the colon.

For breakfast, eat fresh fruit. Eat at least one-half pound of one type of fruit or you may mix a fresh fruit salad consisting of two to four types of fruit from the list below (NO bananas or avocados).

Fresh, raw fruits, organically grown and eaten in season whenever possible may be used: apples, grapes, apricots, cherries, currants, figs, guava, mangoes, papayas, peaches, pears, ripe pineapple, oranges, grapefruit, plums, persimmons, berries, nectarines, etc. Melons of all kinds are permitted, but should be eaten by themselves, *not* mixed in a salad with other fruits. Dried fruits, organically grown and unsulphured and soaked to reconstitute: apples, dates, apricots, figs, peaches, prunes, pears, plums, raisins, mangoes, pineapple and papaya.

No coffee or tea are permitted. For best digestion, do not drink any liquid with meals.

LUNCH

One-half hour before lunch, mix one heaping teaspoon of psyllium seed powder in eight ounces of orange, pineapple or apple juice (use fresh juice when possible).

Fresh vegetable salad: make a chopped salad of fresh, raw vegetables. Use a dressing of cold-pressed olive oil and lemon juice. Oils are not necessary. Use just four of the vegetables listed below. If an individual is not used to raw food, too many different vegetables at a meal can be difficult to digest.

Use fresh, raw vegetables: artichokes, asparagus, beans, beets, brussels, sprouts, carrots, cauliflower, cucumbers, celery, dandelions, endive, eggplant, fresh corn, green peas, green peppers, kale, kohlrabi, lettuce (not iceberg), lotus, okra, onions, parsley, parsnips, pumpkin, radishes, rutabagas, salsify, spinach, sprouts (all kinds), squash (all kinds), swiss chard, tomatoes and turnips (of which you may use the leaves or tops also).

No coffee, tea, milk or beverages at lunch are permitted. Do not eat dessert.

DINNER

One-half hour before dinner, drink two cups of vegetable broth. This can be made up in advance and can be used hot or cold.

Vegetable broth: celery, carrots, beets, zucchini, parsley, onion, green peppers and ½ inch thick peelings of potatoes. Chop fine and simmer for one-half hour in distilled water. Strain and drink. You may add fresh garlic to taste when served.

Fresh vegetable salad: make a salad of fresh, raw vegetables from the list above, using cold-pressed olive oil and lemon dressing.

Steamed vegetables: select two or three vegetables from the list above and steam until crisp tender (about five minutes). Season with oregano, basil, dill, rosemary, thyme, or other unprocessed seasonings.

Bread: one medium slice of whole wheat bread, well toasted, or use unleavened bread (see recipe below). Eat the bread plain with nothing on it.

No coffee, tea or desserts permitted.

Two hours following dinner: mix one heaping teaspoon of psyllium seed powder in eight ounces of orange, pineapple or apple juice (use fresh when possible).

UNLEAVEN BREAD

Soak two or more cups of wheat berries (or rye) in four cups of distilled water for 12 to 18 hours. Strain off water and put soaked wheat into a jar with a stocking, cheesecoth or thin screen to cover the top. Rinse twice daily and leave upside-down to drain properly. On the third day grind sprouted grain in a wheatgrass juicer, meat grinder or a food processor. If desired, mix in onion or garlic powder, kelp, powdered sesame or caraway seeds.

A little ground flax seed or powdered psyllium seed powder can be added to the dough after the grain is ground to help bind the patties together.

Roll out into thin patties and sun dry for four to eight hours. They can also be dried by putting them on top of your radiator or in an oven on the lowest heat possible (below 120 degrees Farenheit) until dry.

After the cleansing diet, if an individual wishes to improve his way of eating, he can follow the directions given on one of the three following diets or slowly change his diet until he is eating only raw foods.

The first diet can be used as the first step toward a raw food diet or one can remain on it. The decision should be left up to the individual. The amount of raw food in this diet should be between 20% to 50%. A person can remain on this diet from four to six months if he decides to make the transition to diet number two.

DIET NUMBER ONE

BEVERAGES

Begin drinking herb teas such as peppermint and spearmint.

BREADS

Use whole grain breads. Try to avoid preservatives and artificial additives. If you are going to make your own breads, use whole grain flours from rye, wheat and corn meal (yellow or white).

CEREALS

Use whole grains. They may be toasted but avoid anything with white sugar or preservatives. Granola, oats, millet, corn meal, barley and wheat can be used. They can be cooked slowly in water or in a double boiler. You can buy them already ground or grind them yourself just before using them. There is a seven grain cereal that can be found in most health food stores.

DAIRY PRODUCTS

Use certified raw milk, cheese and yogurt. Eggs can be used three times per week. It is best to use dairy products only every other day. Whey can be used, added to fruit dishes or in juices.

Desserts

Fresh or canned fruits can be used. Avoid cakes, pies, candy, puddings and ice cream as much as possible.

Fats And Oils

Use unsalted butter and vegetable oils. Safflower, sesame, peanut, soy and sunflower oils can be used. It is best to buy these in health food stores.

Fruits

See the list in diet number two.

Grains

See the list in diet number two. Eliminate processed and refined grains.

Juices

Use unsweetened, frozen, canned or bottled juices. It is good to begin to drink fresh squeezed juices. Black cherry, carrot, concord grape, prune, apple, fig, pineapple and other juices, including vegetable juices, can be purchased in most stores.

Legumes

These can be soaked over night and then cooked slowly. Garbanzos, lentils, lima beans, dried beans, split peas, soybeans and navy beans are examples.

Meat, Fish, Poultry

Chicken, turkey and lean beef is allowed. Bake, broil or roast and only use them four times weekly. Eliminate frozen, canned or smoked meats. White fish, salmon and other ocean fish are good. Avoid canned or frozen fish.

Seeds And Nuts

Use unsalted, raw or roasted nuts, and avoid those sold with preservatives. Almonds, sunflower, sesame, brazil, cashew, chestnuts, pecans, pumpkin seeds and pine nuts are examples.

Vegetables

See the list in diet number two. Begin eliminating canned vegetables.

Salad Dressings

Health food stores have several dressings. Avoid preservatives. Lemon and honey is excellent.

Seasonings

Sea salt, paprika, cumin, cardamon, ginger, thyme, rosemary, basil, garlic, cayenne, oregano, sage, black pepper, dill, celery seed, coriander and tamari are examples.

Soups

Use home made soups made from vegetables and grains. Turkey and chicken can be added.

Sweeteners

Avoid white sugar and artificial sweeteners. Raw sugar, maple syrup, honey, date sugar and blackstrap molasses can be used in small amounts.

DIET NUMBER TWO

This diet is usually 50% to 75% raw food. It is an excellent diet to remain on or use as the next transition step to a raw food diet. An individual can remain on this diet from four to six months using short three to five day juice or water fasts to help purify the body and to prepare for a raw food diet.

Beverages

Herb teas such as mint tea, chamomile, alfalfa, red clover, chaparral, blue violet, rosehip and other natural herb teas; fig or dandelion coffee replacements, non-instant; sesame or nut milk, raw only, may be used. Use also "green drink" (green vegetable juices) and pure water.

Bread

Sprouted grain breads, millet, buckwheat, bran muffins, corn tortillas, any freshly ground or sprouted grains and whole grain crackers may be used.

Cereals

Millet, oats, yellow corn meal, brown and wild rice, whole barley, buckwheat groats, rye and wheat may be used. All should be freshly ground and soaked overnight in pure water or apple juice, then eaten raw or just barely cooked.

Seeds such as flax, chia, sesame, sunflower or pumpkin may be soaked with the grains or used by themselves soaked whole, in fresh apple juice overnight or longer in the refrigerator. They can be eaten raw if the individual has good digestion.

Desserts

Fresh, whole fruits, unsweetened fresh fruit salads may be used. Fruits dried without sulphur dioxide and soaked in pure water to reconstitute may be used.

Seaweeds

The powdered seaweeds can be sprinkled on salads, soups or other dishes. Seaweeds such as hijiki, kombu, wakame, nori, dulse, agar-agar, kelp and irish moss can be prepared by cooking them in soups or just soaking them for one hour and adding them to salads.

Fats And Oils

Avocados, cold-pressed crude oils such as olive oil, soy, sunflower, safflower, corn and sesame oil; all seeds freshly ground or soaked and used whole as cereal (flax, chia, sunflower, sesame or pumpkin seeds) may be used.

Milk

Coconut milk from inside fresh coconut may be used as is, or whizzed in a blender with pieces of fresh coconut and then strained to make coconut milk; keep chilled. Other seed and nut milks may be used.

Nuts

Moderate use of all kinds of fresh, raw, organically grown nuts is suggested. Almonds, filberts, pecans, pine nuts, brazil nuts and walnuts are especially recommended.

Buy fresh nuts in the shell, store in a cool place or freeze, then crack them just before using. Use coconuts, freshly grated only. Use fresh coconut milk in beverages.

Corn

Try the corn raw for a special treat, or lightly steamed.

Salads

Alfalfa, mung beans, radish, lentil or other sprouts, green leafy vegetables, grated or finely chopped raw beets, carrots, celery, potatoes and sweet potatoes, rutabaga, zucchini and other squash, cauliflower, cabbage, brussel sprouts, turnips, chard, kale, chicory, ripe tomatoes, romaine, cucumbers, buckwheat, lettuce (not iceberg), wheat grass (clipped), green peppers etc. may be used. All types of sprouts are recommended.

Potatoes, well scrubbed are best eaten baked, including the potato skins. Use raw slices as crackers with soup or spread with nut butter or avocado. Baked potatoes (eat the skin) or gently steamed with the jacket may be used.

SEASONINGS

Chives, parsley, garlic, sweeet basil and other herbs such as sage, thyme, cumin, savory, oregano, kelp and herb mix seasonings that contain no added sodium chloride are suggested. Cayenne, a healthful red pepper product, may be permitted.

SOUPS

Home made vegetable broths or instant bouillon may be heated, poured in the blender and add any raw vegetable you enjoy. Blend briefly and serve. Soups may be gently simmered using any vegetables.

SEEDS

Use sunflower, chia, flax, sesame and pumpkin.

SPROUTS

Use any fresh, raw or barely warmed sprouts such as alfalfa, mung bean, lentil, black radish, wheat, rye, brown rice, cress, clipped wheat grass and buckwheat (lettuce) sprouts. Add to salads, sandwiches and blender drinks.

SWEETS

Use raw honey and carob in limited amounts and on special occasions only.

VEGETABLES

Use all vegetables, raw preferred. As second choice, carefully and lightly cook with little liquid in stainless steel or ceramic pot with a vacuum sealed cover. Use every drop of the cooking liquid as it contains valuable nutrients. A steamer may also be used. Yams, string and wax beans, corn, leeks, lentils, lima beans and other dry beans (sprouted, then cooked gently below boiling to prevent gastric distress) eggplant, mushrooms (try them raw in salads as well as cooked), squash, artichokes and all vegetables listed for salads above are recommended.

If green vegetables are not in season, use sprouts generously and add to your diet a supplement from "green cereal grass juices" or use alfalfa tablets.

FRUITS

Use fresh, raw fruits, organically grown and eaten in season whenever possible. Apples, grapes, apricots, bananas, cherries, currants, figs, guava, berries, mangoes, papayas, peaches, pears, ripe pineapple, plums, persimmons, nectarines, quince, avocados etc. may be used.

Melons of all kinds are permitted, but should be eaten by themselves for a meal or snack.

Use dried fruits, organically grown and unsulphured. Soak to reconstitute apples, dates, apricots, figs, peaches, prunes, pears, plums and raisins. Fruit leathers (dehydrated fruit) are permitted when made without sugar—but a little honey may be used to sweeten any fruit to make fruit leather. Home-frozen fruits (without sugar) are permitted.

Juices

Use fresh, raw fruit and vegetable juices, made from organically grown products. Carrot with greens or smaller amounts of beet is most popular. You may select from young beet leaves, watercress, parsley, celery, potato, zucchini and other vegetables to be juiced and added to carrot juice for variety and nutrition.

Use no more than two ounces of parsley or beet juice daily. These juices can cause strong cleansing reactions.

Fruits to be used for juices include fresh apple, apricots, peaches, cherries, berries, watermelon (use green part and seeds too). Cranberry juice is especially helpful when made fresh and mixed with apple or other sweet juices. Soak dried fruits in pure water and drain juice to drink. Limited amounts of sweet juices such as grape or prune should be taken.

For weight reduction, use these low carbohydrate vegetables:

artichokes	chicory	mustard greens	spinach
asparagus	cucumber	okra	string beans
beet greens	dandelion	radishes	swiss chard
broccoli	eggplant	rhubarb	tomatoes
brussel sprouts	endive	sauerkraut	turnip tops
cabbage	escarole	(not canned)	watercress
cauliflower	leeks	sea kale	
celery	lettuce	sorrel	
chard	mushrooms	sprouts (mung, alfalfa, etc.)	

Foods to avoid

Beverages: coffee, black teas and other caffeine beverages, cocoa, milk, soft drinks, carbonated drinks and alcohol.

Bread: white bread or any bread made with white flour.

Cheese: avoid all cheese.

Desserts: all commercially canned or frozen fruit. All cakes, pastries, gelatin desserts, junkets, custards, sauces, ice cream and candy.

Eggs: avoid eggs entirely

Fat: any processed or preserved oily foods such as commercial grade nuts, seeds, wheat germ, all margarines of any kind, butter, solid and whipped fats of all kinds, cream and milk substitutes of all kinds. No exceptions. Avoid all iced milk and ice cream.

Meat: avoid all meats.

Milk: avoid milk, liquid and dried; canned or pasteurized. No imitation milk, ice milk or imitation ice cream. No coffee lightener or other chemical milk or cream substitutes.

Nuts: all roasted or salted nuts and nut butters.

Potatoes: french fried, grilled or potato chips.

Corn, rice, noodles and pasta: white rice and white flour noodles and other pastas.

Salads: avoid white macaroni salads, commercial gelatin salads, canned vegetables, cooked salad vegetables.

Seasonings: avoid harsh spices like black pepper, salt and mustard. These can irritate the intestinal tract once an individual becomes detoxed.

Soups: any commercial canned or frozen soups or soup mixes.

Seeds: roasted, rancid or salted seeds.

Sprouts: potato sprouts are poisonous.

Sweets: white sugar, brown sugar, raw sugar, candy, chocolate, maple syrup.

Vegetables: All sprayed and commercially canned or frozen.

Fish: avoid all fish.

Fruits: all commercially canned, frozen or dried fruits. All fruits with artificial coloring or sweetening added. Avoid saccharine or other artificial sweeteners. Avoid all canned juices and juices with artificial coloring or added sweetening. Avoid all "juice drinks".

During times of transition, avoid the foods that cause adverse effects. Eat small amounts of seeds and nuts. Sprouted grains are less mucus-forming than unsprouted. Do not try to make the transition too quickly. The large amounts of waste leaving the body can put undue stress on the liver, heart, kidneys and other organs. Use enemas, hydrotherapy, and teas to aid the body in elimination of these waste materials. An acute condition can be turned into a chronic disease by weakening the body through use of too rapid detoxification methods.

Find a health practitioner that will help you. Have patience, read and study health books and do not be narrow minded or hung up on one method or one person's procedures. Not all therapies work the same on everyone.

Dr. Thurman Fleet, Viktoras Kulvinskas, Professor Arnold Ehret, Herbert Shelton, Ann Wigmore, Dr. Jay M. Hoffman and Dr. Bernard Jensen are just a few who have written books that should be studied. Each of these people have studied the works of many others before them.

RAW FOOD DIET NUMBER THREE

The raw food diet is basically eating all fruits and vegetables raw (uncooked). All seeds and nuts are eaten raw also.

Grains such as wheat, rice, barley, oats and rye are sprouted for three days before eating. Beans such as mung, soy and garbanzos can be sprouted for three days. Seeds that are easy to sprout are fenugreek, alfalfa, radish and sunflower. Legumes like peas and lentils can also be sprouted.

This diet is similar to diet number two, except that the grains are sprouted and nothing is cooked. If there is a question as to which foods can be used in this diet, refer to the lists given in diet number two.

A raw food diet can be difficult for an individual if he or she does not have proper guidance or knowledge. To learn more about this diet, listed below are a few books that can be purchased which will give extensive directions on how to make the transition and give directions on sprouting and fasting which usually accompany a raw food diet.

Survival Into the 21st Century by Viktoras Kulvinskas, 21st Century Publishers, P.O. Box 702, Fairfield, Iowa 52556

Love Your Body by Viktoras Kulvinskas, 21st Century Publishers, P.O. Box 702, Fairfield, Iowa 52556

The Raw Foods Diet by Jim Karras and Carolyn Griesse, New Century Publishers, N.J.

Be Your Own Doctor by Ann Wigmore, Hemisphere Press, Inc. New York.

Off The Stove by Dorothy C. Walker, Westland Publications, McNeal, Arizona.

Add a Few Sprouts by Martha H. Oliver, Keats Publishing, New Canaan, Connecticut.

Mucusless Diet Healing System by Professor Arnold Ehret, Ehret Literature. Publishing Company, Beaumont, California.

The Science and Fine Art of Fasting by Herbert M. Shelton, Natural Hygiene Press, Chicago, Illinois.

Fasting as a Way of Life by Allan Cott, M.D., Bantam Books, Inc., New York, N.Y.

Fasting for Renewal of Life by Herbert M. Shelton, Natural Hygiene Press, Chicago, Illinois.

NATURAL FOOD COMBINING

Without normal digestion, all body defenses begin to weaken. Before any food can be used to build strength, stamina and body immunities, digestion must be normal. You can eat all the best foods, but if they are not properly prepared by the saliva and gastric juices, the body will soon wither and become diseased. Impacted bowels, pebbly stools, colitis, hemorrhoids, bloody stools and gas are just a few problems that exist when the food stagnates and rots if not broken down properly.

Anything that hinders digestive power, whether it slows it down or impairs the stomach's chemical discharges, will favor the growth of bacteria. Eating too fast, overeating, eating on the run, bad combinations or overuse of spices, drinking with your meals, fear, anger, pain, fever—all have hazardous results. Improper cooking and combining of foods can cause an upset stomach, kidney, bowel and skin problems and various deficiencies. Eating good foods does not guarantee health unless the basic rules are followed.

I believe that the most abused practice of eating is wrong food combinations. It seems to be universal and totally ignored because of lack of willpower and education. I have never been in a restaurant that served proper combinations. The new age has brought many health food eating places that are doing their best in proper preparation. I once asked a lady who was really into health and who owned a health food restaurant why she didn't serve properly combined dishes. Her answer was "nobody would eat them." This shows a lack of education.

During diets number one and two, the rules for food combining are not always followed. When foods are cooked, many times they are easier for an individual to digest and some of these rules do not have to be followed. Of course, for the best digestion, it would be advisable to follow them. Health practitioners understand that not everyone is interested in combining their foods properly and that it may not always be convenient. When an individual begins to follow better eating patterns, they can be overwhelmed with too many do's and don'ts and can easily become discouraged. These rules are for people who want to make the extra effort and for those eating a raw food diet. If someone is having digestive problems, gas, nausea, constipation and bloating, these rules should be investigated and practiced to see if improper food combining is the problem.

GOOD FOOD COMBINING HABITS

1. Avoid combining any of the following in one meal:

   Protein rich foods
   High starch content foods
   Fats
   Sugars
   Fruits

2. Combine leafy green vegetables, non-starchy vegetables and sprouts with only *one* other allowed category at one meal:

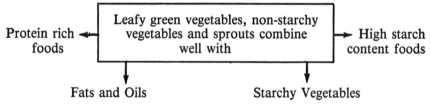

3. Avoid combining fruits and vegetables at one meal.

4. Avoid combining sub-acid fruits with sweet fruits at one meal.

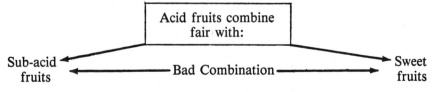

5. Eat melons alone.

RULES TO AID DIGESTION

1. Avoid drinking liquids twenty minutes before meals, during meals and for one hour following meals as liquids dilute the digestive juices and hinder digestion.

2. Avoid drinking liquids which are too cold (out of the refrigerator or with ice) or too hot (close to the boiling point) since the temperature extremes stress the digestive system and may cause indigestion.

3. Since most dessert items do not combine well with foods eaten at meals, it is best to avoid them.

4. Eat only when hungry.

5. Avoid eating immediately before or after strenuous exercise.

6. Avoid eating when under physical or mental distress.

7. Thoroughly masticate and salivate all foods and juices.

8. Avoid overeating.

9. Avoid eating three to four hours before retiring to bed. Especially avoid eating fruit at night as it is very stimulating and can cause a wakeful, unpleasant night's sleep.

The following food lists will help you in proper food combining and indicate whether a food is a protein, starch, fat, etc.

1. PROTEIN RICH FOODS

Combines Best With Leafy Green And Non-Starchy Vegetables

DAIRY[1]

EGGS[1]

FISH[1]

MEAT*

NUTS: (raw)

Acorns, dried	Filberts
Almonds	Hazelnuts
Beechnuts	Hickory Nuts (Carya)
Brazil Nuts	Macadamia Nuts
Butternuts	Pecans
Candlenuts	Pignolias
Cashews	Pine Nuts
Chestnuts, dried	Pistachios
Coconuts	Walnuts

POULTRY[1]

SEEDS: (raw or sprouted)

Chia
Pumpkin
Sesame
Sunflower

FERMENTED FOODS:

All fermented seed and nut sauces,
yogurt or cheeses

MISCELLANEOUS:

Avocados***
Brewer's Yeast$_1$
Dried Beans
Dried Peas
Miso$_1$
Nutritional Yeast$_1$
Olives
Peanuts* (very difficult to digest)
Soybeans$_1$
Tofu[1]

  *Not recommended.

 **Combines well with ripe sub-acid fruit, leafy green vegetables and
   sprouts.

***Combines well with tomatoes, also.

 [1]Use in diet number one only.

2. FATS AND OILS

Combines Best With Leafy Green
And Non-Starchy Vegetables

AVOCADOS**

FATS*:

Butter[1]
Cream[1]
Fat Meats*
Lard*
Margarine, Vegetable[1]
Tallow*

HYDROGENATED OILS*

MOST NUTS: (raw)

Brazil Nuts
Butternuts
Candlenuts
Filberts
Hickory Nuts
Pecans
Pinion Nuts
Walnuts, English

OILS: (cold-pressed oils only)

Cottonseed Oil
Corn Oil
Nut Oils
Olive Oil
Safflower Oil
Sesame Oil
Soy Oil
Sunflower Oil

*Not recommended.

**Combines well with tomatoes, also.

[1]Use in diet number one only.

3. HIGH STARCH CONTENT FOODS AND SUGARS

Combines Best With Leafy Green
And Non-Starchy Vegetables

BREADS (sprouted or Essene breads are best)[1]

CEREALS AND GRAINS: (cooked[1] or sprouted)

Barley
Buckwheat
Corn
Flaxseed
Millet
Oat
Rice, Brown or Wild
Rye
Sorghum
Wheat

DRIED BEANS AND PEAS: (cooked[1] or sprouted)

Azuki Beans
Chick Peas (Garbanzos)
Green Peas
Kidney Beans
Lima Beans
Pinto Beans

PASTAS[1]:

Spinach
Spirulina
Whole Wheat
Vegetable

PEANUTS* (very difficult to digest)

POPCORN

SYRUPS AND SUGARS*:

Brown Sugar
Candy
Cane Sugar or Syrup
Carob, Roasted or Raw[1]
Chocolate
Date Sugar

Fructose
Honey, Raw[1]
Maple Syrup[1]
Milk Sugar
Molasses, Blackstrap[1]
White Sugar

MISCELLANEOUS:

Corn Germ[1]
Wheat Germ[1]

*Not Recommended.
[1]Use in diets number one and two.

4. STARCHY VEGETABLES

**Combines Best With Leafy Green
And Non-Starchy Vegetables**

Cooked or raw:

Mushrooms	Acorn squash
Artichoke	Parsnip
Banana squash	Potatoes
Beets	Pumpkin
Butternut squash	Rutabaga
Carrots	Salsify
Cauliflower	Squashes (winter)
Corn	Sweet Potatoes
Hubbard squash	Yams
Jerusalem artichoke	

5. GREEN, LEAFY AND NON-STARCHY VEGETABLES

Combines Best With Proteins, Fats And Oils, Starches Or Starchy Vegetables

Cooked or raw:

Asparagus	Mint:
Bamboo shoots	Mullein
Beet tops (greens)	Mustard greens
Broccoli	Okra
Brussel sprouts	Onions
Buckwheat lettuce	Parsley
Cabbage (white, red, Chinese)	Peppers (red or green)
Celery	Radishes

Chicory
Chives
Collard greens
Corn (green)
Cow slip
Cucumbers
Dandelion greens
Eggplant
Endive
Escarole
Garlic
Green beans
Kale
Kohl rabi
Leafy greens
Leeks
Lettuces:
 Bibb
 Boston
 Leaf
 Romaine

Radish green
Rhubarb
Scallions
Seaweeds
 Dulse
 Kelp
 Nori
 Wakame, etc.
Sorrel
Spinach
Squashes (summer)
Sunflower greens
Swiss chard
Turnip tops (greens)
Watercress
Weeds
Wheatgrass
Zucchini

SPROUTS (do not cook)

Alfalfa
Cabbage
Fenugreek
Lentil
Mung bean
Mustard seed
Radish
Red clover

6. SUB-ACID FRUITS

Combines Fairly With Acid Fruits

Apples
Apricots
Blueberries
Cherimoyas
Fresh figs
Grapes
Guavas
Huckleberries
Kiwi fruits

Mangoes
Nectarines
Papayas
Pears
Sweet apples
Sweet cherries
Sweet peaches
Sweet plums

7. ACID FRUITS

Combines Fairly With Sub-Acid Fruits Or Sweet Fruits

Blackberries
Grapefruit
Kumquats
Lemons
Limes
Oranges
Pineapples
Pomegranates
Raspberries

Sour apples
Sour cherries
Sour grapes
Sour peaches
Sour plums
Strawberries
Tangerines
Tomatoes**
Ugli

**Combines best with avocado, leafy greens and sprouts.

8. SWEET FRUITS

Combines Fairly With Acid Fruit

Bananas, dried** or fresh
Dates, dried** or fresh
Dried fruits:**
  Apples
  Apricots
  Cherries
  Currants
  Figs

Papaya
Pears
Peaches
Pineapple
Muscat grapes
Persimmons
Prunes, dried** or fresh
Raisins**
Thompson grapes

**Always soak before eating to hydrate.

9. MELONS

Combines Badly With All Other Foods. Best To Eat Alone.

Banana Melon
Cantaloupe
Casaba melon
Christmas melon
Crenshaw melon
Honey balls

ENEMAS

When an enema is properly applied, the benefits will be felt almost immediately. Here are several conditions that can be helped by enemas:

1. Headaches due to reabsorption of fecal matter.

2. Constipation.

3. Gas caused by bad food combinations, overeating or the eating of poisonous foods.

4. Abdominal pains and cramps (warm water should be used).

5. Acute disease, fevers and all mucus conditions.

6. Hemorrhoids. In this case the water that is injected into the bowel will soften the hardened waste and cause an easy release without irritation.

7. All toxic blood conditions. The blood cannot be cleaned if poisons in the bowel are not removed first.

8. To medicate diseased conditions of the rectum, signoid or colon.

The bowel must be clean in order to have a clean bloodstream. Poisons are absorbed into the blood from the bowel and can cause a continuous toxic condition. When toxic blood, kidney, liver and skin conditions are treated without first cleaning the bowel, these conditions will persist because of the toxic absorption. Cleaning the bowels will get to the root of the problems. When the root or the cause of disease is not removed, and only the symptoms are treated, it is called a "palliative" treatment.

Water injected into the bowel softens, dissolves and carries away the hardened mass. As a rule, during fevers, the water used in an enema is cool or slightly below body temperature. In bowel diseases, it can be cool or lukewarm, and during constipation it should be warm.

Distilled water is the best to use for enemas, instead of using chlorinated water from the tap. Herb teas can also be used in enemas to treat specific conditions. Prepare them as you would any herb tea (see chapter on herbal preparations). For example, if there is mucus clinging to the sides of the intestines, astringent herbs in tea form dissolve and strip the mucus from the walls. White oak bark, red raspberry and bayberry are some of my favorites. For heavy mucus conditions another good remedy is to add two tablespoons of apple cider vinegar to two quarts of warm water and inject into the bowel and retain for 15 to 30 minutes.

If gas is a problem, mint, fennel or catnip teas can be used. If the bowel is bleeding, chlorophyll or mucilagenous herbs (such as comfrey root) mixed with astringent herbs are excellent. Liquid chlorophyll can be purchased in most health food stores or freshly made by juicing parsley, wheat grass, spinach or other green grasses and leafy vegetables.

Spasms are very frequently present in a toxic bowel. For this, antispasmodic teas such as black cohosh and chamomile are good. In many cases, a weak bowel is present. Piles, hemorrhoids and prolapsed colons are weak tissue diseases. Cool water and tonic herbs such as white oak bark, red raspberry and yellow dock are used in these cases. After the bowel is cleaned with two or three injections of cool water, inject a cup of cool water in the bowel and sleep with it, retaining the fluid until morning. This will cause the weak tissues to contract and strengthen. Astringent and tonic herbs like witch hazel and red raspberry injected cool and held overnight has produced complete cures in just a few treatments.

Hardened fecal matter that has been stored in the bowel pockets for years is one of the most difficult cases. Here we use two cups of olive oil to one quart of warm water, retained for 15 to 30 minutes, while lying on a slant board, or with the hips elevated. Massage the bowel while lying in that position. The olive oil will loosen and dissolve the hardened mass.

When a liquid is retained in the bowel for any length of time, the therapy is called an "implant" or "retention enema". These can be held overnight if nature doesn't insist on evacuation. One of the most valuable is the wheat grass retention enema (usually the amount of a retention enema is two ounces of wheat grass juice in two cups of water). Anemia and other blood conditions have been cured through chlorophyll, herb tea and juice implants. Always remember: before a retention enema is employed, wash the bowel first with a water injection to eliminate wastes and thus prevent them from absorbing into the bloodstream. While giving an enema you are liquifying the poisonous matter in the bowel which makes it easier for reabsorption, so it must be removed first before the implant.

A two quart enema bag can be purchased at most drug stores. After filling the bag with the liquid of your choice, hang the container about five feet above your body. Put olive oil or an herbal salve on the syringe and rectum. Before inserting the syringe into the rectum, open the clamp on the rubber tubing to release the air until a little water comes out. If this precaution is not taken, the air will cause discomfort in the colon.

The person should assume a knee-chest position during this procedure.

Get down on your knees on a rug, keeping the hips high, lowering your shoulders and head. One shoulder and one side of your face will be touching the rug. Those who are weak or bedridden can lie on their backs with their hips elevated ten to twelve inches higher than their shoulders.

Inject the water while in this position. Two quarts can be injected into the bowel at one time for an adult. If there is discomfort, pains, pressure that is unbearable or cramps, stop the water running into the bowel by clamping it or holding a kink in the hose. If the pain continues, this means you have obstructions and the water that is already in the bowel should be released. Continue this process until the bowel is clean enough so you can get two quarts of water into the colon. Persons who have been eating many animal foods and denatured cereal products (in which case a thick coat of mucus will be adhering to the colon wall) should repeat the enema daily for up to seven days. In these cases, olive oil, apple cider vinegar or flax seed tea enemas can be used which help to loosen the heavy mucus coat. Sometimes three or four enemas will have to be used before two quarts of water can be retained.

Once the bowel is cleaned you can administer and hold two quarts of water from the kneeling position, remove the syringe and lie on your back with your hips elevated. A slant board is excellent for this and especially when working with debilitated organs and prolapses. Massage the bowel for five to fifteen minutes. Rubbing the abdomen helps to break hardened matter loose. Then switch and lie on the right side so the fluid flows into the ascending colon where the appendix is. Here is where much of the trouble begins: appendicitis is due to the long retention of feces putrifying and poisoning the appendix. Return to the toilet and release the water. Repeat the enema until the water released is clear.

The procedures for using enemas to treat specific conditions are presented below.

INFECTIONS, PUS AND GANGRENE

Add thirty drops of myrrh and echinacea tinctures to one quart of warm water. Inject into the bowels and hold as long as possible. Use the teas as injections if the tinctures are not readily available. Take these two tinctures internally also for this condition, fifteen to twenty drops in one-half cup of water three to four times daily. This is a good treatment for any inflammation or pus disease of the intestines but can also be used for these conditions found anywhere in the body. This can be repeated every hour after pain.

Garlic enemas. Oil of garlic can be prepared by peeling and crushing eight ounces of garlic, placing it in a wide mouth jar with just enough olive oil to cover it. Cover it tightly, shake it several times a day. Let it set in a dark place for three days. Press and strain it through an unbleached cloth.

An alternative preparation would be to let the solution set in the sun for four to eight hours. Use this when it is needed in a hurry.

Use four tablespoons or more of garlic oil to one quart of water for worms or other infections and use as an enema. Retain for fifteen to thirty minutes and release.

MUSCLE TENSION AND FEVER

If the body is tense and feverish, add fifteen to thirty drops of lobelia tincture, boneset or pleurisy root tinctures or extracts to the warm enema water or use nervine and antispasmodic teas. If these are given to children, eliminate the lobelia or use one-third the amount.

POOR CIRCULATION

For slow circulation, use warm water enemas (as hot as one can stand), add five drops of cayenne tincture, ten drops of ginger and fifteen drops of myrrh to one quart of water. Repeat every hour if needed.

This enema is also good to raise low body temperatures and help break fevers and bring on a resolution of the disease (including the healing crisis).

APOPLEXY AND CONVULSIONS

During meningitis, lockjaw, apoplexy and convulsions, the enema can be a powerful tool. Use thirty to sixty drops of an antispasmodic tincture (such as lady's slipper) to a quart of warm water. It should be retained for fifteen to twenty minutes and repeated every two hours. Other good nervines can be used. For faster effects, ten to twenty drops can be added to four ounces of water, injected into the bowels and retained for as long as possible. Follow this treatment with warm water fomentations over the stomach and spine, or warm, whole body baths.

INTESTINAL INFECTIONS, DIARRHEA OR BLEEDING

In dysentery diarrhea, pus diseases, bleeding or infections, use astringent herb teas as enemas or add thirty drops of tinctures of bayberry, wild cherry bark, witch hazel or white oak bark to two quarts of lukewarm water. Retain as long as possible. Repeat this every one or two hours if need be. If there is inflammation involved, use twenty drops of echinacea in the water, or make the enema out of slippery elm tea and add suggested tinctures.

Whenever there is pus present coming from open sores or from the intestines, add thirty drops of tincture (or a tea) made from myrrh.

WASTING DISEASES AND ANEMIA

In wasting diseases and anemia, first wash the bowel with an enema made from goldenseal tea or with thirty drops of echinacea tincture added to the enema water. Then put four to eight ounces of wheat grass juice or liquid chlorophyll, herb teas, broths or other juices freshly squeezed into the enema bag. Lie on a slant board, trunk raised so all the juice flows into the colon. Retain for twenty minutes or longer. Check the initial urge to expel juice by applying pressure with the fingers between the anus and the sexual organs. Expel the juice within thirty minutes. These enemas are of benefit in treating all chronic diseases.

Enemas can be used in treating just about every acute or chronic disease. Many times they bring faster results than by taking oral remedies, and they can greatly assist the action of all other herbal preparations.

HYDROTHERAPY

Hydrotherapy (water therapy) is not a modern therapy. Hippocrates 500 years before Christ wrote about his experiences with the water cure. Ancient Egyptians used baths for all illnesses and held them in high regard for their curative effects. The Persians and Greeks built magnificant public buildings where the whole population could come and soak for health maintenance, cleanliness, circulatory disease and other probems.

I have chosen to explain this therapy because it is effective by itself, and is proven to be of great benefit when used along with herbal therapy. Water therapy is simple and can be applied immediately in case of emergency.

The skin is connected to every organ in the body via the nervous system and circulatory system. By changing the skin temperature with water applications that are hot or cold, nerve sensations will stimulate or sedate specific systems and organs. Raising and lowering temperature of the body will help break up congestion and facilitate elimination and circulation.

Disease does not exist without some kind of disturbance in the circulation. All organs receive a certain amount of blood flow. When the flow is interrupted, we have congestion, chills, fevers and disease. Whether using local applications or whole baths, cold water applications reduce the amount of blood, while hot applications draw blood to the surface of the body. If there isn't enough blood in an area (usually caused by accumulation of toxins or mucus) a hot water application is used, and at the same time cold packs can be applied to another area to decrease blood flow. This is often done to help increase circulation in one part of the body.

At this point it is good to remember that a fever is a natural body defense and is not to be suppressed by cool water applications. We use cool water only to bring down the fever if it gets too high (102 degrees and above). This is a general statement because some people are stronger than others and can handle a 104 degree temperature without any problem.

The local areas—legs, lower back, etc. when there is excessive heat and inflammation, cool water treatments are used for immediate relief. Cold water applications, applied locally or to the whole body (baths) will give temporary relief, but afterwards, the opposite reaction will bring blood rushing back to the area, raising the temperature again. Cold water is very seldom used because of this rapid rebound reaction. There are situations when cold water is used and this will be discussed later in this chapter.

When there is congestion in certain areas and lack of circulation, the blood must be drawn to the area to increase activity and elimination. Alternating cool and warm packs (and fomentations) continued for one-half hour to one hour will achieve indicated results. One minute of the cool and ten minutes of the warm, repeated four times twice daily is usually enough. If the individual bring treated is strong, this therapy can be repeated every two hours.

Most painful conditions are caused by overfilled blood vessels and capillaries putting pressure on the nerves. This in turn causes sluggish circulation and a build-up of toxins in the vessels, capillaries and lymphatics. Warm applications will relax the area, increase circulation, release nerve pressure and remove waste accumulations. Taking specific herbs internally will aid this part of the therapy (see the chapter on "Herbs for Specific Diseases"). Once the pain is relieved, switching to alternating cool and warm fomentations will tone the circulatory system and help eliminate any remaining poisons.

When treating a headache, cool water fomentations can be applied to the forehead and back of the neck, reducing the blood flow. At the same time, using warm foot baths will draw the blood downward, away from the congested forehead and back of the neck, reducing the blood flow. This type of therapy can be applied in many congestive illnesses.

To sum up the effects of hydrotherapy, cold water contracts the blood vessels, decreasing the amount of blood flow, followed by a rapid return of warmth and blood. If cold is continued for long periods of time, the area of the body being treated will become bloodless, so use brief cold applications to bring relaxation and warmth. Cool water applications are used for longer periods of time to slightly lessen blood flow, but warmth, relaxation and circulation will return and is not as shocking to the system.

Hot water applications are used to increase circulation and body temperature. They are used when there is not enough blood in an area. As with the cold water, effects differ according to the duration of application. After a hot application the blood is brought to the surface with a fast retreat to the interior. Warm baths increase circulation and have less of a shock to the body and the blood does not retreat as fast from the surface. Warm baths are mild and soothing. Hot baths are stimulating.

Alternating hot and cold applications causes a back and forth return of blood and circulation which can be used to decongest an area.

As can be seen, there are many ways of administering water therapy. This chart will give the specific temperatures, duration of time and effects of hydrotherapy

TEMPERATURE/DURATION HYDROTHERAPY CHART

Temperature	Duration	Effect
Very cold, 32-43° F.	A few seconds, only under supervision	Tonic
Cold, 40-60° F.	30 sec. to 2 min.	Tonic, shocks nervous system
Cool, 60-72° F.	30 sec. to 3 min.	Invigorating; improves circulation
Tepid, 80-90° F.	5 to 7 min.	Cleansing; lowers fevers, cools inflammations
Neutral, 92-95° F.	½ to 1 hour	Refreshes; aids burns
Warm, 90-100° F.	15 to 30 min.	Equalizes circulation; reduces pain, softens skin
Hot, 100-105° F.	8 to 10 min.	Relieves pain; aids neuritis, gout, arthritis, rheumatism and skin eruptions
Very hot, 105-110° F.	A few seconds to a few minutes	Relaxes; reduces muscle pain/spasms, dilates blood vessels, raises blood pressure

This chart was taken from **The Grosset Encyclopedia of Natural Medicine** by Robert Thomson.

RULES FOR HYDROTHERAPY

1. Always use a thermometer to test the water temperature—never guess. The proper treatment depends on the proper temperature.

2. When treating old, debilitated and nervous people, do not use extreme temperatures. Between 80 to 102 degrees are usually the specified limits.

3. Always wait two to four hours after meals before a water treatment.

4. Cold baths (50-60° F.) should always be of short duration. If cold packs or fomentations are used for specific areas, they can be used more often and the treatment can be longer if the patient's condition allows it. The colder the water, the shorter must be the time of employment (see Temperature/Duration Hydrotherapy Chart). The body must be as warm as possible before taking a cold bath. Weak patients should begin at 80 degrees, then gradually reduce by 5 degrees day by day. If you cannot warm the patient before the cold bath or application, warm water should be used first or have them drink warm diaphoretic herb teas.

5. If the patient is chilly after the cold bath, rub them with towels or your hands until warm. Otherwise, no drying is necessary. Have them dress while wet and go to bed so that the natural body heat and circulation will be stimulated to dry the bed clothes.

6. All sick rooms should be well ventilated, but avoid direct drafts.

7. If exhaustion or weakness is felt after water therapy, rest at least forty-five minutes. Otherwise, walk or exercise slightly if indicated.

8. During menstruation, extreme temperatures should be avoided. Use more warm treatments during this time. 98 to 102 degrees is a good range.

Applications Of Hydrotherapy

Sitz Bath. The sitz bath is often called the hip bath. A large tub or a common bath tub can be used for the treatment. Usually the head and feet are out of the tub while the middle body, including the abdomen, is submerged in water. The body parts that are out of the water are usually kept warm by heavy blankets.

If the patient's temperature is above normal, the water should be kept between 90 to 95 degrees Farenheit. If the temperature is normal or the patient is healthy and can stand colder water, the temperature can range from 60 to 70 degrees Farenheit.

This cool sitz bath is used usually twice daily from one to ten minutes. The first thing in the morning and before bed are the suggested times. It is especially good for people who do not sleep well. It is used for all bowel problems, especially for releasing gas. Other uses are for piles, genital and urinary diseases, dysentery, constipation, diarrhea, congestion or infections in the pelvic region, stomach aches, hemorrhoids, uterine complaints and to tone the pelvic organs. If there is poor circulation and congestion in the pelvic area such as constipation, tumors, cysts or urine retention, alternating cool and warm sitz baths may work better than either cool or warm used alone.

Herb teas can be made up first and added to the water. Use the herb that is specified for the condition being treated. Shave grass tea is good for bladder and kidney problems; oat straw tea for gout and hay flowers for stagnant bowels, exterior swellings, ulcers, constipation and spasmodic conditions of the bowel and stomach. Usually one gallon of herbal tea is added to the bath water.

The Cool Whole Bath. A regular bath tub is used for this procedure. The whole body except the head and neck is submerged in the water a half minute to two minutes. The temperature is usually body temperature or slightly below. Whether this bath is given to healthy or sick individuals, ten minutes is plenty. This bath should never be taken when any part of the body is cold or shivering. Beforehand, have the patient walk or exercise to warm the body. If this is not possible because of weather conditions or the person is too sick, use warm baths and diaphoretic herb teas to raise the body heat. If perspiration is present, it is even better. Cool baths given to a warm body only strengthens the individual and its reactions bring more heat into the system.

These baths should be done exactly as the directions specify. Many people have remained cold because of excessive duration of the cool bath.

After the patient is perspiring, or at least the body temperature is raised above normal, the patient goes into the water, trying to cover the whole body except head and neck. Before getting out of the tub, the patient dips his neck into the water, then immediately gets out of the tub and dresses without drying. The person should then begin to walk or exercise to bring the warmth back. A strong constitution will warm without exercise. This is best done outside or in a ventilated room. This bath can be used once a week.

Cool full baths are not only used to strengthen the body, but should be administered during all fevers, such as during typhus, or any mucus or catarrh condition. Vinegar (usually one cup) can be added to the water to increase skin cleansing, help open pores and to strengthen the individual.

Cool baths are used in all hot diseases. Water extinguishes fire, and the whole body is involved when a fever is present. Every time the fever blazes up, the cool bath can be administered. Soon the fire will be under control. Cool baths are used to lower fevers when absolutely necessary.

The Warm Whole Bath. This bath is used for both the healthy and the sick. The tub is filled and the whole body except head and neck is covered. The person may remain for fifteen to thirty minutes. At the end of the bath, the patient quickly dips his body in another tub filled with cool water. The temperatures should be agreeable to the condition. If another tub is not possible, a cool "sponge bath" or shower is rapidly given. The cool water treatment should never last more than one minute. The clothes are put on quickly without drying the body. Exercise is taken to bring warmth back to the body for at least fifteen to thirty minutes in the fresh air. If this is not possible, it can be deleted or the patient may be given a body rub or towel dried.

A second way of taking this bath is by alternating warm and cool baths with two tubs filled—one small tub with cool water for the sponge bath and another one filled with warm water for a whole bath. Three repetitions of each may be used. These are used when there is congestion, energy blockages and slow circulation. The contrasting temperatures are usually hot—100 to 110 degrees and cold—40 to 55 degrees Farenheit.

Ten minutes in warm
One minute in cool
Ten minutes in warm
One minute in cool
Ten minutes in warm
One minute in cool

This therapy is always finished with a cool application. For people afraid of the cool water, shorter times can be used, but should be increased as body stamina builds. Exercise and dressing while wet follows the triple water treatment.

Warm baths alone, without the cool bath following, weakens and relaxes the system, leaving the pores open so as to be sensitive to cold weather. The cool bath closes the pores, brings heat slowly back to the surface and tones the skin. These baths work excellently together for the simple reason that the warmer the bath at first application, the better the body can stand the cool one.

The lukewarm baths are usually recommended for weakened conditions such as gout, cramps, rheumatism, retention of urine and pain in the urethra and bladder. At first when there is pain or infection, start with warm water and as the pain decreases, use cooler water to strengthen the area. The temperature at the start ranges from 98 to 100 degrees Farenheit and the temperature is reduced by 5 degrees every two days until 60 to 72 degrees is reached. Cool and cold water applications are much more strengthening and beneficial.

To the aged and weak, recommended temperatures should be slightly below body temperature (92 to 95 degrees) and the duration of time taken is twenty-five minutes. The individual will feel quite renewed from the stimulation provided to the circulation and increased activity of the skin.

A hot full bath is usually indicated in illnesses such as neuralgia, sciatica, gallstones and colds. This will reduce chills and produce perspiration. Diaphoretic teas are taken immediately before the bath to help induce perspiration. Elder flower, peppermint and yarrow tea taken hot will produce this effect. Remember always to finish with a cool bath or a sponging treatment if the patient is not chilled and has the strength to endure such a measure. Cool compresses on the head and neck are indicated for weak and heart troubled people during the hot water bathing. This will avoid faintness and headaches.

The hot bath is usually taken first thing in the morning and before bed, or whenever needed to induce sweating.

Foot Baths: Cold Foot Bath. A vessel should be used that is deep enough to cover the legs up to the knees. The temperature of the water should be 50 degrees or less and the soaking never lasts longer than one to three minutes.

Cold foot baths are used to treat sprains, swellings of the feet, to stimulate circulation and to act as a tonic to the whole body to help develop resistance to disease. It is proven by reflexology that every organ in the body has nerve endings in the feet. Therefore, foot baths affect the whole system.

The alternating hot and cold foot bath is used for headaches, toothaches, colds, head and sinus congestion, ovarian congestion, suppressed menstruation, poor circulation to the pelvis and abdomen, infections of the feet, old foot injuries and insomnia. During these conditions, cool packs can also be applied to the area that you are trying to decongest.

Warm Foot Bath. Many times I have seen individuals who could not tolerate herbs or other cold water remedies and were forced to turn to warm foot baths. Excessive drug ingestion or illness can leave a person very sensitive to other methods of healing.

Temperatures to be used are between 90 to 100 degrees and followed by a cool application for one minute. The warm foot bath is used to overcome congestion in the upper part of the body, to prepare for a cold bath or cold water treatments and for circulation problems.

The hot foot bath leads the blood to the feet and helps to draw out impurities. It is excellent for painful menstrual periods, pelvic pains and suppressed menstruation. For blood poisoning, sore feet, gout, corns and tumors a handful of epsom salts can be added to the hot water for drawing, cleansing and dissolving purposes. When trying to draw the blood to the feet with hot or warm baths when trying to decongest the upper body, never follow the warm with the cold. Remember the cold drives the blood away from the area and you would only be undoing your purpose of the treatment. But for cleansing and stimulating, alternating warm for three minutes and cold for one minute is suggested. Always finish with a cool bath. In the case of drawing out impurities when using epsom salt, the soaking time is usually twelve to twenty-five minutes, finishing with a cool bath.

Leg Baths. This bath is useful in treating ulcers of the legs, swollen ankles and knees, varicose veins, heart palpitations, head congestion, neckaches and headaches.

Standing in water up to the calves or kneeling, are the two ways this bath is taken. If the patient is too debilitated to stand or kneel, have them sit on the edge of the tub or put a small stool in the tub. Have them sponge their legs with cool water for one to three minutes. Use the same rules as with the rest of the baths.

Eye Bath. The face is usually dipped in water with the eyes open for fifteen seconds and repeated four to five times.

The cold eye bath is excellent to strengthen the eyes for people who do much studying and eye exertion. Jethro Kloss in ''Back to Eden'' suggests using cool or cold applications when the membrane that covers the eyeball is inflamed and to use warm washes if the cornea or pupil is troubled. Herb teas such as eyebright, fennel and goldenseal as eye baths amplify the results.

A general cool or cold bath three times weekly strengthens and rebuilds both exterior and interior eye parts.

Here is a treatment for drawing mucus out of the eyes, such as with boils, sores or styes. Two vessels are needed—one vessel with cold water and the other with a warm tea. The face is kept in the warm water for thirty seconds to a minute; then dip in the cold water for a few seconds. Repeat this ten times, two or three treatments daily.

Sinus Bath. The temperature of sinus baths should be tepid warm. Never force water with a syringe into the nose; this could push substances into the eustacian canal.

In chronic catarrh, colds or thick mucus congestion, warm water or herb tea is put into a teaspoon or the palm of your hand and drawn up into the nose while keeping the mouth shut. Goldenseal tea is excellent for this. Sometimes a little lemon juice or salt is added to the water. This application can be repeated three to five times daily, depending upon the condition or sensitivity. The water or tea is usually kept around 70 degrees Farenheit. Once this liquid has been snorted up through the nostrils, it will usually end up in the mouth and can be ejected.

Ear Baths. The ear baths are taken to remove hardened wax and other substances—inflammations and abscesses. Ear injections are usually given with a small rubber syringe, holding the ear while the head is tilted over a tub or vessel. Be sure not to insert the syringe into the ear too far, and only use this therapy when absolutely necessary.

Tea is sometimes used between the temperature of 70 to 84 degrees Farenheit, four to six applications daily. The injection should not be used with too much force so as to damage the eardrum. Chamomile and goldenseal teas are used in case of inflammation. Dr. John Christopher often suggested warm, distilled water mixed with apple cider vinegar (10 parts water to one part vinegar) as a remedy to clean out infections and wax. Three to six drops of sweet almond or olive oil have been used as ear drops twice daily and the ears flushed with warm water and apple cider vinegar on the third day. This is good for cramps in the ears, sharp pains in the ears and humming in the ears.

HYDROTHERAPY USING BANDAGE TO TREAT HEAD, NECK, KNEES, ANKLES, CHEST AND LEGS

Bandages are used to treat specific areas when baths are not possible, or when treating invalids and when a water therapy is needed to be applied to an area over a long period of time.

A suitable vessel is filled with water or an herb tea. The herbs used are usually cleansing herbs, tonic, stimulants, nervines or a combination of your choice.

A piece of linen, soft cotton, muslin or wool is used. Cut the material into strips wide enough to overlap the area being treated by at least two inches on all sides. Make the wrap long enough to go around the area three to six times. Pin or tie the wrap in place, then cover with a large plastic bag or heavy blanket to keep the heat in, if you are using warm water therapy. This is usually indicated when wraps are left on for one-half hour or longer. Remember to use the proper temperature and duration of time as indicated on the chart.

Oils, tinctures and volatile oils can be added to the water to increase the activity. A good example is one that I have seen work several times for arthritic joints. Boil two quarts of water, then turn the stove off. Add fifteen to twenty-five drops of stimulating wintergreen or eucalyptus oil to the hot water. Soak the bandage in the water and wrap the area in need. Cover this with a heavy woolen towel. Change it when it gets cool. If warm wraps are indicated, don't let them get cold.

After the wraps are removed, massage the area with rapid movement if it is not too tender. Do not expose the area to extreme outside temperatures and rest until the circulation is normalized.

This wrap will reduce inflammation, pain and swelling. If the body part is feverish and hot, use cool water wraps.

All bandages and water therapy are intended to prevent excessive blood flow to certain areas or to increase blood flow (depending upon the temperature used). They are also used to reduce heat and to draw blood away from congested areas. The wonderful thing about using bandages and other modes of hydrotherapy is that warm bandages around the body part will draw blood to that area, while at the same time a cold wrap applied to another body part will decrease the flow to that area. This is used when you want to direct the blood flow toward specific areas. For example, during kidney inflammations, cool water packs applied to the kidneys, while at the same time warm wraps are applied to the lower extremities (legs, thighs, etc.) will draw the blood away from the kidneys to help reduce pain and congestion.

For information on the proper temperature and duration of time see the previous hydrotherapy chart when using bandages and wraps.

BANDAGES

Body Part	Indications
Head	Circulation to the scalp
	Dandruff
	Eye and ear diseases
	Head ulcers
	Dry scalp eruptions
	Head colds
	Deafness
Neck	Throat inflammations
	Difficult swallowings
	Infections
	Fevers
	After singing and lecturing

Chest and Back	Remove chest mucus
	Bronchial congestion
	Pneumonia
	Sore breasts
	Fevers
	To draw blood away from head and sinus areas to decongest them
	Good for headaches
Foot	Remove heat during fevers
	Cold feet
	Gout
	Sweaty feet
	Tired feet
	Athlete's foot
	To draw blood from the upper part of the body
Knee and Leg	Drawing heat away from the upper body
	Tired legs
	Intestinal gas
	Circulatory problems
	Edema
	Ulcers

HOMEOPATHY

Homeopathy is a therapeutic system of medicine developed by Dr. Samuel Hahnemann in Germany around the year 1796. Homeopathy, from the Greek words "homoios" and "athos" means similar affections. This therapy is based on the principle that any drug which is capable of producing symptoms of disease in healthy individuals will remove similar symptoms in a diseased individual. Thus we have the theory that like cures like, also referred to as the "law of similars."

Medicinal activity is a distinct property of all drugs. Whether the drug extract comes from plant, mineral or animal, each has stored within substances that, when prepared and taken internally, produce characteristic effects. These effects are discovered when the medicine is given to a healthy person in varied large doses. Both physical and mental symptoms produced by the drug are important in homeopathic medicine. Varied quantities of the same medicine produce different effects. A teaspoon of ipecac causes vomiting, while a drop will cure the same. Large doses of opium cause constipation, small doses have the opposite effect. This antagonistic physiological effect between large and small doses is made use of in homeopathic medicine.

Hahnemann found that a very small dose of a remedy prescribed according to the law of similars produced better results than larger doses. He found that larger doses were more aggravating to the sickness, which led him to the theory of potentization. Potentization is a controlled process of successive dilutions alternating with shaking, which may be continued to the point where the resulting homeopathic remedy contains no molecules of the original substance. Lesser dilutions are called "low potencies," greater dilutions are called "high potencies." The higher the dilution, the greater the potency. Thus, "potency" refers to the number of times that the remedy is diluted and shaken or triturated. An example of this is arnica, which is an extract from leopard's bane, a somewhat toxic plant. The standard plant extract is known as the "mother tincture"; it is mixed with *nine* parts of water/alcohol mixture and shaken ten times with sharp downward motions. The result is a 1x potency. 1x indicates the number of times the remedy was diluted by a factor of ten and shaken. Then one part of this 1x solution is taken, mixed with *nine* parts water/alcohol mixture, shaken ten times; it is called 2x potency. This process can be continued until the medicine contains only trace amounts (minimal essence) of the substance and is referred to as "energized medicine." A substance may be potentized 200 times. Higher potencies are considered more powerful and work at deeper levels than lower potencies. The potency to be used depends on the condition of the patient.

If the medicine is insoluble in water, the pharmacist grinds the substance to powder, called trituration, mixes one part powder with *nine* parts lactose or "milk sugar ' It is ground for *one hour* to produce 1x potency. One part of this mixture is added to *nine* parts milk sugar, ground for *one hour* are marked 2x. This process is then continued as necessary to produce the desired potency.

Homeopaths believe that the body is always striving for balance and a healthy state. When the body is threatened by harmful factors, the vital force within the body produces symptoms of pain, fever, mucus, etc. The purpose of these symptoms is to restore balance. Symptoms are always changing; this is referred to as a dynamic condition. Homeopaths determine the treatment on the basis of the symptoms, not the disease. This is contrary to the orthodox medical view, where disease is looked at as an entity unto itself, separate from the power within the body, and the symptoms are considered as products of the disease. Both in naturopathic and homeopathic medicine, it is believed that the same power within the body produces health and produces disease (symptoms) which is the curative process. All body parts are interrelated, therefore the whole body is treated, not just an individual organ or tissue.

In prescribing homeopathic remedies, all the symptoms, both mental and physical are grouped. These symptoms are matched as closely as possible to the symptoms that were produced in healthy persons by large doses of the best chosen remedy. In the Homeopathic Materia Medica, each remedy is described by a list of the symptoms it produces, and hence the symptoms it treats.

Standard dose in acute ailments is usually every two to four hours. Following accidents and during painful periods the intervals of taking the remedy is shortened, depending upon the urgency of the situation. In violent acute conditions such as severe neuralgia or tissue inflammations, it may be necessary to repeat the dosage every few minutes. During an earache, the dose may be every fifteen minutes. The remedy is given until improvement is noted and then stopped, or the intervals between doses may be lengthened. If the remedy is the right one and is given in the appropriate potency, an effect on acute ailments is usually noticed within fifteen to thirty minutes. It is of paramount importance to learn to wait for the action of the remedy. Excessive use of a remedy may result in aggravation, producing the symptoms once again after it has cured them.

If the patient reports improvement and a sense of well being, even though painful symptoms are not completely relieved, the remedy is acting curatively and should not be changed. A short aggravation (healing crisis) followed by improvement indicates that the remedy is well chosen and is acting curatively. A prolonged aggravation with slowly developing improvement is a sign that the patient is borderline and still has the reactive power but the potency was too high and the initial stimulus too strong. A brief amelioration followed by aggravation denotes the wrong remedy. A prolonged aggravation with decline of the patient may mean too high a potency or that the case is incurable.

Aggravation following a certain remedy should include only symptoms that have already existed. The appearance of new symptoms is noted when the remedy is the wrong one, when the potency is too high, too low or too frequently repeated. The remedy should be discontinued. Homeopaths usually give single remedies in order not to confuse the symptomology.

In taking remedies, put the medicine directly under the tongue and let it dissolve. Only the person taking the remedy should touch it. Eliminate coffee and tobacco; these may neutralize the remedy. Take the remedy in a clean mouth free from food, toothpaste, drink, mints, mouthwash, etc. Some practitioners use homeopathic remedies and herbs together during treatments for specific ailments. This is usually an accepted practice by many skilled physicians.

In the chapter on remedies for specific ailments, I make mention of homeopathic remedies. If there is any question on the application of these, refer back to this chapter or to other sources on the subject.

COMPREHENSIVE THERAPIES FOR COMMON AILMENTS

In the preceeding sections of this book, I have explained to you the methods of diagnosis and therapy that can be applied to any individual. I almost always recommend combining the different types of therapy: diet, enemas, hydrotherapy, homeopathy, and internal and external applications of herbs, in order to achieve a quick, and reliable resolution of the disorder. In this chapter, I supplement the general suggestions with some specific examples of therapies that have proven to be greatly successful through years of experience. In many cases, I list several alternatives that you might use, and you can choose among them on the basis of availability of the materials and convenience of application. Also, should one method prove unsuitable for your particular case, an alternative can then be tried.

Among the ailments mentioned in this chapter are some which are quite severe, including cancer, apoplexy, peritonitis, and heart disease. It is understood that the person interested in using these natural therapies for such ailments will also remain in close consultation with a competent health practitioner. Many people, after consulting with their physicians are told that there is nothing that can be done ("you have to live with it"), or are provided with simple palliative treatments which have no curative effects. In such cases, the use of the natural remedies described here is particularly appropriate. Other times, medical intervention is essential, but naturopathic remedies can be utilized simultaneously, or afterwards during the recovery phase (and to prevent recurrence).

ABSCESSES

Principal Therapy - blood purification.

Use the cleansing diet in this book. Clean the bowels with an enema once weekly. Continue on a vegetarian diet avoiding meat, dairy products, refined food and heavy starches. Three day juice or water fasts once monthly are indicated.

A. *Internal:* Take one of the following:

Echinacea - capsules or tablets
Chaparral - capsules or tablets

Take two echinacea *or* two chaparral capsules every two hours until the inflammation subsides. Then reduce dosage to two capsules, three times each day.

Drink three cups of red clover tea daily.

B. *External:* Make a poultice out of powdered:

2 parts slippery elm
1 part comfrey leaves
1 part plantain
½ part cayenne

Mix herbs with warm water and make a paste. Spread on the affected area and cover with a natural fiber cloth (cotton). Apply a heating pad, if desired.

Another good poultice is slippery elm and bran poultice. Make a slippery elm poultice by mixing slippery elm and warm water together. Then mix powdered bran with water, then add to slippery elm. Apply to boils and cover with hot towels. This can be left on for hours or overnight.

C. *Hydrotherapy:* Take alternating warm and cool showers morning and evening. Dry brush the skin daily. If showers are not possible, take whole cool baths at 20 minute durations in the evenings.

ACIDITY

Principal Therapy - blood purification.

Use the dietary, herbal and hydrotherapy suggestions under arthritis. Between meals drink a strong tea made from goldenseal or agrimony. These teas will regulate stomach acidity and tone the digestive organs. If needed, use digestive enzymes.

A. *Internal:* Take 6 to 10 alfalfa tablets with every meal.

3 parts dandelion
1 part sassafras
1 part celery seed
¼ part ginger

Add a teaspoon of this mixture to one cup of boiling water. Cover and steep for 20 minutes. Strain and drink. Three cups daily will aid the liver and kidneys in ridding the body of excess acids.

Eat plenty of ripe oranges, beets, celery, okra, cucumbers, apples, coconut milk, green vegetables, turnip greens, carrot juice and liquid chlorophyll.

Note: Study tonification therapy in this book, and see the use of this therapy under Allergies.

ACNE AND SKIN DISEASES (See Dermatitis, Eczema)

Principal Therapy - blood purification, stimulation.

This problem is caused by eating too many refined starches, fried foods, high protein consumption, dairy products and the use of sugar. The skin is being used to throw off the excess waste which the kidneys and liver aren't able to handle.

Use the cleansing diet in this book for 7 to 14 days with an enema for the first three days in the diet. Drink celery, carrot, beet and apple juices. These juices should be made fresh and taken three times a day in 8 ounce measurements. Drink distilled or purified water. Study the section in this book on foods to use and foods to avoid. Remain on a low fat, low protein diet, high in complex carbohydrates, avoid canned and refined foods. Keep the bowels moving twice daily with fruits and high fiber foods.

A. *Internal:* Mix the following herbs together:

> 2 parts red clover
> 1 part echinacea
> 1 part nettles
> 1 part burdock root
> 1 part dandelion root
> ½ part licorice root
> ½ part ginger

Powder herbs and put into #00 capsules. Take two capsules three times each day, or make an infusion and drink one cup three times each day. Get plenty of fresh air and vigorous exercise to induce sweating.

When first starting on a cleansing program, it is good to drink some kidney purifying teas to assist the body in eliminating toxic acids. Buchu, parsley, celery seed and goldenrod are good.

Also use teas made from sassafras, dandelion, sarsaparilla and burdock seed. Combine or use individually.

B. *External:* Facials using clay, carrot poultice, avocado skins or raw honey are good.

Eucalyptus, thyme and wintergreen can be used in steam. Boil 2 quarts of distilled water and add 2 ounces of herbs. Cover head with a heavy towel and lean over the container. Caution—always turn stove off before leaning over the container.

C. *Hydrotherapy:* Take hot and cold showers daily. Three times a week soak for 20 minutes in a hot tub with 2 to 4 pounds of epsom salts or kosher salt added to the water. Rinse well and rest when finished. Keep the skin stimulated with skin rubs, massage, exercise, sunlight and fresh air. Steam and sauna baths are excellent.

HERPES SIMPLEX, HERPES ZOSTER (Shingles)

Principal Therapy: - blood purification, tranquilization

A. *Internal:* Make a tincture using:
   2 ounces oregon grape root
   1 ounce chaparral
   1 ounce echinacea
   ¼ ounce prickly ash bark

   Mix the four ounces of herbs in one pint of vodka. Let it stand in a cool, dark area for fourteen days, shaking twice daily. Strain on the fourteenth day through a fine cheesecloth. Put the tincture in a dark, tightly capped bottle.

   Dosage: Take one teaspoon three times a day in warm water, or one tablespoon morning and night.

B. *Internal:* (for pain)

   Make a tincture using four ounces of kava kava to one pint of vodka. Follow the same directions as given above.

   Dosage: One teaspoon three times daily. The night dose is most important to help relieve pain during sleep. Also paint the sores with this tincture at night to relieve any irritation.

   Note: If nervousness persists, take one teaspoon of valerian root tincture in one cup of warm water when needed. Also drink herb teas made from hops, lady's slipper, vervain, or other antispasmodic herbs.

   Note: If the first tincture mentioned cannot be made, take two chaparral tablets, and alternate them with two goldenseal tablets every two hours.

C. *External:* Boil two ounces of uva ursi for five minutes in a gallon of water. Let cool. Add this to bath water which should be cool, about 70 degrees or lower. Soak one-half hour morning and night.

D. *External:* The eruptions can be painted with black walnut tincture, or a strong decoction made from equal parts of marigold and kava kava. Then soak a wool or cotton cloth in the decoction and foment the area.

E. *External:* Ice packs will also relieve pain and itching.

F. *External:* (Salve)

   Make a salve out of marigold, goldenseal and myrrh. Use equal parts of each herb. (See directions on how to make salve in section "How to Use Fresh and Dried Herbs".) Cover skin eruptions with salve.

If the eruptions are not bothersome, do not apply anything, just keep them dry.

Note: Once in a while, some people may be sensitive to one of the above treatments. This is why I have suggested a few different ways to treat this disease.

Diet: It is most important to use a cleansing diet (see cleansing diet) and short three-day fasts, using green drinks like parsley, spinach, wheatgrass, spirulina, and green magma. Carrot juice is also good for all nerve problems. Dilute carrot juice with 25% distilled water. Too much sugar will irritate the nerves and cause fatigue.

Remain on a vegetarian diet which will aid in preventing the recurrence of infections. B vitamins are necessary for the proper functioning of the nerves. Taking calcium will help relax the system and alleviate pain.

Keep the bowels clean daily with a warm water enema every day for the first five days; then once a week until the condition clears.

Foods to Avoid: Refined sugars and starches, jams, ice cream, eggs, red meats, fish, fowl, foods which have preservatives in them, fats, oils, fried foods, milk, cheese, all white flour products, nicotine, coffee, tea, alcohol, etc.

Foods to Include: Parsley, sprouts, bee pollen, brewer's yeast, sunflower and sesame seeds, garlic, apples, celery, carrots, lemons, wheat germ, coconut, oats, carob, onions, kelp, dulse, chives, limes, wild rice, watercress, millet, sprouted grains, almonds, all ripe fruits and melons.

Caution: Use only small amounts of citrus—and it must be tree ripened or avoid them.

Note: With venereal herpes, refrain from sexual intercourse and do not wear tight pants, pantyhouse or synthetic underpants. Wear cotton clothing, especially to bed at night.

ADDISON'S DISEASE

Principal Therapy - blood purification, tonification. Follow the dietary, herbal and hydrotherapy suggestions under Hypoglycemia.

A.   *Internal:* Two cups of celery juice daily will supply the needed sodium and help eliminate excess uric acid. Make vegetable broths made from vegetables that are high in sodium and magnesium. Eat foods high in B-complex. Sprouted grains, wild rice and rice bran syrup are excellent. Siberian ginseng, or a good panax ginseng extract (ten drops morning and night) are two botanicals that are excellent toners to the adrenal glands. Usually four siberian ginseng capsules daily (two twice daily between meals on an empty stomach) is sufficient. Give one day rest from all supplements.

Raw glandular therapy has been very successful using both raw pituitary and adrenal gland. Consult a qualified therapist to help determine the proper dosage and duration of time if glandulars are used. These are not supplements that should be taken over long periods of time.

Note: It is good to rest as much as possible and avoid all kinds of stress.

ADENOIDS (Swollen) (Tonsilitis, Quincy)

Principal Therapy - blood purification.

Do a three to five day fast on diluted citrus juices (25% distilled water). Then use the cleansing diet in this book until all symptoms disappear. Clean the bowels with an enema three consecutive days.

A.   *Internal:* Drink herb teas such as red clover, sassafras, and burdock root, three cups daily.

Take myrrh/goldenseal capsules, two every two hours until symptoms subside. Then maintain a dose of two capsules three times daily. Echinacea or chaparral can also be used.

Gargle several times daily with goldenseal tea. For all glandular swelling, echinacea and myrrh tinctures are specific, fifteen to twenty-five drops every two hours until swelling subsides. Poke root tincture, five to ten drops three times daily is excellent.

B.   *External:* See neck bandages.

AFTER BIRTH PAINS

Principal Therapy - tranquilization therapy.

A.   *Internal:* Fast on vegetable broths and freshly squeezed juices until the pains are gone. Use herbal formula B under Menstrual Cramps. Also see antispasmodic tincture. If this tincture is available, take twenty-five drops in one cup of warm water every one-half hour.

> Wild yam, cramp bark and black haw are specific remedies for after birth pains and cramping throughout the pelvic area. It is best to use these in tincture form fifteen drops every hour. A decoction of one or more of these with 1/5 part ginger added to them taken in two ounce doses every hour or two will also work, although tinctures will work much faster.

B.   *Hydrotherapy:* Use warm, whole baths until the pain subsides. Hot fomentations put over the area after a warming liniment has been rubbed into the skin works very well.

Reflexology given immediately will relax the patient and relieve the pain. Once the pain is relieved, use a castor oil pack for one hour.

AGE SPOTS

Principal Therapy: blood purification. Deobstruent (use liver [hepatic] herbs to clean out liver obstructions).

Use the cleansing diet in this book. Continue on a vegetarian diet using plenty of raw foods (60% of diet), raw fruit and vegetable juices. Clean the bowels weekly with an enema. The main objective is to keep the blood clean and restore normality to the liver.

A. *Internal:* Use formula A under Arthritis, Gout and Rheumatism. Use formula B under Liver Problems, Indigestion, Jaundice, Hepatitis.

If these combinations cannot be made, drink three cups of tea daily made from dandelion, goldenseal, red clover, parsley root or burdock root. Combine these in equal parts or use them separately.

B. *Hydrotherapy:* Use cold, whole baths.

ALCOHOLISM

Principal Therapy - blood purification, tonification.

The patient should be put to bed and kept away from his habit. The use of enemas and diaphoretic teas followed by warm, whole baths which should last twenty minutes should be utilized. Bed rest should follow the bath. This will cause the body to sweat off the toxins. Keep the skin active with cool baths and alternating hot and cold showers. Brush the skin before baths and showers. Use towel rubs after to dry the skin.

Use a cleansing diet of fruits and vegetables—plenty of broths and distilled water. Alcohol robs nutrients from the body and weakens digestion. Keep the food easy to digest. Steamed and baked fruits and vegetables are good. Berries of all kinds are excellent blood and liver cleansers—use them freely. Carrot, beet, celery and apple juices will help clean the liver. Use foods, juices and herbs that cleanse and stimulate the liver functions.

A. *Internal:* Alcoholism causes many vitamin and mineral deficiencies so the use of nutritive herbs should be employed. Infections could develop because the body resistance is low, so keep close watch on the patient.

Chaparral tablets or capsules will help clean the liver; two every two hours until the alcohol craving is gone. Alterative herbs (blood cleansers) such as plantain, red clover, oregon grape, sassafras and yellow dock can be put into combinations. These teas should be taken freely to stimulate elimination.
2 parts plantain
1 part parsley leaves
1 part yellow dock
1 part fennel

Boil one pint of distilled water, turn stove off and add one ounce of herb combination. Steep for twenty minutes. Strain, drink three to six cups daily. Counseling is sometimes necessary in chronic cases of alcoholism.

ALLERGIES

Principal Therapy - blood cleansing, tonification (stomach). Clean the bowels with an enema weekly. Go on a three to five day fast using carrot, beet, celery, and apple juice. Then continue with the cleansing diet in this book for one to three weeks. After this avoid meats, wheat, any refined foods, salt and other toxic substances.

Use one tablespoon of bee pollen from your home town daily. Take digestive enzymes before meals.

A. *internal:* Use formula A under Acne and Skin Diseases. Use several of these herbs in tea form if all of them cannot be found. Drink three cups daily.

Tonification Therapy. After the cleansing diet, use bitter stomach tonics to help build the system. Wormwood, goldenseal or gentian are excellent. Add honey and small amounts of licorice root if the bitterness cannot be tolerated.

> 1 part wormwood
> 1 part goldenseal
> ¼ part licorice root
> ¼ part ginger

Simmer one ounce of herbs for ten minutes in one pint of water. Strain, drink one-half cup three times daily on an empty stomach.

B. *Hydrotherapy:* Use alternating hot and cold showers for five minutes morning and night. Also use nose baths or head bandages (see hydrotherapy).

AMENORRHEA

Principal Therapy - blood purification, stimulation, dietary.

By amenorrhea we understand the suppression of the menstrual discharge after it has once appeared.

Use the same cleansing and dietary suggestions as mentioned under menopause. Drinking two ounces of beet juice mixed with apple and carrot juice will help bring on the menses. It is important to use foods high in iron which will act as a tonic to the system. All green drinks, especially fresh parsley juice daily (two to four ounces), are excellent.

A. *Internal:* If the problem is chronic and has existed for some time, the whole system must be toned and purified. Use the dietary suggestions under menopause, along with cool, whole baths and alternating hot and cold showers daily. The formula suggested under menopause is excellent for chronic conditions. Drink ginger tea whenever cold, or just to increase circulation and tonicity. Be sure to exercise outside every day.

If nervous symptoms manifest, study the formulas under Nervousness and Insomnia. Warm, whole baths are good for all nerve problems.

If the problem is acute, brought on by sudden shock, coldness or a sickness, use warm foot baths and a tea made from equal parts of boneset and pennyroyal, taken hot while the feet are soaking. Hot ginger foot baths are excellent for this.

B. *Internal:* another good formula is as follows. Mix together the following:

> 2 parts pennyroyal
> 1 part rue
> ½ part mugwort
> ½ part ginger

Pour one pint of boiling water over one ounce of mixed herbs. Steep for twenty minutes. Drink hot, one-half cup three to four times daily.

C. *Internal:*The following is a corrective tonic for all female problems:

> 1 part blue cohosh
> 1 part helonis root
> 1 part squaw vine
> 1 part cramp bark
> 2 parts goldenseal
> 1 part ginger

Mix the powdered herbs and put them into #00 capsules. Take two, three times a day between meals. Although bitter, make a decoction and drink two ounces every two hours or three times daily.

D. *External:* Use ginger fomentations over the stomach and ovaries. Refer to Arthritis, Gout, Rheumatism formula C.

ANEMIA

Principal Therapy - tonification.

Keep the bowels moving freely daily. Use an enema if needed. Avoid refined foods, meats, salts, white bread etc. Use the cleansing diet in this book. Suggested foods are sprouts, raisins, kale, dried prunes, spirulina, parsley, dandelion greens, beets, blackberries, bee pollen (one ounce daily). Take dulse and kelp tablets with meals. Seaweeds such as hiziki, hukame and dulse can be added to your salads.

A. *Internal:* Mix together the following:

> 1 ounce alfalfa
> 1 ounce parsley root
> ½ ounce dandelion root
> ½ ounce burdock root
> ½ ounce comfrey root
> ½ ounce yellow dock root
> ½ ounce nettle leaves
> ½ ounce dulse

Simmer for twenty minutes in a quart of water in an uncovered pot. Let cool and strain. Return liquid to a pot and simmer uncovered for one hour until it is reduced to half the amount. Stir in one cup of unsulphured blackstrap molasses and store in the refrigerator. Take one tablespoon three times daily. The above combination (powdered) can be put into #00 capsules and two to four can be taken with every meal.

Yellow dock, dong quai, ginseng, peony and watercress are excellent tonics to the blood.

Fresh beet juice (2 ounces daily), parsley (2 ounces daily) mixed with fresh apple juice (8 ounces) can be taken once or twice daily.

B. *Hydrotherapy:* Use cool, whole baths if the body is warm. Alternating warm and cool showers morning and evening can be used two hours after or one-half hour before meals. Do deep breathing exercises and dry brush the skin daily.

ANEURYSM

Principal Therapy - blood purification.

Bed rest until relief has been achieved is the first line of defense. Use a 48-hour fruit juice fast with an enema each morning of the fast. Then follow the cleansing diet in this book for seven days, keeping the bowels moving twice daily with enemas, fruits, psyllium powder (one teaspoon in juice three times daily) and soaked dried figs, raisins, etc. Return the person to a vegetarian diet low in protein and fats, high in whole grains and sprouts. Drink two ounces of liquid chlorophyll in juice twice daily.

A. *Internal:* Alfalfa, nettles, comfrey, watercress, kelp and dulse can be used daily in broths, salads or soups. Take hawthorn berry tablets three at three times a day between meals.

> 2 parts St. John's wort
> 1 part arnica flowers
> 1 part yarrow
> 1 part comfrey leaves
> 1 part prickly ash bark

Use as many of these herbs as you can find. Take an ounce of this mixture to one pint of boiling water. Steep for one-half hour. Strain, drink one cup three times daily on an empty stomach.

ANGINA PECTORIS

Principal Therapy - blood purification, tonification

It is best to rest to decrease the load on the heart. Because heavy meals put a stress on the heart, eat light meals, salt free. The cleansing diet is excellent for all heart diseases.

Detoxify the body with short fasts, fruit diets and keep the bowel clean with enemas. Use a low protein, low fat and starch diet. Intestinal gas should be avoided so use carminative herb teas taken hot for this purpose. Avoid smoking, alcohol, extreme temperatures and overindulgence in food and negative thinking.

Dulse, kelp, prunes, peaches, wheat germ, bananas, sprouts, apricots, dates, figs, bee pollen, chives, tomatoes, endive, dandelion greens, beets, melons and lemons are excellent foods for this condition.

A. *Internal:*"Arnica 30x" ten drops in water sipped throughout the day is good when arteriosclerosis is present. Tincture or syrup of hawthorn berries will strengthen the heart muscles and relieve cramping. Take five to ten drops of tincture every half-hour to relieve stabbing pains. Black walnut tincture is good to clean and build arterial walls and for heart pains.

Use chaparral and goldenseal tablets daily to clean the blood and kidneys. Cayenne is an antispasmodic, stimulant, astringent and tonic, and can be taken in doses of ¼ teaspoon two times daily for three days per week in juice or water to strengthen the heart and stimulate the circulation to move out deposits. Other heart tonics are lily of the valley, ginseng, motherwort, eleuthero and rehmania.

> 3 parts hawthorn berries
> 1 part borage leaves
> ½ part cayenne
> 1 part black cohosh
> 1 part valerian root
> 1 part anise

Powder herbs and put into #00 gelatin capsules. Take two capsules every four hours during cramping and pain. For maintenance, one capsule every four hours will be sufficient or two before breakfast and retiring at night.

B. *Hydrotherapy:* Draw the blood from the arms by using arm baths. This is done by bathing the arms in warm water for twenty minutes, or hot water for a shorter time. Soak towels in hot apple cider vinegar and wrap the arms. This is an old folk remedy that has been successful in Europe. This will relax the nervous system and relieve the cramps.

ANKLE (Sprained)

Sprains and strains in any part of the body can usually be treated the same way.

1. For immediate relief take the whites of five eggs, beat them until stiff while adding ¼ teaspoon of cayenne, some thyme or eucalyptus leaves. Powder the leaves of these herbs first. They will act as a stimulant to the circulation. One ounce of the powdered leaves will be enough. Spread

the paste in a natural fiber cloth (cotton or wool) and bandage tightly over the wound. Leave it on all night. In the morning soak the ankle or bruised area in comfrey tea; massage while in the tea. Repeat this procedure until healed.

2. Clay poultice. Make an infusion of thyme or juniper berries and add clay until you have a thick consistency. Spread in linen and bandage tightly. Then follow the same instructions as given above (number 1).

3. Make a poultice of crushed cabbage leaves and clay and apply as directions indicate above.

4. Apple cider vinegar compresses are good for sprains—soaking the sore area with a linen soaked in apple cider vinegar. This is usually wrapped tight and left on for a few hours or overnight. Then soak in comfrey tea between compresses.

5. Burdock leaf poultice is also excellent for sprains. Make an infusion, soak a clean linen in the tea and wrap the wounded area. Follow above directions.

6. A liniment to rub in as needed for sprains:

> 1 tablespoon cayenne
> ½ teaspoon wintergreen oil
> 1 pint apple cider vinegar

Mix the cayenne and apple cider vinegar together. Bring it to a boil and turn off immediately. Steep for twenty minutes. When cooled, add the wintergreen oil. Never boil the oil. Store in a dark bottle. Use when needed.

See hydrotherapy for sprains and strains.

ANUS ITCH (Pruritis) (Worms)

Principal Therapy - blood purification.

Use the cleansing diet. Eat a handful of raw pumpkin seeds daily. Use a tea of equal parts plaintain leaves and catnip and use it to wash the lower bowel with an enema. Enemas of cold water are excellent to relieve itching. A cotton ball soaked in witch hazel inserted into the rectum will remove the trouble.

A. *Internal:* Take chaparral tablets to clean the blood, kidneys and liver, two tablets every four hours till itching stops, then one tablet every four hours for one week.

> Parasites or worms:
> 2 parts wormwood
> 1 part powdered garlic
> 1 part cascara sagrada
> 1 part thyme
> ½ part lobelia
> 1 part fennel
> 1 part slippery elm

Powder these and mix together. Put them in #00 capsules. Take one capsule every four hours making sure to take one after every meal.

A three day fast using this combination and drinking three to six cups of fennel tea daily will remove worms or parasites. Stay away from heavy grains, meats and dairy products—they produce a perfect soil for the multiplication of worms. Wormwood taken alone in capsule form with a little powdered licorice added (1/10 of the mixture) will usually do the job.

Use black walnut tincture daily—ten drops in water every couple of hours and wash the anus with it also. Other herbs that could be used are buckthorn bark, sage, tansy, wood betony, male fern, mandrake, myrrh and southernwood.

For children with worms, clean the bowel with the enema suggested above. Cut up two raw onions and let them soak for 24 hours in one quart of distilled water. Strain, and teaspoon the juice to the child throughout the day. It can be added to a little water to dilute the taste. If the child will not take it, add honey to taste. Also use black walnut tincture in the proper dosage.

All treatments to rid the body of worms should continue for seven to fourteen days to make sure the eggs are destroyed. A month later, repeat the treatment for one week to prevent the spreading of other parasites. If the constitution is weak, or you are working with an elderly individual, the duration of treatment can be one to five days and repeat in one month.

B. *External:* Make a salve out of burdock root, plantain and goldenseal equal parts and apply externally several times daily (see salves). Aloe vera gel is widely known to heal burns and rashes. Spread the gel in linen or gauze and let it remain all night.

C. *Hydrotherapy:* Take cool water sitz baths daily with 12 drops of thyme oil added to the bath water.

APOPLEXY

Principal Therapy - tranquilization, tonification.

A. *Internal:* Use the cleansing diet in this book for one week; then add seeds, nuts, small amounts of tofu and yogurt and sprouted grains. Drink chlorophyll juice daily, but start with one ounce daily and increase to four ounces.

Use the following formulas. Mix together equal parts of the following:

> Valerian
> Spearmint
> Lemon balm
> Lady's slipper
> Scullcap

Drink as an infusion when needed, using one ounce to a pint of boiling water. Steep for twenty minutes.

Use the following as a cough syrup, for stomach spasms, and to relax the solar plexus:

> 3 teaspoons ginger
> 1 teaspoon licorice

Simmer in two cups of water for ten minutes. Remove from heat; stir in two teaspoons of coltsfoot and horehound. Cool and strain. Add four tablespoons of honey or vegetable glycerine.

Dose: Two tablespoons when needed.

Read through tonification therapy and choose some nervines to tone the nervous system.

Remain on a vegetarian diet. An enema taken weekly for several months is advisable.

B. *External:* Hot and cold fomentations over the spine for five minutes, two or three times daily. Use the all purpose liniment on the spine. Mix together the following:

> 1 quart rubbing alcohol
> ½ ounce oil of eucalyptus
> ½ ounce oil of wintergreen

Mix all ingredients together. Use for arthritis, rheumatism, sprains, backaches, etc.

Brush the skin daily and obtain acupuncture treatments and spinal manipulations.

APPENDICITIS (Chronic)

Principal Therapy - heat dispelling, tonification.

A. *Internal:* Undertake a water fast immediately. Use myrrh/goldenseal capsules two every two hours. Take echinacea tincture (twenty to forty drops in one cup of warm water) four times daily. Alternate hot and cold fomentations over the appendix area. Clean the bowels with an enema made from warm water or slippery elm tea. Drink a comfrey root decotion, two ounces every hour until the inflammation subsides.

Break the fast with two days of a fruit diet, then use the cleansing diet in this book. Grapes, melons, apples, fresh ripe pears, and other seasonal fruits are excellent. Take one teaspoon of psyllium in juice or water three times daily for two weeks after appendicitis has ceased.

B. *External:* Use a cold castor oil pack. Materials needed:

> Wool flannel cloth. Cotton flannel may be substituted, though wool is much preferred. Old wool socks, wool blankets, or woolen underwear may also be used. The size depends on the size of the area to be covered. When the material is folded into four thicknesses, it should be large enough to cover the area involved.
>
> Piece of waterproof material (wax paper, cellophane, plastic). Size should be a little larger than the area to be covered by the flannel.
>
> Hot water bottle.
>
> Bath towel. (Use an old towel, as castor oil may leak onto it).
>
> Sleeping bag or heavy blanket.

Procedure: Place the folded wool flannel in a pyrex glass or enamel baking pan. Pour castor oil over the cloth until it is well saturated. Heat the pan and pack in an oven about 225 degrees Farenheit, being careful to get the pack no hotter than you can touch. The flannel tends to heat up quickly (5 to 10 minutes) and you may burn it if you are not careful. You may put the pack on and apply a heating pad to avoid placing it in the oven. Lay down in a comfortable position and apply the heated pack to the area to be treated. Next, apply a waterproof covering over the pack. On top of this place a hot water bottle semi-filled with very hot water. Cover the hot water bottle with a bath towel wrapped around the body to secure the water bottle and pack in place. Cover everything with a sleeping bag or heavy blanket to insulate the heat.

The pack should usually remain in place for one hour, and preferably from one and one-half to two hours.

The skin should be cleansed afterwards to avoid a rash, which affects some people, and because the oil will leave your skin very greasy. To clean castor oil from your body (or any surface where it is spilled) use a solution of two teaspoons baking soda to one quart of water.

Store the pack in a baking pan or a plastic bag and reuse. A pack must *never* be washed! Castor oil is impossible to wash out of cloth. To reuse, just add additional castor oil as it dries out from use. A pack can last for six weeks. Use your pack only on yourself.

For general use it is desirable to use the pack three or four nights consecutively and then not use it for three nights. Then begin the cycle again.

Castor oil packs are a fairly simple procedure when done carefully and methodically. Be very careful not to spill the castor oil on sheets or rugs. If you should spill any, however, a concentrated solution of baking soda and water is the best way to clean it up.

See cabbage leaf poultice and formula B under Abscesses for other external treatments.

APPETITE (Weak or loss of) (Anorexia)

Principal Therapy - tonification.

If the problem is due to depression, vomiting, or schizophrenic tendencies, professional help should be considered.

A. *Internal:* Use easily digestible foods such as steamed foods, spirulina, bee pollen, etc. Raw fruit and vegetable juices are advised. A limit of four or five foods may be used at a meal, and never combine fruits and vegetables at the same sitting. Take digestive enzymes before meals until the stomach tone returns.

Use the cleansing diet in this book with short three to five day juice fasts which relax and help the return of nerve energy.

Tonification. Use stomach and liver tonics in tea or tincture form. They are bitter and should not be sweetened. The stomach tonic mentioned under allergies is excellent for this condition.

Use tincture of oregon grape root. Take twenty drops in warm water three times daily.

For liver tonification, mix the following together:

    1 part barberry root
    1 part wild yam
    1 part dandelion
    ½ part licorice root

Simmer one ounce in a pint of water for ten minutes; strain. Drink two ounces three to four times daily.

Barberry can be added to the formulas or taken separately in very small amounts (see proper dosage). This herb does not dry up the stomach secretions, but promotes them and tones and stimulates circulation. If the body becomes cold, use stimulation therapy.

B. *Hydrotherapy:* Use cool, whole baths if the body is warm; and warm, whole baths if cold. Also, alternating hot and cold showers and foot baths are recommended.

ARTERIOSCLEROSIS

Principal Therapy - blood purification, stimulation.

Limit the fat, protein and cholesterol intake. It is better to eat foods from plants rather than from animal sources. Use the cleansing diet in this book and continue on a vegetarian diet. Avoid dairy products, meats oils, heavy starches and tap water. Drink only distilled water.

A. *Internal:* Take twenty to thirty alfalfa tablets or wheatgrass tablets daily. Eat plenty of high fiber foods like whole grains, sprouts, raw celery, carrots, beets and cabbage. To reduce deposits in the arteries, roast alfalfa seeds and take six teaspoons daily. They can be eaten alone or added to salads. Read the section under Constipation and use the three seed combination made from chia, flaxseed, psyllium and raisins. Two ounces of liquid chlorophyll twice daily is an excellent cleanser for this condition.

Chaparral and garlic capsules taken daily will help dissolve deposits and congestion in the body. Add plenty of seaweeds to the diet, such as kelp, dulse and wakame. Rutin, present in buckwheat, will help build weak vessels and arteries. The diet outlined here is also good for all heart diseases.

Clean the bowels weekly with a warm water enema. Drink one pint of freshly squeezed carrot or orange juice daily. Squeeze one lemon in a cup of warm water and drink upon rising in the morning.

Cayenne, ginger, cumin and cardamon can be added to warm vegetable broths. Short fasts of three to five days will aid in cleansing. See the section on diuretics for herbal teas.

Read stimulation therapy and use the formula suggested or use the following. Mix the following herbs together:

    4 parts chaparral
    2 parts yucca
    1 part dandelion
    1 part sassafras
    1 part prickly ash bark
    1 part black cohosh
    1 part ginger root
    1 part burdock root

Powder herbs and put into #00 capsules. Take two, three times each day.

Drink teas made from burdock, sassafras, red clover and other alterative herbs.

B. *External:* Get plenty of fresh air and exericse. Obtain massage and spinal manipulations. Take sweat baths or the cold sheet treatment as explained under Colds, Fevers and Flus. Drink diaphoretic teas while trying to produce sweating.

Dry brush the skin daily and take sun baths. Soaking in the ocean and taking salt baths will relieve the kidneys and draw excess fluid from the body.

C. *Hydrotherapy:* Use warm, whole baths three to four times weekly. The all purpose liniment can be used on stiff, congested areas. Alternate warm and cool showers for ten minute durations morning and night. Dry brush the skin morning and night to increase the circulation.

ATHLETE'S FOOT

Principal Therapy - blood purification.

Let the feet breathe. Sandals are excellent for this condition. Take apple cider vinegar and spread in the sores three or four times daily.

A. *Internal:* - Use the cleansing diet. Stay away from tea, coffee, meats and other cooked high acid foods. Fruit juice fasts are excellent. Drink green juices daily.

B. *External:* Use wheatgrass juice daily. Soak the feet in this juice or soak cotton in the juice and place the cotton between the toes and let the cotton remain overnight. Expose the feet to the sun as much as possible.

Dr. Devrient of Berlin says that "whey concentrate preparation is the quickest and most reliable remedy." Powdered whey can be mixed with water and slippery elm to make a paste. Use only enough slippery elm to thicken. Spread on a linen and wrap the feet. Leave on overnight. Rinse the feet in the morning with apple cider vinegar and water, half and half.

Thyme oil, six drops to a cup of water, rubbed on the feet five times daily is an excellent remedy.

Garlic oil mixed with equal parts of olive oil is good. Rub into feet five times daily. Make the oil yourself. Peel eight ounces of garlic and pulverize it. Cover with olive oil just enough to cover the garlic. Shake it daily, let it set for three to five days. Strain and add a teaspoon of wheat germ oil to it and preserve it. Rub on the feet before bed. Cover with a sock. Repeat nightly.

Black walnut tincture is good. Soak the area several times daily.

Make a salve or oil from equal parts of:

Agrinomy
Balm of Gilead
Echinacea

Take two chaparral tablets every four hours. Then return to two tablets three times daily for a maintenance dosage.

C. *Hydrotherapy:* Alternating hot and cold foot baths three times daily will sometimes cure this fungus alone.

ARTHRITIS, GOUT, RHEUMATISM

Principal Therapy - blood purification, stimulation therapy.

Use the cleansing diet in this book, then continue on a vegetarian diet. Avoid meats, dairy products, coffee, tea, tobacco, and refined foods. A three day fruit fast monthly will aid in cleansing the blood and joints. Eating just grapes for two weeks is excellent to overcome this condition. Clean the bowels weekly with an enema.

Drink distilled water and fresh juices made from carrot, orange, kale, wheatgrass, parsley and apple. Juice one raw potato and dilute with 25% distilled water or vegetable broth for a morning cocktail.

Two ounces of liquid chlorophyll can be taken daily mixed with apple or carrot juice.

A. *Internal:* Mix the following herbs together:

> 4 parts chaparral
> 2 parts yucca
> 1 part dandelion
> 1 part sassafras
> 1 part prickly ash bark
> 1 part black cohosh
> 1 part ginger root
> 1 part burdock root

Powder herbs and put into #00 capsules. Take two, three times each day.

B. *External:* All purpose liniment

> 1 quart rubbing alcohol
> ½ ounce oil of eucalyptus
> ½ ounce oil of wintergreen

Mix all ingredients together. Use for arthritis, rheumatism, sprains, backaches, etc.

C. Ginger fomentation

For painful joints, grate five ounces of fresh ginger root and simmer in two quarts of distilled water for ten minutes. Use as a fomentation—dip natural fiber cloth into hot liquid and cover body part. Cover this with heavy wool blankets and keep heat in. Repeat procedure when fomentation cools off.

D. *External:* Fomentation for pains, sprains, and rheumatism:

> 2 parts ginger root
> 1 part slippery elm
> 1 part cayenne
> 1 part lobelia

Make into a fomentation and apply to affected area.

E. *External:* Dry brush the skin daily and get plenty of exercise. Massage and spinal manipulations will aid circulation.

F. *Hydrotherapy:* Morning and evening take alternating warm and cool showers for ten minute durations. Take warm, whole baths three to four times a week.

ASTHMA (Bronchitis)

Principal Therapy - deobstruent (expectorants), stimulation.

Use a cleansing diet for seven to ten days using an enema daily. Avoid dairy products, meats, eggs, refined foods, coffee, tea, etc. Spices such as ginger, cardamon, cumin and cayenne should be added to soups and salads.

A. *Internal:* Horseradish syrup

Finely grate two cups of fresh horseradish and soak in enough honey to slightly cover horseradish. Soak for four to eight hours; then strain. Add a little water to the strained out horseradish and simmer for ten minutes. Strain and add this to the honey mixture. Take one teaspoon three times daily.

Also use for gall bladder congestion, respiratory problems and sinus congestion, colds, chills and poor digestion.

B. *Internal:* Spasmodic coughs, lung congestion, asthma

2 parts wild cherry bark
1 part lungwort
1 part mullein
1 part prickly ash bark

Simmer one ounce of herbs in one pint of distilled water for ten minutes. Strain. Drink one-half cup three times daily.

Put powdered herbs in #00 capsules. Take two capsules three times daily.

C. *External:* Mustard pack for mucus conditions of the respiratory tract for chills, colds, flu.

Stir one tablespoon of mustard powder in a quart of warm water, and saturate a towel in this liquid, cover lungs, stomach, etc. Rub olive oil over body part first. Mustard packs can irritate skin. Cover pack with heavy blankets. Renew pack when it gets cold. Leave on for 20 minutes to one-half hour.

D. *External:* See Spasmodic Coughs and Lung Congestion, formulas A and B.

E. *Hydrotherapy:* Alternate hot and cold fomentations over the lungs ten minutes two to three times daily. Take cool, whole baths in the mornings. Get plenty of fresh air. Deep breathing exercises will aid elimination of mucus congestion.

BACKACHE

Principal Therapy - blood purification, stimulation.

Use the cleansing diet in this book. Flush the bowels out weekly with an enema. Discontinue the use of meats, coffee, tea and other kidney damaging foods.

A. *Internal:* Drink infusion of:

> 2 parts uva ursi
> 1 part dandelion root
> 1 part marshmallow
> 1 part ginger
> 1 part plantain

Simmer two ounces of herbs in one quart of distilled water for ten minutes with top on tightly. Steep for ten minutes; strain. Drink one cup three times daily.

B. *External:* See castor oil pack under Appendicitis, external treatments. See also ginger fomentation under Arthritis, Gout and Rheumatism, formula C. Obtain spinal manipulations.

BAD BREATH (Halitosis)

Principal Therapy - purgation, carminative.

Purification of the intestinal tract and keeping the teeth clean will improve this condition. Use the cleansing diet in this book and use an enema weekly. Take two tablespoons of liquid chlorophyll in warm water or juice four times daily between meals. All raw fruits, vegetables and juices will improve this condition. Chew whole cloves when the breath is offensive. Parsley juice is excellent. Do deep breathing exercises and use an emetic to remove the foul putrifying food waste left in the stomach.

A. *Internal:* Use aperient (light laxatives) foods and herbs to keep the bowels clean (see purgation therapy). One hour before meals, drink a bitter cup of tea made from equal parts of goldenseal root powder, myrrh and peppermint leaves. One hour after meals, drink another cup of the tea. Also see the formulas under Gastritis, Indigestion and Gas. Tinctures of goldenseal or myrrh can also be used—twenty drops in one-half cup of warm water taken three to four times daily.

Gargle daily with rosemary oil, thyme oil or peppermint oil several times. Use only two drops of one of these oils to one cup of warm water.

BALDNESS

Principal Therapy - blood purification.

The bloodstream is the soil for the hair. I have seen several individuals grow thick beautiful hair after changing to a pure vegetarian diet. Use the cleansing diet in this book, then add seeds, nuts, raw juices, sprouts, seaweeds and sprouted grain to your diet. Wash the hair with a pure herbal shampoo. Once weekly, rub pure cold-pressed olive oil into the scalp and sit in the sun for one hour or use hot towels on the scalp, sit in a steam room or use a heating pad. Jojoba oil is also excellent for this. Massage the scalp and brush it daily. Make sure you get plenty of foods that have iodine in them to aid the thyroid gland: kelp tablets should be taken after every meal. Exercise and get plenty of fresh air.

A. *Internal:* Drink blood purifying teas like red clover, burdock root, parsley, nettle, alfalfa, sassafras, etc. in the amount of three cups daily. See vitamin and mineral tonic for weak debilitated conditions.

B. *Hydrotherapy:* See head bandages and alternate them using hot and cold to bring circulation to the scalp. Lay on a slant board or hang upside down for twenty minutes daily.

BED WETTING

Principal Therapy - blood purification, tonification.

Clean the bowels with an enema and avoid stimulating drinks like coffee, pepsi cola, tea and hot spices. The diet should be vegetarian style avoiding salt, meats, milk and other dairy products.

Eat plenty of asparagus (steamed), spinach, bee pollen, parsley, endive, dandelion and beet greens. Do not use liquids two hours before bed.

Never scold the child or person that is bed wetting. If the problem is emotional, go to the proper counselor. The nervous system is affected strongly when negative emotions are expressed.

A. *Internal:* Tinctures made from plantain or pipsissewa are good. See the formulas under Kidney and Bladder Infections and Stones. They will tone and clean the kidney. Ginseng extracts will tone the digestive system, kidneys, spleen and liver.

B. *Hydrotherapy:* Use cool water sitz baths or cold, whole baths. Alternate hot and cold fomentations over the kidneys every morning. Obtain acupuncture treatments and/or spinal manipulations.

BED SORES

Principal Therapy - blood purification.

Use the cleansing diet in this book. Clean the bowels with an enema made from myrrh or goldenseal tea to disinfect the area. Keep the body stimulated by hot and cold baths or packs over the spine accompanied by massage. Stay away from meat and dairy products. The diet should be a natural one. Use plenty of carrot juice, parsley, spinach, sprouts, wheat germ, sprouted grains, almonds, lemons, oranges, onions, raisins and figs. Vitamin A and D foods are important.

A. *Internal:* Alternate chaparral tablets with echinacea capsules, two every four hours. This will clean the blood and lymphatic system. Eat plenty of garlic and onions along with this.

Another good remedy is to take the homeopathic remedy "silica 12x" internally. It is very good for the skin and connective tissues. You can sprinkle it on the wound and take five tablets five times daily until the sore ripens. It also improves the hair and nails.

A tincture made from horseradish is excellent to wash wounds. Make a paste out of crushed comfrey leaves and slippery elm and cover the sores. Take powdered comfrey leaves and slippery elm in equal parts, mix with water to make a paste. Spread on a linen and tie it over the sore. It can be left on overnight.

B.   *External:* Make a tea from witch hazel, myrrh or goldenseal and wash the sores three or four times daily. While dry, sprinkle some powdered goldenseal or echinacea over the sores to disinfect the area and cover with a natural linen (wool or cotton).

An excellent remedy is a wheatgrass poultice using the juice which a cloth has been soaked in or the pulp left a little juicy. This can be left on all day. Use liquid chlorophyll from the health food store. It is a natural disinfectant and healer. Not enough can be said about the healing qualities of chlorophyll.

A cabbage poultice, clay poultice or a raw potato grated up and mixed with milk and applied are excellent external treatments for sores and wounds. These can be left on for hours at a time.

A salve made from balm of gilead (disinfectant), burdock root and comfrey is excellent for both a healing and disinfectant salve.

BILIOUSNESS

Principal Therapy - blood purification and deobstruent therapies (cholagogue).

Do a three to seven day fast on grape or carrot juice. Use them separately and be sure to dilute them with 25% distilled water. Clean the bowels with a warm water enema for five consecutive days.

Drink plenty of green juices (parsley, wheatgrass, etc.) Use the cleansing diet in this book and avoid dairy products, meats, salt and other toxic, congestive foods.

A.   *Internal:* See formulas under Liver Problems, Indigestion, Jaundice and Hepatitis.

B.   *Hydrotherapy:* Cool, whole baths or alternating hot and cold fomentations.

BLEEDING (Internal)

Principal Therapy - hemostatic

Fast until bleeding stops and the severity of the condition is over. Choose herbs that are specific for the area bleeding. Shepherd's purse, white oak bark and marshmallow root are for the kidneys and intestines. Bethroot is a specific for the uterus; cranesbill, white oak bark and comfrey are for the lungs. These herbs can be taken as tinctures or decoctions—twenty to thirty drops of the tinctures to two ounces of decoction every two hours.

If the bleeding is from the bowels, inject one pint of the decoction of white oak bark in the bowel and retain as long as possible while lying in a slant position, head lower than legs. Any one astringent herb would be good for this. See astringent herbs. Astringents can be used as douches if bleeding from the uterus is present. Retain as long as possible.

The following is a combination for all internal bleeding problems:

> 1 part bayberry
> 1 part cranesbill
> 1 part comfrey root
> 1 part shepherd's purse
> 1 part licorice root
> 1/8 part cayenne
> 1 part goldenseal

Boil an ounce of this combination for fifteen minutes in one pint of water. Let it cool and strain. Drink two ounces every two hours. The powdered herbs can be mixed and put into #00 capsules and taken two every two hours.

Any one of these astringent herbs can be used separately if all are not available.

Liquid chlorophyll is also good taken internally or used as a douche (diluted with 50% water) and the same dilution as an enema. Two drops of liquid chlorophyll put up the nose will stop nose bleeds. Also for nose bleeds, put a cold water pack on the nose area.

When external cuts are bleeding, cover the cut with powdered cayenne. It will immediately stop the bleeding. When an artery or vein is severed, apply powdered cayenne or tincture immediately, then apply direct pressure and seek a physician or go directly to a hospital.

When the bleeding is over and the problem is cured, for several weeks drink two cups of a demulcent tea. Flaxseed, slippery elm, mullein are some of my favorites. Two or three cups a day is sufficient.

BLOOD POISONONG (Septicemia)

Principal Therapy - blood purification.

A. *Internal:* A fast on fruit juices is necessary. Orange, lemon, grapefruit are the best. Clean the bowels with a flaxseed tea enema.

Dr. Vogel in his book, "Swiss Nature Doctor", says "lachesis 12x" (homeopathic) is a good remedy for malignant diseases, blood poisoning, septicemia, scarlet fever, gangrene, chronic ulcers, boils, carbuncles, and small pox. Even in cases of gangrene and typhus, this remedy has worked when no other one has.

Echinacea is one of the best herbs for blood diseases. Drink as many cups of this herb daily as possible. The warm tea will penetrate the blood system faster than powders in capsules. Switch to echinacea in capsules once the condition is under control. Goldenseal and chaparral are also good remedies for this condition.

Mix the following:

¼ part poke root
1 part garlic
1 part chaparral
1 part echinacea
½ part licorice root

Mix all powdered herbs together or get as many as possible. Put into #00 capsules and take two every hour until symptoms subside. Take two to three times a day.

Other herbs that may be used include chickweed, goldenseal, myrrh, bloodroot and charcoal poultice.

BLOOD PRESSURE (Hypertension)

Principal Therapy - blood purification, tranquilization.

Avoid meats, dairy products, fried foods, salt, etc. Use the cleansing diet in this book and clean the bowels with an enema once weekly for a month. Then continue on a vegetarian diet. Get plenty of fresh air and light exericse.

A. *Internal:* Liquid chlorophyll, two ounces twice daily mixed in apple or freshly squeezed orange juice. Make vegetable broths including large amounts of onions, garlic, leeks and celery.

Drink blood cleansing herb teas like sassafras, alfalfa and red clover. Mistletoe (viscum album), hawthorn berries, leeks, garlic and arnica are specific herbs to clean the veins and arteries and lower the blood pressure (see antispasmodic tincture).

6 parts hawthorn berries
3 parts ginseng
2 parts comfrey root
2 parts mistletoe (viscum album)
1 part valerian root
1 part cayenne

Make a tincture of this combination or put the powdered herbs in #00 capsules and take two, three times daily. Twenty drops three times a day of the tincture is plenty.

Avoid beet juice, bee pollen, and carrot juice. They are much too stimulating.

Siberian ginseng tincture, twenty-five drops morning and evening in one cup of warm water is a popular remedy for high blood pressure.

B. *External:* Spinal manipulations and acupuncture are advised. Dry brush the skin daily and obtain massages.

C. *Hydrotherapy:* Warm, whole baths. Take alternating warm and cool showers morning and night.

BLOOD PRESSURE (Low)

Principal Therapy - blood purification, tonification, stimulation.

Use the cleansing diet in this book while drinking carrot, beet, and apple juice. Also use prickly ash bark, hyssop or goldenseal tea. These herbs and juices will stimulate circulation, raise the red blood cell count and help to overcome fatigue.

Do not change the diet rapidly at this time. After the cleansing diet add rye, barley, wheat, wild rice, millet and sprouts to the diet. Sometimes fish is needed to help keep the blood pressure normal until the body is toned up in some elderly people. Use kelp, dulse and other seaweeds to stimulate glandular output, especially if the reproductive system is involved.

A. *Internal:* Use a good ginseng extract (ten drops morning and night in one-half cup of warm water). Four ounces of liquid chlorophyll a day can be taken in small doses added to juice or water. Spirulina is excellent for this condition. Study the section on tonification and use nerve tonics to increase body activities.

B. *External:* Acupuncture is excellent for all blood pressure conditions.

C. *Hydrotherapy:* Cool, whole baths or alternating cool and warm showers, foot baths or sitz baths.

BOILS AND CARBNCLES

Principal Therapy - blood purification, stimulation.

Use the cleansing diet in this book along with the use of enemas for seven straight days in the morning.

A. *Internal:* See the formulas under Abscesses and Acne and Skin Problems.

B. *External:* Get plenty of fresh air, sweating and exercise. Remain on a vegetarian diet and drink red clover tea daily.

C. *Hydrotherapy:* Cool, whole baths and alternating hot and cold showers morning and night.

BONE DISEASES

Principal Therapy - tonification

Use the cleansing diet in this book. Short two day fasts on vegetable or fruit juices are good. Clean the bowel with enemas or laxative herbs. The vitamins that are important are A, C, D, and minerals calcium, bone meal, magnesium, manganese and phosphorus. Sprouted grains and nut butters made from almonds and brazil nuts will supply the above vitamins and minerals. Use wheatgrass juice (one ounce daily, increase weekly to four ounces). Dilute this juice in distilled water; it is a powerful cleanser. Spirulina is another good nutritive algae. Take it daily, capsule or powder form. Eat as many green vegetables as possible. Drink carrot juice combined with green vegetable juices like endive, parsley, spinach, etc.

A. *Internal:* Homeopathic aconite (Aconitum hapellus) is one of the best remedies for pain and inflammation, especially when the skin is hot and dry. Take homeopathic dosages (3x or 4x) five drops in a glass of water at hour intervals till the pain is gone, then stop the aconite treatment. It is mainly used to ease the pain.

> 4 parts comfrey root
> 6 parts horsetail grass
> 3 parts oat straw
> 1 part lobelia
> 3 parts nettles

This is an excellent calcium formula to rebuild weak bones. Take three to six cups daily or mix powdered herbs in #00 capsules and take two, three times daily or nine daily if desired. It will also help relieve the pain. See alterative herbs for other blood cleansers.

Plenty of nutrients are needed in bone diseases. These herbs can be used for this purpose: comfrey, irish moss, iceland moss, kelp, dulse, alfalfa and watercress.

Boneset is an herb that relieves aching of the bones. Drink an infusion of the leaves (one teaspoon to one cup of boiling water) three to four cups daily.

Comfrey encourages the healing process of new bone cells. It contains 0.8 to 1% allantoin. It is excellent for healings of the dense fibrous coverings of the bones.

Dr. Scheussler's biochemical cell salts for bone diseases:
Calcarea Phos. Use for weak, soft bones in children, rickets, bowed legs, slow dentition and fractured bones.
Calcarea Flour. Disturbance in the surface of the bones or bruises of the covering of the bone (periosteum).
Silicea. Ulceration of the bones, thick yellow offensive pus.
Ferrum Phos. Early stages of bone disturbances and when red, swollen, hot inflammed areas are present. Give five tablets 12x potency every hour when in pain.

B. *External:* Take warm baths, followed with a stimulating towel rub. Hot and cold showers are beneficial.

Inflammations. Wrap a cold, wet compress around the swollen, tender area. Cover it with a flannel cloth and leave on all night. To help ease the pain, simmer flaxseed, one teaspoon to a cup of water for five minutes. Spread the seed and some of the tea (liquid) on a cloth. Wrap it around the swollen joints. Cover with flannel cloth. Keep on all night. Also use the all purpose liniment in this book.

BOTULISM

Principal Therapy - blood purification.

Immeditely a lobelia emetic should be administered to empty the stomach. Lobelia is not needed if one can cause himself to vomit by sticking his fingers down his throat after drinking a quart of warm water with one tablespoon of salt added to it.

Follow this with a cup of peppermint tea to settle the stomach. Use hot packs over the stomach if there is severe cramping. Take hot baths and drink a combination of nerve herbs—hops, chamomile, catnip and peppermint is good to settle the stomach and relieve cramping.

Next an enema should be administered to empty the bowels. Take two echinacea capsules every two hours until symptoms subside. Chaparral can also be used. Do not take medicines that suppress symptoms and impede the body's functions.

Fast until all symptoms are gone. Drink clay water. Use white or yellow clay—a teaspoon of clay to a small glass of warm water to which has been added ten drops of echinacea tincture or lobelia tincture. Take this drink three to five times daily.

This condition will usually clear up within three days. Eating will only burden the digestive functions and delay elimination of the poison. If one begins to vomit bile, use dandelion tea with a little honey or peppermint added to it to soothe and clean the liver. When a fever is present, use the process in this book under fevers. If the urine is hot and burning, horsetail grass, buchu, parsley and marshmallow root are herbs that can be used. On all kidney problems, add marshmallow root or some other demulcent to soothe the area.

When the patient's appetite returns, grated apples and fruit juices can be used for forty-eight hours after the crisis; then return to the cleansing diet.

Other herbs to cleanse the blood are burdock root, sassafras root bark, plantain, dandelion root, nettles, and juniper berries.

BREAST TUMORS

Principal Therapy -blood purification.

See cancer treatment. Use the cleansing diet in this book. Keep the bowels clean with herbal laxatives or enemas. Poisoning waste from the bowels is constantly being absorbed into the blood and lymphatic system. This will cause the tumor to grow and remain. Three to seven day fasts can be used, alternating with a vegetarian diet. Do not use dairy products, fried foods, heavy starches or high protein foods. Keep the diet simple and use cleansing foods.

A. *Internal:* Internally the alterative herbs should be used. Chaparral tablets are excellent—two tablets four times daily. Sassafras, red clover, chickweed and burdock root are good teas to drink to cleanse the blood along with the chosen formula.

Homeopathic silica is excellent for all tumors and swelling caused from a toxic lymphatic system. Silica is found in plants, usually in the stalks or grains or grasses. Hepar. sulph. 4x should be used first to encourage the elimination of pus. Silica will promote the healing process. It is excellent for all suppurations (discharge of pus). Take five tablets of 12x five times daily.

B. *External:* Use hot and cold water packs over the tumor to bring circulation to the breast. Exercise to maintain good circulation. Skin brush daily. Once the blood is purified, the tumor will begin to dissolve.

Prickly pear cactus (optunia species) makes an excellent poultice for sore breasts. Slash the leaf and apply the pulp over the swelling.

Combine clay and macerated cabbage leaves and mix together with powdered flaxseed and water. Make a thick paste, add a pinch of cayenne and spread on a linen and apply. This can stay on for several hours.

Make a drawing, soothing poultice using equal parts of powdered plantain leaves, comfrey leaves, lobelia. Mix these leaves with wheat germ and castor oil to a thick consistency. Spread it ¼ inch thick on a linen and apply to the tumor. Keep this on from four to six hours daily.

Ichthammol and vegetable glycerine mixed together in equal parts as a poultice is very good for all tumors. Ichthammol is found in drug stores.

Soak a cloth in castor oil and place inside a bra. This can be worn during sleep or daily activities. Poke root oil is also excellent for this. Poke root tincture is a powerful lymphatic cleanser for all tumors and swelling. Take five drops in ⅓ cup of water three times daily.

The Red Clover Combination carried by Nature's Way Products is similiar to Hoxey's formula which he used for most of his cancer patients. Take four tablets three times a day.

The tumor may get larger at the very beginning of detoxification, simply becuase there is so much toxic poison being released by the cells. This is not a time to panic; once the body gets cleaner and the organs can handle the waste elimination, the tumor will shrink.

It is important to use a low sodium, high potassium diet so the fluids will not be held up in the tissues. Study the potassium foods listed under Tumors and Cancer Therapy.

Chlorophyll enema implants are very important during this therapy. Use wheatgrass or parsley juice freshly squeezed and study the section "Nutrient Implant" in the chapter on Enemas. Drink two to four ounces of liquid chlorophyll juice mixed with water taken straight or with juice (celery or apple) twice daily.

St. John's wort oil or a salve made from this plant applied daily to tumors, swellings, bruises and caked breasts is excellent. The tincture, ten to fifteen drops three times daily, can be taken internally.

It is very important to keep the iodine level of the blood normal for both the thyroid gland and tissues to have proper cell oxidation. Eat plenty of seaweeds and take kelp or dulse capsules daily.

BRIGHTS'S DISEASE (See Prostatitis)

BRONCHITIS (See Asthma)

BRUISING

Use the cleansing diet in this book. Eat plenty of vitamin A and C foods such as red peppers, dandelion greens, carrots, apricots, kale, spinach, mustard greens, collard greens, watercress, parsley, swiss chard, beet greens, endive, soybeans, all sprouts, wheat germ, nutritive herbs, kelp, dulse, whole grains (best when sprouted), chives, rose hip tea, all fruits except citrus.

Eat an alkaline, light food diet. Heavy proteins and starches put excess stress on the organs and blood vessels. Fruits, greens, seeds and nuts are good. Do not overeat the seeds and nuts.

Clay poultice will reduce swelling. Mix white or yellow clay with horsetail grass or lobelia tea. Make a thick paste and spread it ¼ inch think on a linen. Apply wet area over the wound.

Cabbage leaf poultice is cleansing and drawing. Beat the leaves until the juice runs, spread them over the wound and tape a linen over the top to hold it on.

Potato poultice can be used with raw potatoes or baked. Pulverize raw potatoes with a mixture of bran, slippery elm, milk, honey or wheat. Spread the mass on a linen and cover area. Bake the potatoes in their jackets. Mash them up with bran, slippery elm and a little water to a thick consistency. Apply same as above. Keep these poultices on for several hours.

Marshmallow root powder mixed with equal parts lobelia and 1/5 part cayenne is an excellent poultice or fomentation for wounds, swellings, insect and snake bites and bruises.

Aloe vera gel, wheat germ oil and safflower oil can be rubbed on the aggravated areas.

BURNS

First degree burns are mild and can be treated with the application of cold water and aloe vera gel. If the burn is second and third degree, it must be treated with caution.

As soon as the blisters appear they can be punctured and drained. Dust the wounds with myrrh or goldenseal powder. This formula can be used topically:

    ½ part slippery elm
    3 parts comfrey leaves or root
    1 part lobelia
    ½ part wheat germ oil
    ½ part honey

Combine all ingredients and bottle. Spread the combination on a linen and bandage. Leave it on for three days. New skin will develop. After this, aloe vera gel can be put on it daily until healed. The honey is a naural antiseptic and will prevent infections.

For first and second degree burns, hold the affected area under ice water until the pain stops. Then spread vitamin E oil over the burn to reduce redness and blistering.

A comfrey ointment or poultice made from comfrey leaves can be applied to first and second degree burns.

For third and fourth degree burns, a poultice of goldenseal - 6 parts; comfrey - 3 parts and cayenne - 1 part should be applied externally.

If the burn is chemical, echinacea and chaparral tablets should be taken internally, two tablets every four hours. Wheatgrass juice internally is good to remove toxic substances from the body. A wheatgrass pulp mixed with the juice can also be applied to burns.

The diet should be kept alkaline and the blood stream clean to prevent scarring and poor healing.

Raw potato pulverized and mixed with powdered flaxseed or slippery elm and spread on a linen and bandaged on burns is excellent.

Wheat germ oil or vitamin E oil alone or mixed with comfrey root powder or slippery elm as a poultice is another good remedy. If there is pain, add lobelia or lady's slipper to your poultice and drink nervine teas to help relieve the excitability.

Calendula flowers (marigold) and plantain leaves in equal parts mixed with honey and glycerine into a paste and used as a poultice is excellent for painful burns and sprains. Used as an oil or salve, it can be used to stop bleeding and soothe pain.

BURSITIS (See Arteriosclerosis and Arthritis)

CANKER SORES (Mouth)

Principal Therapy - diet and blood purification.

Go on a three day carrot juice fast or just a plain distilled water fast. Use an enema every morning while on the fast. Then go to the cleansing diet in this book for one week.

A. *Internal:* Take goldenseal capsules, two every four hours. Gargle four to five times daily with an herb tea made from goldenseal and myrrh.

Another good gargle is using three drops of rosemary, thyme, or juniper berry oils to one cup of warm water. Wheatgrass juice or liquid chlorophyll can be used as a gargle and drink two ounces three times daily to purify the stomach and intestines. Paint the sores with lobelia tincture several times a day.

CHEST CONGESTION (See Asthma, Coughs and Colds)

CHICKEN POX (See Measles)

Principal Therapy - blood purification, diaphoresis.

Keep the child out of direct sunlight and use a fruit juice diet for three days. Freshly squeezed lemon juice (1 lemon) in two cups of warm water with honey added can be taken copiously throughout the whole period of the pox. Clean the bowels daily with a catnip tea enema.

A. *Internal:* Prepare herb teas made from chickweed, red raspberry, yarrow and peppermint. Mix them in equal parts and drink them throughout the day.

If the fever gets over 103 degrees, ferrum phos. 3x, 6x, 12x, two tablets taken in a teaspoon of warm water or juice every hour will help lower the inner heat.

B. *External:* If the sores begin to itch, use aloe vera or comfrey salve on them. The best therapy for it is to take a warm bath with ½ cup of apple cider vinegar and one cup of baking soda added to the water. The hot bath will help bring out the poxes. After ten minutes in the bath, dress the child while still wet, put them to bed and apply diaphoresis therapy using the tea mentioned above. The pox can be painted with black walnut tincture or witch hazel bought in drug stores.

C. *Hydrotherapy:* If the itch gets fierce, use cool baths with chaparral tea (1 gallon) or ginger tea added to the water.

When this condition is over, use tonification therapy using easily digestible foods, broth and juices to assist the cleansing of left-over waste.

CHILBLAIN (Frostbite)

In the early stages, rub the feet with cold towels that have been soaked in the snow or ice water. When there is relief, hot, followed by cold foot baths will improve the circulation. In hot water, the area should be soaked for two minutes, in cold, only five to ten seconds. Repeat this six to ten times. Finish off with a cold dip and towel dry. Rub lemon juice into the skin.

Another remedy after the water treatment is to mix together two ounces of cayenne mixture with one pint of olive oil and rub on the affected area. Use two teaspoons of cayenne and one teaspoon of powdered ginger, mix with one pint of rum whiskey or pure alcohol. Rub on the area several times daily.

CHILLS AND POOR CIRCULATION

Principal Therapy - blood purification and stimulation therapy, diaphoresis therapy when cold.

This condition usually means the body is overloaded with poisons and the circulation is impaired. The blood stream must be purified for normal circulation.

Never let the body chill. Use warm baths, hot packs, electric blankets and foot baths to keep the body warm.

Immediately clean the lower bowel with an enema and take some herbal laxatives to clean the whole intestinal track. Use the cleansing diet in this book for one week. Plenty of citrus juices, carrot, beet and celery juices and distilled water should be used. Stay away from high proteins, starch, dairy products and mucus producing foods. All green vegetables will help clean the blood. Exercise will increase the circulation. Use deep breathing exercises and brush the skin daily. Hot and cold alternating showers are good. Eat plenty of foods that contain calcium. Plants rich in iodine such as dulse, kelp, watercress and seaweeds will supply the body with proper minerals. Garlic, cayenne, leeks, onions and horseradish will improve circulation.

Avoid a high fat diet, especially animal fats, high protein foods such as cheese, meats and eggs. Alcohol is also harmful to the capillary walls. The following guidelines may be used: 1) use a cleansing diet; 2) fast one day weekly; 3) eat only two meals daily when the patient returns to eating; 4) exercise every day; 5) take cool morning showers and massage; 6) take steam, vapor or sauna baths; and 7) use blood cleansing (see alteratives) and stimulating herbs.

A.   *Internal:* Drink red clover, sassafras and burdock tea to clean the blood. Practice deep breathing and drink teas made from prickly ash, ginger, cumin, peppermint and other stimulants. Cayenne tincture added to hot water (five to ten drops) is also very good. Cayenne capsules may be taken daily, two every four hours. If cayenne is disturbing in any way, discontinue.

Mix the following herbs together:

   4 parts peppermint
   1 part angelica
   1 part prickly ash bark
   1 part mullein

Pour one pint of boiling water over one ounce of herbs. Steep for twenty minutes; strain. Drink one-half cup whenever needed or sip continuously. See horseradish syrup described under Asthma. Use ginger foot baths described under Colds, Flu and Fevers.

B. *Hydrotherapy:* Whole, warm baths are used at first, then slowly change to cool, whole baths. Exercise after baths. Morning and evenings take alternating hot and cold showers for five minutes. Brush the skin daily from head to toe.

Pennyroyal tea taken warm helps the circulation and should be taken after warm baths.

CHOLESTEROL (High)

Principal Therapy - blood purification.

Use a low protein, low fat, non-processed diet. Fat is the worst enemy of the liver. All heated fats should be avoided—no fried foods. Avoid beer which supplies the body with carbohydrates which in turn produce fatty deposits.

Use sesame seeds, sunflower seeds and flaxseeds. Suggested foods are bee pollen, green leafy vegetables, apples, all citrus fruits and juices, garlic, onions, pears, peaches, watermelon and its juice, sprouts, lemons, cabbage (red and green), spinach, dates and leeks.

Use the cleansing diet in this book for ten days and clean the bowels with an enema for five consecutive days. Exercise daily to increase circulation. Take one tablespoon of liquid chlorophyll in apple juice four times daily.

Short two day fasts every eight to ten days will remove fatty deposits quickly. Use citrus juices or carrot, apple and spinach juices for this purpose. Vegetable broths made from leeks, garlic and onions will purify the blood. Remain on a vegetarian diet.

A. *Internal:* Take six hawthorn berry capsules and six chaparral capsules daily, alternating three every four hours. The circulation is most important when the cholesterol is high. Warm and cool alternating showers every morning followed with a brisk walk or jogging, is excellent. Don't evereat. Prickly ash tea will improve your circulation (see also stimulants). Siberian ginseng is used to reduce cholesterol. Take two capsules three times a day between meals and first thing in the morning. If they cause nervousness, reduce the dosage. Ginseng is not to be taken if there is inflammation, or fevers anywhere present in the body.

B. *Hydrotherapy:* Take cool, whole baths and warm and cool showers daily.

COLIC (See formulas under Gastritis, Indigestion and Gas)

Principal Therapy - carminative therapy.

Food should be withheld until the symptoms disappear. The quickest way to relieve gas is a warm water enema, retaining the water while in a slant position. Adding one tablespoon of apple cider vinegar per quart of warm water and injecting it into the bowels gives fast relief. Teas made from catnip, chamomile and fennel and used as the liquid for the enema will relieve gas, bloating and nausea. Use these teas or a strong tea of ginger and apply them as a fomentation over the lower stomach area. This can be used before, after or during the enema. Fomentations will usually relieve the gas without further treatment.

Use proper food combinations, do not drink with meals or eat late at night. Colic means that there is putrification in the intestines. A short one to two day fast or warm water or antispasmodic or carminative teas will break up the intestinal gas.

A. *Internal:* See formulas under Gastritis, Indigestion and Gas. Drink warm carminative teas or use twenty to thirty drops of catnip and fennel combined as a tincture in a cup of warm water. Adjust the dosage for a child. Lemon squeezed in warm water and honey is another good remedy. All mint teas are good for colic.

When the symptoms have passed, use warm vegetable broths, mint teas, enemas, and fresh juices to clean the intestines.

B. *External:* Warm fomentations or alternate hot and cold over the stomach and lower spine. Use sitz baths or warm whole baths.

COLITIS (See formulas under Constipation and Ulcers)

Principal Therapy - heat dispelling, demulcent therapy.

A liquid diet is advisable for three to seven days, using carrot juice and demulcent herb teas like slippery elm, comfrey root and mullein. Avoid high fiber foods with thick skins, seeds, and popcorn. Blend the vegetables to make them soupy and thick before eating. Use soups, but never hot liquids.

For intestinal bulk, use a tablespoon of powdered psyllium and flaxseed soaked with raisins and prunes overnight. Eat this in the mornings. Grate apples and pears and combine them with soaked figs and prunes. This will cause normal bowel movements without griping and drying of the intestines.

Emphasis is on foods that contain little fiber until the condition clears. Yellow fruits, cantaloupe, pears, watermelon, kelp, agar agar, prunes, olives, tomatoes, plums, cucumbers, berries and mushrooms are a few.

A. *Internal:* See formulas under Constipation and Ulcers. Make a comfrey root decoction and drink two ounces four times a day. Take an enema using white oak bark or bayberry mixed with equal parts of slippery elm or mullein. Chlorophyll enemas (one cup to one quart of water) is also excellent for retention enemas.

B. *External:* Warm fomentations over the lower spine and stomach.

C. *Hydrotherapy:* Use warm, whole baths.

When this condition clears, take comfrey tablets, ten to twenty daily with meals.

CONJUNCTIVITIS

Principal Therapy - blood purification.

If it is simple conjunctivitis, the blood must be thoroughly cleansed. Clean the bowels with an enema. A fruit or carrot juice fast for three days will clean the blood. Drink one pint of carrot juice daily. Put one drop of castor oil in each eye three times daily.

A. *Internal:* Use the formulas under Acne and Skin Problems and drink red clover, red raspberry and sassafras teas. Ferrum phox. 12x and kali. sulph. 12x will relieve inflammation. Take five tablets of each five times daily.

B. *External:* Make an infusion of eyebright or goldenseal and wash the eyes out several times daily with the use of an eyecup.

   A cabbage leaf poultice over the eyes will reduce inflammations. Take fifteen drops of echinacea tincture three times daily, or the capsules two to four times a day.

C. *Hydrotherapy:* Use alternating hot and cold fomentations over the eyes several times daily.

CONSTIPATION

Principal Therapy - purgation.

Take an enema with hot water or red raspberry leaf tea, slippery elm or bayberry bark. If the waste is hard, inject two cups of olive oil into the bowel and retain as long as possible. Go on a fruit fast for three to seven days, eating soaked prunes and figs. Do not drink with your meals. Eat your food dry as possible and chew until all the flavor is gone. Saliva is a natural laxative. Most people don't realize how long they should chew their food. There are no teeth in the stomach. Drink plenty of raw fruit and vegetable juices, especially apple, beet and carrot. Apples, figs, peaches, berries, oranges and prunes are excellent. Study proper food combinations.

Get plenty of outdoor exercise—walking, running, yoga, swimming, etc. is most important for sluggish bowels. Nervous tension can cause constipation and exercise will calm the system and relax the bowels.

Avoid starchy grains (unsprouted), potatoes, white rice, meats, cheese, eggs, cakes, pastries and all dairy products. Use only fruits, vegetables, raw juices, sprouts and sprouted grains, seeds and nuts. Never overeat; this is one of the main causes of constipation.

First thing in the morning, drink a glass of warm water. Soak prunes overnight and eat them for breakfast. Take a tablespoon of olive oil before bed. Warm hip baths in the evening will relax the intestines and promote morning evacuation.

Eating before bed, drinking with meals, avoiding nature's call to evacuate, high protein diet, overeating, tension, etc. all can cause constiptation.

Research your activities and find your cause of sluggish bowels. The longer the waste is retained, the more of the poisons are being absorbed into the blood. It has been said that over half of all sicknesses start in the colon. The waste is absorbed and recirculated in the blood and is deposited in the joints, liver, gall bladder, etc. The lungs, skin and kidneys have to filter the excessive waste that has been absorbed into the blood from the colon. This is one of the causes of skin disease, urinary infections, blood poisoning, gout, etc. Almost any disease can be caused by reabsorption of colon waste. The bowels must get first consideration in all diseases, including everyday sicknesses like the common cold, flu, fevers, measles, mumps, etc.

The bulk laxatives can be used for long periods of time. Avoid mineral oil and other purgatives. They can cause inflammation and bleeding of the bowels. Try to regulate the bowels with natural fruits and a better way of living. Do not become dependent on any laxatives. This will weaken your whole system. If your digestion is bad, use a tonic for the stomach and liver. Do occasional fasts; this will strengthen the system. Eat light; the body only needs about one-half the food an average person eats. Be happy and use your God-given will to overcome deadly habits.

A. *Internal:* Children's constipation. Mix the following herbs.:

> 1 ounce raspberry leaves
> 1½ ounce flaxseed

Pour one quart of boiling water over herbs. Let steep for one-half hour; strain. Take two tablespoons three times daily.

B. *Internal:* Dr. Christopher's Lower Bowel Tonic by Nature's Way:

> Cascara sagrada bark
> Bayberry root bark
> Turkey rhubarb root
> Goldenseal root
> Red raspberry leaves
> Lobelia
> Cayenne
> Fennel seed

C. *Internal:* Take cascara sagrada capsules at a dosage of two to four before bedtime with a cup of warm herb tea or water.

D. *Internal:* Grain extract. Use whole, organic grain. Powder grain in a coffee mill, add three tablespoons to one pint of water, boil for one hour. More water may need to be added for proper absorption to make a gruel. Strain through a fine cloth. Add one tablespoon or more to juice (apple, fig, grape or prune). If the baby is constipated, use an oat gruel; if the bowels are loose, use barley or wheat.

> Another baby formula: pulverize ripe pears and apples together. Add cooked figs and prunes. Use teaspoonfuls several times a day.

C. *Internal:* Mix together equal parts of the following:

> Flaxseed
> Chia seed
> Psyllium seed
> Raisins

Soak in distilled water or apple juice overnight. Just cover them with liquid. Drain off any excess fluid. Take one tablespoon three times daily.

CONVULSIONS

Principal Therapy - tranquilization

The bowels should be emptied immediately with an enema. Take some laxative herbs to clean out the small intestine. Fast on fruit juices, water or nervine teas until all symptoms subside. Keep the body warm at all times.

A. *Internal:* See the formulas under Cramps and Spasms, and the the antispasmodic formulas under Spasmodic Coughs and Lung Congestion. This tincture can be taken every fifteen minutes using twenty drops in one-half cup of warm water. Two cups of valerian root may be taken every two hours following the convulsions. Tinctures, of course, work faster in a condition like this.

If parasites are the cause, see garlic enemas. Take one teaspoon of black walnut tincture in water three times a day. Drink one cup of wormwood tea three times daily between meals. Eat garlic, onions and apple cider vinegar. A good therapy for worms is to fast for three days on pumpkin seeds. Cut up two raw onions and soak them for twelve hours in one pint of water. Strain while squeezing out the juice. Drink a cup of this three times daily. Along with this, use garlic enemas. One teaspoon of apple cider vinegar in one cup of water three times a day will aid expulsion of worms.

Powdered tansy, wormwood, balmony and bitteroot can be put in capsules, combined or used individually. Take two capsules four times a day.

For children, make an infusion of senna tea, strain it, then add enough raisins to soak up the tea. Give the children a teaspoon of raisins two to five times daily. The more they weigh, the more raisins. Use garlic enemas and put a garlic clove up the rectum before bedtime.

Another effective remedy is to crush garlic in milk and drink it throughout the day. Use a garlic enema every morning during these treatments.

Following the worm treatment, the diet should be meatless, plenty of raw carrots and greens, garlic, onions, horseradish and no potatoes or bread products. Drink plenty of papaya juice.

Tape worm remedy:

> 1 ounce valerian root
> 1/6 ounce powdered aloe

1/6 ounce wormwood
2/3 ounce senna
1/3 ounce black alder bark
1 ounce spearmint

Mix the above herbs together and make an infusion using one ounce to one pint of water. Drink two ounces three times a day while on a three day fast.

B. *External:* Take a hot bath to keep the nerves relaxed and put the patient to bed. Use a warm ginger fomentation over the spine. Use reflexology and acupuncture for all spasmodic problems.

C. *Hydrotherapy:* Warm, whole baths can be taken for long lengths of time. Lobelia tincture, fifteen drops in one cup of warm water while the patient is soaking in the bath is wonderful.

CORNS, CALLUSES AND WARTS

Principal Therapy - blood purification

Internally the blood must be purified. Take echinacea, garlic and chaparral daily.

Externally, here are some good remedies:

A. Put a few drops of citric acid on the area. In the morning use emery board or pumice stone and rub off the dead skin.

B. Thuja, wintergreen oil, thyme oil or sassafras oil can be used the same as above. Do this every night. Pumice the area in the morning.

C. Rub the fresh juice from any of these on the callus or wart: jojoba oil, dandelion juice, milkweed, wheatgrass juice or garlic oil. These methods might take a while, but with persistence, they will work. Use emery board or pumice stone every day to skim off the dead skin.

D. Massage with castor oil twice daily. This will cause the corn to peel off in layers. Use emery board or pumice stone.

E. Soak the area in a mixture of oil of wintergreen, witch hazel and black walnut tincture daily. Use pumice stone and emery board. This is good for warts, calluses and corns.

F. Fry poke root in grease (hard). Paint the wart, callus or corn with this four to five times daily.

G. Put a drop of iodine on the wart daily. This has been known to rid the body of the problem in a few weeks.

H. Soak a piece of cotton in freshly squeezed lemon juice or pineapple. Bandage the cotton over the wart, corn, or callus. It will dissolve it. Be persistent.

I.   Any sweet oil rubbed on warts, corns or calluses several times a day with the use of emery board or pumice stone to skim off the dead skin is good.

COUGHS, SORE THROAT, LUNG CONGESTION

Principal Therapy - blood purification, deobstruent, stimulation.

Clean the bowels with a warm water enema. Go on a raw fruit and vegetable juice fast for a few days. Avoid high protein foods, starches and dairy products. These foods create mucus and congest the bowels and respiratory organs. Milk is the worst offender of the lungs and intestines. If the stomach and system were kept in good order there would be no coughs. Exercise outside and do deep breathing exercise. This will help expel mucus.

Drink freshly squeezed lemon juice with a little honey, cayenne and ginger sprinkled in the mixture. Sip this every hour. Hold a piece of garlic in your mouth. This is good for coughs and sore throats.

Suggested foods are leeks, onions, garlic, figs, flaxseed, honey, horseradish, apricots, asparagus, comfrey, dandelion greens, mustard greens, beet greens, cabbage, endive and peaches.

A.   *Internal:* Here are some cough and cold remedies that are easy to use.

   1. Homeopathic coccus cacti—whooping cough 3x or 6x.

   2. One ounce of horehound, one ounce of elecampane root, one ounce of comfrey root, one ounce of wild cherry bark. Boil in 2½ quarts of water down to one quart. Strain and add eight ounces of honey. Take a tablespoon every one-half to one hour when needed.

   3. Take two ounces of elecampane root and pour one quart of boiling water over it. Steep it for one hour on low heat, do not boil. Strain, add one cup of honey and one teaspoon of cayenne. Take one tablespoon five times a day.

   4. For all chest and cough afflictions, take one ounce of the following: horehound, Irish moss, flaxseed, boneset and licorice root. Simmer in a gallon of distilled water down to one-half gallon. Take ¼ cup four times daily.

   Other suggested herbs are chickweed, slippery elm, angelica, elder flowers, St. John's wort, plantain, eucalyptus, anise and catnip.

B.   *Hydrotherapy:* Tincture of benzoin may be added to steam to be breathed into the lungs. Massaging the sides, front and back of the neck in a clockwise motion using ice and then followed by cold, wet compresses is effective. When renewed every thirty minutes for at least four times the cough becomes modified, expectoration is eased and breathing becomes easier. This treatment may be continued until cough disappears. The compresses may also be applied on the chest.

COLDS, FEVERS AND FLU

Principle Therapy – blood purification, heat dispelling.

These conditions are usually caused by the body being overloaded with poisons. Months of eating improperly, coupled with bad habits such as using coffee, tea, soft drinks, etc. can force the body into a healing crisis. The immune system is put under stress, the energy is low and the mucus membranes throughout the body, in the nose, throat and intestines are forced to eliminate these toxic substances that have built up.

A short fast is a necessity; usually three to five days. Keep in mind that the body is eliminating poisons and not absorbing nutrients. Eating will only prolong the condition. There is no greater fallacy than thinking that the person inflicted needs nourishment to sustain his or her strength. The stomach and intestines are throwing waste matter out from the interior of the body and this process should not be interrupted. The fast can be a juice fast, using apple, citrus juices or just lemon in water, or you can use herbal teas. If you are dealing with a child, red raspberry leaf, catnip, peppermint or nettles can be used. Adults can use goldenseat leaf or root, elder flowers, myrrh or bonset. If the joints are sore coupled with a high fever, bonset is excellent. If there is stomach pain present, goldenseal leaf tea or tincture is good.

Clean the bowels with an enema whenever necessry during the fast, or at least once at the beginning and once at the end. If a fast is not possible, then use a fruit diet but avoid avocadoes and bananas. Juicy fruits are the best. If constipation is present, use cascara sagrada before bed. Your health food store should carry this herb. Laxative herbs should never be used for long periods of time.

After the fever has subsided, a few days should be allowed for healing and restoring of the tissues. Easily digestible foods should be eaten. Fruits and sprouts would be an excellent choice. Avoid all dairy and flour products for two to four weeks after the fast or eliminate them entirely from your diet.

While in its cleansing mode, the body is usually in an acid state which means that the urine and body secretions are acid. You want to use alkaline foods and juices to bring the body back to its normal pH, particularly after the fast. A fast way of doing this is to use a product called Green Magma (dried juice from young barley plants) or Kyo-Green (a powdered drink of concentrated juice from young barley and wheatgrass plants, chlorella, kelp and brown rice). Green Magma has been in health food stores for several years and is excellent to help restore alkalinity and can be used as a daily supplement. It is a complete protein, contains 22 of its own enzymes and an array of vitamins and minerals. It is excellent for weight loss. You can purchase the product in most health food stores but if you have trouble finding it, write to: Green Foods Corp., 620 Maple Ave., Torrance, CA 90503.

Kyo-Green is a relatively new product on the market but it is excellent as a daily supplement and to use during and after fasting. Recent research from Lomalinda College has shown Kyo-Green to stimulate the immune system. I have personally used this product for four consecutive months and have noticed less hunger and more endurance in my athletic events. This is an excellent product for athletes. You can find this product in health food stores. If not, encourage them to carry it. You can get more information on this product by writing to Wakunaga of America Co., Ltd., Mission Viego, CA 92691.

CROUP (See Coughs, Sore Throat, Lung Congestion)

CRAMPS AND SPASMS

Principal Therapy - tranquilization, blood purification.

Calcium is very important when cramps are present. Use high calcium foods and raw juices. Carrot juice is excellent. Other suggested foods are green leafy vegetables, sprouts, sunflower seeds, sesame seeds, pecans, peas (sprouted), cashews, garlic, almonds, figs, oranges, soybeans (sprouted), onions, millet and brewer's yeast.

Avoid high protein foods, flour products, sugar and starches. These foods plug the intestinal tract and hinder absorption of vitamins and minerals. Always keep the bowels active. At least two bowel movements a day or as many as meals you eat daily. Use herbal laxatives if needed. Keep the circulation normal with plenty of fresh air, exercise and alternating hot and cold showers.

A. *Internal:* Drinking a juice combination made from two ounces of parsley juice, two ounces beet juice, one pint of carrot juice and four ounces of cucumber juice also relieves cramps. Sip it slowly and hold each mouthful until it is mixed with saliva. Avoid overeating; masticate your food properly, do not drink with meals, and use proper food combinations and the cleansing diet.

Mag. phos. 12x taken five tablets every one-half hour till cramping subsides is excellent. The blood must be kept clean and the pH normal. Use alkaline broths made from fresh vegetables.

Herbal teas that will clean the blood are sasssfras, burdock root, dandelion, red clover and other alteratives. Other suggested herbs for cramping are fennel, cayenne, rue, thyme, wood betony, pennyroyal, valerian, lobelia, mistletoe and lady's slipper.

B. *Internal:* Mix together the following herbs:

> 1 part scullcap
> 1 part mistletoe
> 1 part valerian root
> 1 part vervain
> ½ part ginger

Steep one teaspoon of mixed herbs in one cup of boiling water; strain. Take two ounces every one-half hour until cramps stop.

C. *Internal:* Mix together the following herbs:

> 3 ounces of powdered cinnamon
> 1 ounce of cardamon seeds
> 1 ounce of nutmeg

Mix herbs together in a blender. Dosage: ¼ to ½ teaspoon steeped in one cup of boiling water for ten minutes. Take cold for nausea. Drink hot sweetened with honey for cramps and spasms.

Take calcium tablets daily.

See also antispasmodic formula and castor oil packs.

D. *Hydrotherapy:* Warm hip baths with an infusion of chamomile or hayflower added to the tub is excellent. The temperature of the water should be just above body temperature. The duration of the bath can be one-half hour. These baths are good for cramps, colic, menstrual problems and leucorrhea. The abdomen areas which contain all the vital organs become congested and irritated when there is poor blood, overweight and not enough exercise.

A hot shower for fifteen minutes followed by a cabbage leaf poultice will quickly relieve cramps. An onion poultice placed over the stomach is also very good.

CYSTITIS (See Kidney and Bladder Infections)

DANDRUFF AND HAIR LOSS

Principal Therapy - blood purification and stimulation therapy.

The diet should be low protein, low fat, high complex carbohydrates and fibrous foods. Use the cleansing diet in this book. Give an enema every day for seven days. Three day fasts every month using carrot juice and liquid chlorophyll (four ounces daily) will clean the blood. Remain on a vegetarian diet. Avoid oils and fried foods.

Only shampoos made from herbs should be used followed by a hair rinse made from an infusion of nettles, rosemary and sage. Add one tablespoon of apple cider vinegar to one quart of hair rinse.

A. *Internal:* Eat all seaweeds and take kelp and dulse tablets with your meals. Drink nettle, sage and rosemary teas daily.

B. *External:* Put one cup of sage leaves in a quart of boiling water. Simmer for one-half hour, strain and add one teaspoon of borax. Wash the hair three times weekly with this. Brush the hair daily.

Take four ounces of olive oil and five drops of rosemary oil mixed together. Massage scalp with this every night. Wash the hair in the mornings. Wheat germ oil and olive oil are also excellent scalp oils.

C. *Hydrotherapy:* Put hot towels over the scalp or take a steam bath with these oils massaged into the scalp.

For stimulation, alternate hot and cold towels on the scalp three to four times weekly for two minute durations for ten minutes is sufficient.

DENTITION

Principal Therapy - tranquilization.

Other problems may be present that can contribute to this painful malady such as eye or ear inflammations, respiratory infection or intestinal disturbances. These should be checked for and taken care of immediately.

Remedies for teething babies are as follows:

1. Yarrow flowers soaked in brandy for a few days. Strain and rub on the gums.
2. Mullein oil or lobelia tincture rubbed on the gums several times daily.
3. Cayenne tincture and lobelia tincture combined equal parts and rubbed on the sore area several times daily.
4. Rub peppermint oil or clove oil on the tender area. These are strong so just a drop is needed.
5. Holding finger pressure on the area will sometimes relieve the pain.
6. Cajaput oil, calendula powder and vervain tincture are others for sore gums and teeth.
7. Hops and valerian tincture or the anti-spasmodic tincture rubbed on the gums and taken internally is very good.

Note: During this time from six months of age to twenty-four months, the child needs the proper amount of calcium for growth of bones and teeth. Diluted fruit and vegetable juices can be given to the child. They should be made fresh and taken within the hour. Herb teas such as nettles, alfalfa and comfrey will also supply the needed calcium. Freshly squeezed carrot and grape juice diluted to 50% distilled water may be used.

Homeopathically, calcium fluroaticum alternated wtih calcium phosphate 6x or 12x, two tablets, taken three times a day.

DERMATITIS (Eczema) (Erysipelas)

Skin conditions usually indicate poor elimination through the bowels and kidneys. If the kidney function is impaired, see formulas under Kidney and Bladder Infections. Drinking kidney herbs such as horsetail grass, corn silk, cleavers and buchu in combination or individually will help eliminate the excess acid. Remember, if the kidneys are not functioning properly, the skin will be used to eliminate the excess acid which is one of the main causes of all skin conditions. Clean the bowels with an enema and use laxative herbs if absolutely necessary. The diet should be kept alkaline. Mainly fruits, vegetables and sprouts should be used in raw and fresh juice form. Carrot juice is excellent. Use the cleansing diet in this book for one week, with an enema every morning for five consecutive days. Avoid meats, sugar, starches and especially salt which is highly toxic. Get your proteins from soybean sprouts, almonds and sesame seeds. Sesame seeds are especially good for the content of vitamins A, B, E, unsaturated fatty oils, phosphorus and calcium. Make it into a cream by powdering the seeds and mixing them with water. Some good foods for skin conditions are parsley, spinach, sprouts, bee pollen, brewer's yeast, green leafy vegetables, celery, pineapples, grapes, melons, kelp, garlic, seeds and nuts (unsalted), onions, chives, papayas, pears and peaches.

A. *Internal:* Use the treatment suggestions under Acne and Skin Problems. Homeopathically there are some good remedies that can be taken with herbal therapies. If there is a pus discharge, heper sulph 3x or 6x; if the condition is a highly acid one, rhus tox 4x or 6x. Along with this use a calcium supplement.

   Echinacea tincture ten drops every two hours will purify the blood and stop itching.

B. *External:* Skin maladies are either dry or wet conditions. In both cases, plenty of distilled water, fresh air and exercise is of paramount importance. If the skin is dry, lanolin cream or herbal salves made with lanolin are good. St. John's wort oil dabbed on dry sore areas will bring relief. In the evenings, the skin can be powdered with powdered calcium. This will disinfect the areas and give relief from itching.

   Fomentations made from comfrey, plantain, burdock, dandelion, black walnut and periwinkle are all excellent. They should be applied cool or body temperature and can be kept on for one hour periods a couple of times daily. The extract of pansy is especially good for external treatment as a fomentation. Take cool baths with chaparral tea added to the water.

DIABETES

Principal Therapy - blood purification, tonification.

There are two kinds of diabetes. Diabetes mellitus is characterized by increased urination where excess sugar is found. This is usually neurologically based. Diabetes insipidus is unassociated with sugar (glucose) which is not continually being found in the urine, but excessive urination is present (polyuria).

It is generally understood that the digestive organs are impaired in this disease, especially the pancreas, liver and stomach. The diet should be kept simple and avoid stress and stimulating foods. Heavy starches, animal products, soft drinks, tobacco, starches, dairy products, eggs, all denatured foods must be eliminated.

The diet should consist of sprouted grains, watercress, non-starchy vegetables, fresh fruits, sprouts, bee pollen, millet, garlic, onions, chicory, dandelion, endive, all berries, grapes, beets, greens, leavy green vegetables, and small amounts of raw seeds and nuts.

Dr. Henry Beiler in his book "Food is Your Best Medicine" says that he has relieved many diabetics with the use of a mucusless diet with the addition of a broth made from zucchini and string beans taken several cups daily. Fresh fruits are a good addition to this because they contain natural sugar called fructose, which does not require insulin in order to be assimilated.

Fasting will help rid the body of the excess sugar. Short fasts should be used because the patient is usually in a weakened state but prolonged fasting will enhance the emaciation. Use. Dr. Beiler's broth during the fast.

Keep the bowels clean with enemas. Brush the skin daily to activate the nervous system. Exercise is important for proper elimination and oxidation of the excess sugar in the blood. Walking, bicycling, roller skating, yoga, and deep breathing are suggested. Do not overdo.

A. *Internal:* If diabetes mellitus is the problem, give special attention to the nerves. Avoid stress. The diet and herbal therapies can be basically the same for both kinds of diabetes. If the pituitary gland is not functioning properly and there are hormone imbalances, raw pituitary extract can be used. For those who would prefer herbal remedies for the pituitary glands, alfalfa, ginseng, and gota kola can be used. Chinese herbs that have been successfully used in diabetes and to tone the whole system are don sen, fu ling (nutritive herb for pancreas), ho shou wu (this herb is good for hypoglycemia and diabetes) and pai shu.

Dandelion root and cedar berries have an excellent reputation for relieving diabetes. Dandelion tea will strengthen the digestive system and detoxify the liver, spleen, blood and pancreas. An important formula for all pancreatic problems is as follows:

    1 part uva ursi
    1 part goldenseal
    1 part elecampane
    2 parts dandelion root
    2 parts cedar berries
    1 part fennel
    ½ part ginger

Mix the powdered herbs and put them in #00 capsules. Take them after every meal. Drink gentian or goldenseal tea between meals to strengthen digestion. Take digestive enzymes with every meal. Make sure pancreatin, bromelian, lipase, amylase and chymotypsin are in the enzyme formulas.

Huckleberry leaf tea has been known to cure diabetes by itself. One cup three times daily.

B. *Hydrotherapy:* Hot and cold packs over the pancreas and kidneys will help insulin production and kidney elimination. Hot showers will help stimulate the pancreas. Take these showers two or three times daily.

DIARRHEA AND DYSENTERY

Principal Therapy - purgation (aperients)

Fast for two to three days. Take an enema on the morning of each day of the fast made from a decoction of bayberry bark and slippery elm tea in equal parts. If a child is effected with diarrhea, wash the bowels with a catnip tea enema. Feed the child a gruel made from slippery elm or fresh ground oats. Grated apples will prevent diarrhea in children and adults. Drink carrot juice diluted with 25% distilled water.

A. *Internal:* Drink one teaspoon of yellow or white clay in water three or four times a day. Drink teas made from huckleberry leaf, bistort, white oak bark, bayberry, gentian or cranesbill. Usually one-half cup three or four times daily of any of these herbs will be sufficient. (See proper dosages.)

Tormentilla tincture twenty drops in one-half cup of warm water four times daily for adults of three drops for children may be taken. Give children clay water also.

One teaspoon of psyllium seed mixed with three tablespoons of bentonite in juice three times a day is excellent. Take this every day until seven days after the problem has stopped. Eat only fruits and vegetables until this condition clears.

Diarrhea in babies and adults can be stopped by boiling slowly, one-half cup of wild rice in six cups of water for one and one-half hours. Strain, add an equal portion blackberry juice to the strained water. Take teaspoonfuls several times daily.

Dysentery can be treated the same, except for enemas. Use garlic water injections. Use the herbal treatment under parasites and worms under Convulsions. If there is bleeding from the bowels make a decoction of equal parts comfrey root and bayberry bark and drink two ounces every two to four hours until the bleeding stops.

B. *External:* Hot and cold fomentations over the stomach.

C. *Hydrotherapy:* Use cool water sitz baths mornings and evenings.

After the treatment, use tonification therapy to help build the digestive organs and intestines. Eat homemade yogurt and drink bifidus (toppers) twice daily to build up the natural bacteria. Eating seaweeds will aid in this therapy.

DIPTHERIA

Principal Therapy - blood purification, stimulation.

Give the patient an enema every morning and evening. Bayberry, white oak bark or red raspberry enemas are excellent for this condition. Fast on carrot juice or citrus juices freshly squeezed. Bed rest and a well-ventilated room is most necessary. Avoid the chills by using warm baths. An emetic is usually necessary to empty the stomach of putrifying material or high fevers will result (see emetics). If there is choking during the night, give the patient a warm herbal tea made from prickly ash, bayberry bark and red raspberry. These can be mixed in equal parts and sipped slowly until the condition is relieved. Bayberry is an herb that should be considered in all cases of throat or stomach mucus conditions.

If the patient insists on eating, stewed dates, raisins, figs, bananas and oranges are the only foods that should be taken. When the disease has passed, have the patient return to a vegetarian diet.

All clothing and bed linens should be cleaned by boiling them and changing daily.

A. *Internal:* After the bowels have been washed out properly as mentioned above, they should be kept moving regularly by herbal laxatives if necessary.

A gargle made from red sage tea or equal parts myrrh and goldenseal with a pinch of cayenne added to it should be prepared and used every one-half hour to clean the mucus and germs out of the throat. Drinking a cup of red sage tea every hour will purify the blood and cause sweating. Keep the patient in bed during this time. Add ten drops of lobelia tincture to each cup of tea. If nausea is caused by the lobelia, cut down on the dosage.

Ephedra, an herb sometimes called mormon tea or Brigham tea, should be discussed here. It is an excellent herb for the mucus membranes of the lungs and nasal passages. Its active ingredient, ephedrine, has an anesthetic action wherever it is absorbed. When spasms or coughing is persistent, mormon tea dialates the bronchial tubes which bring relief. It stimulates the heart and nervous system. When the heart or lungs are affected by diptheria, mormon tea helps strengthen and relax these areas. Hawthorn berry tablets should also be taken every two hours if the heart is affected.

Good remedies to cure this infectious disease are two echinacea or myrrh/goldenseal capsules every two hours or one-half cup of the herbs in tea form. Use a tincture of these herbs if a child is being treated. An especially good tincture is myrrh, goldenseal and cayenne (¼ part), fifteen drops every hour for an adult; four to eight drops for a child, depending upon weight. Put these drops in an herbal tea or juice if need be.

B. *External:* Use hot and cold fomentations over the liver, stomach, kidney and spine to keep the circulation normal. This disease effects the lymphatic system where the toxins have accumulated and by stimulating this system by water treatments, light exercises and stimulating herbs, it will detoxify rapidly.

If there are symptoms of heart failure, use one-half teaspoon of cayenne in hot water. Have the patient drink it down immediately. Repeat this if necessary. A teaspoon of brandy or whiskey will do the job if cayenne is not available.

This disease usually lasts from a week to ten days if properly taken care of.

DIVERTICULITIS (See Colitis)

Principal Therapy - heat dispelling, demulcent.

This is a condition where the pouches or sacs of the mucus membrane of the large intestine become inflamed and infected.

Take fenugreek and comfrey tablets, two every two hours and follow the same treatment as colitis. With severe inflammation take two myrrh/goldenseal capsules every two hours.

DROPSY

Principal Therapy - stimulation, diaphoresis.

Use the cleansing diet in this book and avoid meats, sugar, flour products, pastries, dairy products, salt and fried foods. Foods should be eaten as dry as possible, chewed well and in proper combinations. Avoid eating after 6:00 p.m. Some suggested foods are citrus, tomatoes, beets, parsley, grapes, celery, asparagus, onions, cucumbers, sprouts, endive and watercress.

Drink only distilled or purified water, wheatgrass juice and celery juice and apple juice combined in equal parts. Monthly do a 48-hour fast using small amounts of herb teas or freshly squeezed juice. Many times a three day watermelon fast clears several pounds of excess water from the body. Only drink when thirsty to avoid putting undue stress on the kidneys and heart. Use an enema weekly and keep the bowels moving freely.

A. *Internal:* See the formulas under Kidney and Bladder Infections and under Urine Retention.

    If there is gravel or stones in the kidney, use the formula found under Kidney Stones.

    Whenever there is suspected heart problems, use one tablespoon of hawthorn berry syrup or tincture three times daily. The capsules can also be taken in the amount of twelve daily.

    Pipissewa (prince's pine) is excellent for dropsy and rheumatism. Take twenty drops of tincture three to four times daily or three cups of the tea.

B. *External:* Use a ginger fomentation over the kidneys or hot and cold alternating water fomentations for stimulation.

DYSENTERY (See Diarrhea)

See the section on Anus Itching and the section on Diarrhea. The treatment under diarrhea combined with the herbs used under anus itching and worms will cure the worst dysentery.

DYSMENORRHEA

Principal Therapy - tranquilization, blood purification.

Dysmenorrhea is painful and difficult flow of menses. During the painful period, a fast should be adhered to until the symptoms pass. Then continue on with the diet and cleansing suggestions as listed under menopause. Make sure to clean the bowels immediately with a warm water enema. Use hot baths or hot fomentations over the abdomen and lower spine.

A. *Internal:* Use a douche made from one tablespoon of lady's slipper, one-half tablespoon of lobelia, one teaspoon of goldenseal. Steep for ten minutes in a quart of warm water.

Drink the tea that is suggested under menstrual cramps or the female corrective tonic under Amenorrhea.

Neuralgic Dysmenorrhea. When the nerves are affected the herbs that should be used are pulsatilla, black cohosh and black haw. A teaspoon four times daily of any one of these tinctures or ten to twenty drops every fifteen minutes will decrease pain and cramping. They also can be taken in tea form individually or combined. Also see the antispasmodic formula in this book and use the same dosage as suggested above. If none of these herbs can be found, use lobelia tincture fifteen drops every twenty minutes in one-half cup of warm water. Cut back on the dosage if nausea is felt.

After the symptoms subside, read carefully the section in this book on tonification therapy. Choose some nervine herbs and take them daily to help overcome this condition. Especially take them one week before the menstrual cycle, along with a good egg or oyster shell calcium supplement.

DYSPEPSIA (See Gastritis, Indigestion and Gas)

Principal Therapy - carminative.

A. *Internal:* Make an infusion of the following:

> 2 parts angelica
> ¼ part fennel seed
> ¼ part anise seed
> ½ part ginger

Make an infusion of a teaspoon of herb to one cup of boiling water. Drink one-half cup four times daily between meals.

EAR INFECTIONS

Principal Therapy - blood purification.

Drink the juice of an orange or lemon diluted with 25% water until the infection and pain is gone. Fast until the infection subsides. Clean the bowels with a warm water enema.

A. *Internal:* Put three to four drops of lobelia tincture, mullein oil or garlic oil in each ear three times day. If the ear has abscessed and broken, use peroxide to wash the ear out. Repeat this until the ear is clean.

   Take ten drops of a tincture made from echinacea or plantain every three hours until the infection is gone. The teas of these herbs can be taken also. Myrrh/goldenseal or chaparral taken in capsule form is good for the infection. The dose is two every two hours.

   A good homeopathic procedure is five drops of belladonna 4x every two hours with two tablets of ferrum phos. 6x or 12x every two hours. These should be alternated so every hour the patient is taking medication. Hepar sulph 4x, two tablets every hour is used when there is excessive discharge. Use silica 12x after the pain is gone to help clear up the pus.

   Take calcium supplements after the problem is cleared.

   Chamomile, calendula and St. John's wort oil can be used to wash the ears out or as drops put into the ears. Always remember to treat both ears even though the infection is just in one ear.

B. *External:* A warm fomentation over the ear made from lobelia, wild lettuce, chamomile or catnip teas may be used. To relieve pain, bake a large onion until soft, cut it in halves and apply over the ear and wrap it tightly. It is also successful to apply this behind the ear. A cabbage leaf or clay poultice is also very effective.

C. *Hydrotherapy:* Neck bandages which are soaked in cool water, along with hot foot baths with one tablespoon of mustard or cayenne added to the water will reduce pain and swelling by drawing the blood away from the upper body.

ECZEMA (See Dermatitis)

Principal Therapy - blood purification, stimulation, tonification (kidneys).

Use the cleansing diet in this book and proper food combinations. The diet should be kept alkaline—mainly sprouts, fruits, vegetables eaten raw. One pint of carrot juice or two ounces of chlorophyll juice should be taken daily. Parsley juice is excellent for all skin conditions. Avoid meats, sugar, refined foods, salt, etc. Protein foods that can be eaten in small amounts are almonds, soybean sprouts, tofu (small amounts), walnuts, brazil nuts and sesame seeds.

Suggested foods are spinach, bee pollen (from your area), nutritional yeast, celery, melons, grapes (all kinds), kelp, seaweeds, garlic, chives, peaches and papayas.

Clean the bowels with an enema once weekly until the condition ceases. Do a three day juice fast (preferably the juices mentioned above) at the end of every month. Expose the nude body to fresh air and sunlight twenty minutes daily.

A. *Internal:* See the formulas listed under Acne and Skin Problems.

Tinctures of burdock, bittersweet, coneflower, rhubarb, dandelion or goldenseal are specific remedies for skin diseases. These tinctures can be combined, ten drops of three of them taken together in a cup of warm water three times or more daily.

The treatment that I have suggested for Abscesses is also very good. Drink plenty of blood purifying teas like red clover, burdock, calendula and sassafras. Thirty drops of echinacea tincture four times daily has been successfully used by itself.

Homeopathically, for pus discharges heper sulph 3x or 6x is good taken along with calcium supplements. Usually four tablets four times a day of both of these remedies will suffice. Heper sulph can be used along with tincture of myrrh for all pus discharges.

B. *External:* Mix together the following:

> 1 part calendula flowers
> ½ part plantain leaves
> ½ part wormwood
> ½ part chickweed

Mix two ounces of herbs in one pint of olive or linseed oil. Bake in the oven in a closed container at 300 degrees Farenheit until the leaves become crisp (approximately two to four hours.) Stir every 45 minutes. Strain. Add one to one and one-half ounces of beeswax and one teaspoon of lanolin. To preserve it, add the oil of two vitamin E capsules or one-half teaspoon of gum benzoin. These are added while the solution is hot. Put in jars and wait until it hardens.

For dry skin, lanolin cream or herbal salves made with lanolin are good. St. John's wort oil dabbed in dry areas is good. Powdered calcium sprinkled on itchy areas in the evening will give relief.

Fomentations made from comfrey, plantain, burdock, dandelion, black walnut or periwinkle are all excellent. They should be applied cool and kept on for at least one hour. The extract of pansy is good for external applications.

C. *Hydrotherapy:* Cool baths with one pound epsom salts or one gallon of chaparral or chamomile teas added to the water will stop itching and infections.

Note: During all skin disease the kidneys should be properly cared for. The kidneys and skin work together in the process of removing toxic fluid wastes from the body. Teas made from corn silk, cleavers, uva ursi, goldenrod or buchu are all excellent. Here is a formula that will clean the blood and kidneys:

    1 ounce dandelion root
    1 ounce parsley root
    1 ounce agrimony
    1 ounce red raspberry leaves
    ½ ounce ginger

Boil in three quarts of water down to three pints, strain and let cool. Drink three to four ounces three times daily.

During severe skin disease like erysipelas, take belladonna 4x, five drops in four ounces of water and taken three to four times a day will stop the most severe eruptions. Many times this remedy coupled with echinacea tincture (thirty drops) every four hours is all that is needed. See a competent physician for severe skin conditions.

Aconite (3x or 4x) five drops in a glass of water taken at one hour intervals is also good for fever coupled with severe skin conditions.

EMPHYSEMA (See Asthma)

ENDOMETRIOSIS

Principal Therapy - blood purification.

Follow the dietary suggestions under Menopause. Use castor oil packs along with the "Ichthammol and vegetable glycerine" pack mentioned under Ovarian Cysts. Take chaparral and goldenseal capsules. Alternate them two every four hours.

During the inflammation stages, use echinacea tincture twenty drops every two hours until pain subsides, then use the same dosages three times a day.

To tone the reproductive organs, use the female corrective tonic under the section on Amenorrhea or the formula under Ovarian Cysts.

EPIDIDYMITIS (Swollen, inflamed testicles)

Principal Therapy - heat dispelling (demulcent).

Do a three day carrot juice fast using water and slippery elm tea enemas every morning. Return to a low protein, low fat diet high in fruits, raw vegetables and liquid chlorophyll. The diet under Arthritis would be appropriate for this condition.

A.   *Internal:* Take twenty drops of echinacea tincture every hour during the day. Drink four cups of mullein tea daily.

B.   *External:* During the night, apply a pack made from equal parts of slippery elm and clay. A cabbage poultice can also be used. Add two tablespoons of St. John's wort oil to the slippery elm and clay. Mix with water until a thick paste is made. Spread this on gauze and tie around the testicle. Put a pair of underwear on or a jockstrap to hold in place. Do this before bed.

C. *Hydrotherapy:* Take cool, whole baths twice daily for ten minute durations.

EPILEPSY (See Convulsions)

GALLSTONES (To remove)

Principal Therapy - deobstruent.

Use the following formula:

> 1 part wood betony
> 1 part dandelion root
> 1 part wild yam
> 1 part parsley root
> 1 part licorice root

Simmer one ounce of this formula in one and one-half pints of water for forty-five minutes, strain. Drink one-half cup three times a day. This tea should be taken during a three day apple juice fast.

Before the fast the patient should first empty the bowels with a warm water enema. The bowels should always be emptied first before attempting to flush out the gallstones. Then begin the three day fast using apple juice and the above tea. Clean the bowels with another enema after the fast. Drink a cup of tea made of one part goldenseal, two parts dandelion, one-half part peppermint every two hours the day before you are going to flush out the gallstones. This will liquify the bile.

Put a castor oil pack over the liver and gall bladder area for one hour. Immediately after using the pack, drink four ounces of cold-pressed olive oil mixed with four ounces of freshly squeezed lemon juice. Take a strong herbal laxative after the drink. A cup of senna tea with a little ginger added is good. Lie down on your right side with your hips elevated by a pillow. This position will cause the oil to run down into the gall bladder. Place a hot castor oil pack or a fomentation of hops and lobelia over the liver while in this position. The stones will pass freely within a two to six hour period.

After the stones are removed, the patient should remain on a fruit diet for three days, while taking two tablespoons of olive oil mixed with two tablespoons of lemon juice once daily. Then return to a cleansing diet.

When the cleanse is over, the patient should include in his or her diet, plenty of figs, prunes, raisins, dandelion greens, chicory, beets and tops, carrot juice, cold-pressed olive oil, grated apples, flaxseed, sesame seeds, lemons, oranges, grapes, celery, garlic, onions, tomatoes, dates, melons, pineapples, etc.

Liver And Gallbladder Flush
(Detoxification)

The liver and gallbladder flush is an important detoxifying agent which will help restore the normal functional capacity of these organs. It is not recommended for patients under 25 years of age or patients with known large stones. Listed below are the steps that should be followed:

1. Monday through Saturday noon, drink as much apple juice or apple cider as your appetite will permit in addition to regular meals and any supplements that may have been prescribed. The apple juice should preferably be purchased from a health food store to assure there are no additives.

2. At noon on Saturday, you should eat a normal lunch.

3. Three hours later, take two teaspoons of disodium phosphate dissolved in about one ounce of hot water. The taste may be objectional and may be followed by a little citrus juice (freshly squeezed if possible).

4. Two hours later, repeat step 3.

5. You may have grapefruit juice, grapefruit or other citrus fruits or juices for your evening meal.

6. At bedtime, you may have one of the following:
   a) ½ cup of unrefined olive oil followed by a small glass of grapefruit juice; or
   b) ½ cup of warm, unrefined olive oil blended with ½ cup of lemon juice.

   Unrefined olive oil can be purchased from any health food store. It is best to use fresh citrus juice, but canned or bottled are permissible.

7. Following step 6, you should go immediately to bed and lie on your right side with your right knee pulled up close to your chest for 30 minutes.

8. The next morning, one hour before breakfast, take two teaspoons of disodium phosphate dissolved in two ounces of hot water.

9. Be sure to continue with your normal diet and any nutritional program that has been prescribed for you.

Some patients have occasionally reported slight to moderate nausea when taking the olive oil/citrus juice; this nausea will slowly disappear by the time you go to sleep. If the olive oil induces vomiting, you need not repeat the procedure at this time. This occurs only in rare instances. A cup of strong peppermint tea will help relieve the nausea. This flushing of the liver and gall bladder stimulates and cleans these organs as no other method.

Patients who have chronically suffered from gallstones, billiousnesses, backaches, nausea, etc. occasionally find small gallstone-type objects in the stool the following day. These objects are light green to dark green in color. They are very irregular in shape, gelatinous in texture, and vary in size from grape seeds to cherry seeds. If there seems to be a large number of these objects in the stool, the liver flush should be repeated in two weeks.

GANGRENE

Principal Therapy - stimulation, blood purification.

The diet should be vegetarian using high fiber, complex starches, low protein and low fat diet. Clean the bowels daily with an enema. Take one teaspoon of powdered psyllium seed in eight ounces of juice three times daily to assure proper bowel movements.

Drink raw carrot juice daily, and eat 80% of your food raw. Avoid meats, refined foods, alcohol, salt, etc. Use dulse, kelp and other seaweeds daily to assist the thyroid gland.

A. *Internal:* Take vitamin A emulsion 50,000 units daily with proteolitic enzymes. If the lips crack or blurred vision is experienced, stop the vitamin A for one week. Then continue with 30,000 units. The enzymes will eat the dead flesh and the vitamin A will kill the infection. Divide the vitamin A up into three doses daily.

Use the blood purifying formula under Acne and Skin Problems. Chaparral and echinacea either capsules or tinctures can be used, taken every three hours. Alternate the two if possible.

Drink stimulating teas like prickly ash and ginger to assist elimination. If there is excessive sweating, cut back on stimulation therapy. If the kidneys are not functioning properly, drink uva usi or celery seed tea. Other diuretics can be used. Dr. Vogal strongly suggests a homeopathic remedy called lachesis 12x for this condition along with large doses of calcium.

Echinacea tincture fifteen drops taken every two hours is an excellent remedy. Baptisia (wild indigo) tincture ten drops several times a day is an old remedy used by the famous eclectic physicians.

B. *External:* If the skin is dry, a mixture of equal parts of olive oil, wheat germ oil and castor oil can be rubbed on to prevent cracking. When pus is oozing, bathe the affected areas with warm peroxide and wipe it off carefully. Whenever possible, walk or massage the legs to help stimulation.

Fomentations made from goldenseal, chamomile and chaparral are excellent several times daily. When there is pain, add five to ten drops of arnica to the fomentations and poultices.

Make a paste out of equal part powdered myrrh, goldenseal, lobelia, flaxseed and flour. Add water and apply to infected areas. Add arnica tincture to the poultice if pain is present.

C. *Hydrotherapy:* Use cool leg baths or whole, cool baths whenever possible. Chaparral or tea can be added to the water or apple cider vinegar (one tablespoon to one quart of water).

Alternate hot and cold foot baths or fomentations to increase circulation.

Tonification therapy. The patient should use easily digestible foods and plenty of raw juices. Study tonification therapy.

GASTRITIS (Indigestion, Gas, Gastroenteritis)

Principal Therapy - tranquilization, demulcent.

Inflammation of the mucus membrane of the stomach wall is caused by stress, alcohol, coffee, tea, high protein diets, excessive dairy products and fried foods. Go on a carrot and cabbage juice fast for three to ten days. Four parts carrot juice, one part cabbage juice should be taken four ounces at a time every four hours. Clean the bowels with a slippery elm tea enema three consecutive days.

If there is constant gas and bloating in the stomach, use a lobelia emetic (see emetics) followed by a cup of equal parts peppermint and slippery elm tea. Between drinking juices, vegetable broths with the addition of large amounts of barley and oats can be taken. The broth should be somewhat thick and slippery to bathe the inflamed intestines. Add more oats or slippery elm to produce this effect. Two ounces of liquid chlorophyll juice daily is also excellent. With the juice, broth, and chlorophyll, this treatment is nutritious enough to continue for two to three weeks until the symptoms subside.

A. *Internal:* Make an infusion of the following:

> 2 parts angelica
> ¼ part fennel seed
> ¼ part anise seed
> ½ part ginger

Make an infusion of one teaspoon of herb to one cup of boiling water. Drink one-half cup four times daily between meals. Do not use the above for gastritis; use for gas and indigestion.

B. *Internal:* Use myrrh/goldenseal capsules. Take two after every meal.

C. *Internal:* Mix together the following:

> 1 part slippery elm bark
> ½ part licorice root
> 1 part marshmallow root
> 1 part comfrey root
> 1 part goldenseal

Use as a decoction and drink two ounces every two hours until the condition clears. Then reduce to three times daily for one week. Or, put powdered herbs in #00 gelatin capsules and take two to three times daily after meals and before bed on an empty stomach. Take two comfrey tablets or capsules every hour during inflammation and burning; then reduce to two every four hours.

D. *Internal:* Drink the fresh juice of one potato in a cup of warm water first thing every morning. This will reduce the acid in the stomach and intestines.

Formulas B, C and D are to be used for gas, indigestion or gastritis.

E. *Internal:* A tea made from equal parts of agrimony, red raspberry and meadow sweet is excellent for all digestive problems. Drink a small cup every three hours. Meadow sweet alone can be used (one and one-half ounce to one pint of boiling water). Steep for fifteen minutes. Drink four ounces three to four times daily. It is best to drink these teas between meals and during a fast to clean the stomach.

To help cleanse the stomach and soothe the irritation, a strong tea made from slippery elm and red raspberry is excellent. When there are chills and fevers see stimualtion therapy and chills.

A quick remedy that will handle this problem is equal parts of the following:

> Red raspberry
> Slippery elm
> Goldenseal
> Myrrh
> Peppermint

Use one teaspoon to one cup of boiling water. Steep for twenty minutes. Strain. Drink one-half cup every hour. This tea should be taken hot.

Other good herbal teas are flaxseed, comfrey root, mullein and marshmallow root.

F. *External:* Fomentations can be put over the stomach. A ginger fomentation or alternating hot and cold packs will relieve the pain and excess gas. They can be kept on for one to two hours if necessary. The alternating water treatment usually is used from one-half to one hour.

GLANDULAR ENLARGEMENTS (See Adenoids and Abscesses)

GOITER

Principal Therapy - stimulation, blood purification, tonification.

Use the cleansing diet in this book and continue on a vegetarian diet. Clean the bowels once weekly with an enema or colonic. Drink juices from freshly squeezed parsley, wheatgrass, celery or spinach. Combine these with a small amount beet and apple juice. Four ounces of liquid chlorophyll daily is excellent. Add seaweed such as dulse and kelp and use spirulina daily. Bladderwrack is a good remedy for all thyroid problems, capsule or extract is suitable.

A. *Internal:* Drink a tea made from equal parts red respberry, red clover, nettles and alfalfa. This tea will add iodine and iron to the diet and clean the blood. Chaparral or echinacea tablets or tinctures taken daily (two or three times daily) will clean the lympatic system. Exercise every day to increase circulation.

Use the following to build the blood. Mix together:

> 1 ounce alfalfa
> 1 ounce parsley root
> ½ ounce dandelion root
> ½ ounce burdock root
> ½ ounce comfrey root
> ½ ounce yellow dock root
> ½ ounce nettle leaves
> ½ ounce dulse

Simmer for twenty minutes in a quart of water in an uncovered pot. Let cool and strain. Return liquid to a pot and simmer uncovered for one hour until it is reduced to one cup. Stir in one cup of unsulphured blackstrap molasses and store in the refrigerator. Take one tablespoon three times daily. The above combination (powdered) can be put into #00 capsules and two to four can be taken with every meal.

Oregon grape root tincture, ten drops three times daily will also activate the thyroid gland.

Take calcium supplements between meals and kelp tablets with meals.

B. *External:* Alternate hot and cold fomentations over the thyroid gland using one minute durations of each for ten minutes, three times daily.

GONORRHEA (Venereal Diseases)

Principal Therapy - blood purification, heat dispelling.

The stomach should be kept empty during the acute symptoms. A short fast on fruit juices should be used until the most severe part of the infection is gone. Drink two ounces of freshly squeezed parsley juice three times daily mixed with four ounces of apple juice. See the formulas under Infections and Kidney and Bladder Infections. After the fast, use the cleansing diet in this book.

A. *Internal:* Take echinacea and chaparral capsules. Alternate them, two of each every two hours until the infection is gone. Make a tea of the following:

> 1 part of uva ursi
> 1 part cleavers
> 1 part goldenseal
> 1 part kava kava
> 1 part buchu
> 1 part slippery elm
> 1 part ginger

Pour one pint of boiling water over one ounce of these herbs. Steep for twenty minutes. Strain and drink one-half cup four times daily. A tincture of oregon grape root, twenty drops, three times a day can be added to this treatment. Echinacea tincture is another good remedy.

Poke root tincture is another good remedy. It should be used discriminately. Ten drops in water three times daily may be taken.

If there are sores, they can be washed with tincture of myrrh or one quart of warm water with five drops of juniper or rosemary oil added to it. Juniper berry oil can be taken internally for this condition. Take three drops mixed in a teaspoon of honey three times a day. For pain take one teaspoon of kava kava tincture internally, mixed in a cup of herb tea or water.

B. *Internal:* Specific remedy for syphilis:

> 2 parts oregon grape root
> 1 part red clover
> 1 part burdock seed
> 1 part cascara sagrada
> 1 part blue flag
> 1 part prickly ash bark
> 1 part blood root

Make a tincture of these herbs. Dose: twenty to forty drops in one cup of water three times daily. It can be taken in tea form or capsules, but it seems to be more effective in tincture form. Use a menstrum of 50% in making the tincture.

C. *External:* Use warm, whole baths with fifteen drops of juniper oil, wintergreen, peppermint or rosemary oil added to the bath. These baths can be taken three times a day.

Note: Many times taking calcium every hour will help relieve pain.

GOUT

Principal Therapy - blood purification.

See formulas under Arthritis, Gout and Rheumatism. A three day carrot and apple juice fast is excellent for this condition. Take an enema every morning. After the fast use the cleansing diet in this book for seven to ten days. It is mandatory that we change from an acid-producing diet to one of alkalinity. Avoid all meats, poultry, fish, dairy products, refined foods, coffee, tea, sugar, salt, etc. Drink the juice of a potato in warm water every morning. Use spirulina and seaweeds like kelp and dulse daily.

A. *Internal:* Drink a tea combination of two or more of these herbs: uva ursi, buchu, dandelion root or goldenrod. Take chaparral tablets two every three to four hours. Twenty drops of echinacea or pipsissewa tincture four times daily will clean the kidneys, blood and ease the pain.

Twenty to forty wheatgrass or alfalfa tablets should be taken during the day with meals or on an empty stomach to help produce alkalinity.

B. *External:* Use the all-purpose liniment in this book for painful areas. Warm fomentations or ginger fomentations are also good.

C. *Hydrotherapy:* Use alternating hot and cold baths or showers to stimulate circulation. Whole, warm baths are used with two pounds of epsom salts added to aid elimination and to ease pain. Taking the baths in the evening or during times of pain is indicated.

HALITOSIS (See Bad Breath)

HAY FEVER

Principal Therapy - blood purification, tonification stimulation.

Use the cleansing diet in this book for seven days with an enema every morning. Avoid all meats, dairy products, salts, sugar, refined foods, etc. Drink green juices like wheatgrass, parsley, celery and spirulina daily. Get plenty of exercise and fresh air. Do not overeat. Use enzymes with all meals, and the last meal should never be after 6:00 p.m.

A. *Internal:* Use the formulas found under Colds, Fevers and Flu. Mix together the following:

> 2 parts brigham tea
> 1 part sage
> 1 part mullein
> 1 part boneset
> ½ part ginger

Make an infusion out of these and drink three cups daily.

If the body is cold and there is a lack of circulation, use stimulating herbs like cayenne, ginger and prickly ash bark. Also see the formulas under Colds, Chills and Poor Circulation.

Take one to two ounces of bee pollen from the same area the patient lives. Honey is also good if it is raw and from the patient's home area.

Oftentimes the adrenal glands are weak, which results in low calcium and blood sugar. Licorice root, two capsules three times a day, plus calcium tablets will sometimes cure the most stubborn hayfever problems. Raw adrenal gland is also excellent for this. If the blood is clean and the adrenal glands strong, there will be little allergies and hayfever. Echinacea, six capsules daily, will help build immunity.

B. *External:* Brush the skin daily both morning and evening. Alternate warm and cool showers or baths. In the mornings take cool, whole baths for stimulation.

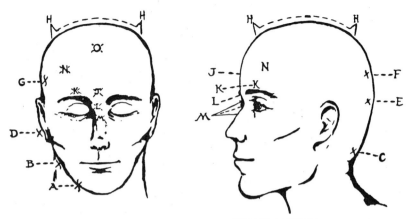

PAIN IN THE HEAD - HEADACHES

As headaches are always warning symptoms of an underlying condition, the cause must be removed. The use of headache pills and powders might give you relief but it is a dangerous proceeding. Study the above pictures and from the location of the headache marked with letters you may readily determine the possible underlying cause.

A - Pain and aches at the upper side of neck and lower jaw may indicate pharyngitis, laryngitis, diptheria or trigominal neuralgia

B - Aches below and lateral of C may indicate nervous disorders, stomach troubles, spinal irritation, impending rheumatism or disease of cervical vertebra.

C - Ache at back of neck, near base of brain may indicate nervous disorders, nephritis, diseases of spinal cord or middle ear disease.

D - Ache at mastoid processes may indicate mastoid troubles, pus, etc.

E - Ache near and below F may indicate constipation causativeness.

F - Ache at center back of head may indicate eye trouble - refraction myopia, etc.

G - Ache at back side of head over ears may indicate poor blood or uterine trouble.

H - Ache over entire top of head may indicate female disorders, bladder trouble, hysteria, neurasthenia, anaemia, chlorosis, epilepsy, ovarian trouble.

J - Ache in center of forehead just above L may indicate trouble with nose, eyes or intestines.

K - Ache over and around each eye may indicate dyspepsia, stomach trouble or occular disturbance.

L - Ache above bridge, between eyebrows may indicate constipation, stomach trouble, faulty refraction or decayed teeth.

M - Ache around eye and bridge of nose may indicate stomach, eye or nose trouble.

N - Ache of bandlike character around forehead may indicate anemia.

O - Ache in upper center of forehead may indicate catarrh of nose or throat.

HEADACHES

Principal Therapy - tranquilization.

The most prominent cause of headaches is constipation and a toxic blood stream. Study the sections in this book under Digestive Disorders, and Constipation. These treatments will take care of most of the headache problems in the world today.

If the patient is anemic, give him wheatgrass, spirulina, parsley juice, beet juice, yellow dock, nettles and fruits. If the problem is eyestrain, the eyes should be checked. If there are liver problems see the section of this book on Liver Problems, Indigestion, Jaundice and Hepatitis. If the patient is weak and is suffering from headaches, detoxify him slowly using vegetable juices and fruit juices for your cleansers.

Many times the spine is out of line and it can be relieved by a manipulation by a myopractor or chiropractor.

Diet is so important it cannot be overstressed. Food eaten too fast, in wrong combinations, overeating, eating unnatural foods, all cause fermentation in the stomach and intestines. This putrifactive process develops gases, which enter the liver through the portal circulation and then into the blood. These gases irritate the brain and nerve tissues and cause headaches.

Clean the bowels with a catnip or warm water enema. Go on a fast or just eat fruit for a week. Avoid bright lights, air pollution, toxic foods, stress. If the stomach has gas and a sour taste or coated tongue is present, take an emetic (see emetics). Follow this with a cup of peppermint tea. A hot foot bath with a tablespoon of mustard in it will draw the blood from the head area. Along with this put a towel dipped in cool water around the neck. Drink a cup of sage, peppermint, scullcap, valerian, spearmint, catnip or black cohosh tea while taking the foot bath. After this, lie down in the fresh air. Sometimes just a shower with warm water being sprayed on the back of the neck will relieve headaches.

Boil two quarts of water, turn the stove off and add fifteen drops of eucalyptus, wintergreen or peppermint oil to the water. Cover your head and the pot with water in it and inhale the fumes.

Mistletoe extract is a specific for vertigo, dizziness and headaches—fifteen drops every one-half hour while in pain. Maintenance is fifteen drops three times a day.

Get on a cleansing diet, purify your system, keep the bowels clean, fast on a regular basis and avoid hostile tempers. In any case, avoid the use of drugs whenever possible for this condition.

A. *Internal:* Mix together equal parts of the following:

    Scullcap
    Rosemary
    Peppermint

Make as an infusion. Drink warm. Drink one cup whenever needed.

B. *External:* Fu-sho oil and Tiger Balm can be rubbed on the forehead. Along with this, hot foot baths with cool towels around the neck will draw blood to lower body parts.

C. *External:* Use ginger foot baths.

Simmer one-half pound or more of grated fresh ginger in one quart of hot water; then dilute to needed amount. Soak feet in water and keep water hot.

HEART DISEASES

Principal Therapy - blood purification, stimulation.

Follow the diet and cleansing suggestions under Arteriosclerosis. The main emphasis here is on cleaning out the blood stream, normalizing circulation and using a natural, high fiber diet.

A few other suggestions that I might add concerning the heart, are the use of hawthorn berries or hawthorn berry syrup, along with wheat germ oil. Two teaspoons of wheat germ oil daily, taken for fourteen consecutive days out of every twenty days should be enough. Take three teaspoons of hawthorn berry syrup daily. Mistletoe (viscum album) abstract, fifteen drops three times daily or three cups of the tea daily is a specific for lowering blood pressure and taking the strain off the heart.

A. *External:* Brush the skin daily, every morning and evening. Use alternating hot and cold baths or showers every day and get plenty of exercise. If the person has a cold condition, use only warm water therapy until circulation improves. Reduce the temperature of the water slowly, until warm and cool water can be used. Use diaphoretic herb teas to increase circulation. Angelica, ginger and prickly ash bark are excellent to stimulate circulation.

HEMATURIA (See Bleeding)

Principal Therapy - heat dispelling (demulcent).

A three day carrot juice fast or fruit fast is indicated. The fruit must be ripe and in season. Avoid citrus fruits. Carrot juice is excellent. Clean the bowels in the mornings for three consecutive days, then use the cleansing diet for six days.

Avoid coffee, high protein diet, sugar, alcohol, tobacco, salt, fried foods, meats and dairy products.

A. *Internal:* Mix together:

    2 parts comfrey
    2 parts mullein
    2 parts slippery elm
    2 parts peppermint

> ½ part lobelia
> 2 parts cleavers
> 1 part marshmallow root

Take one ounce of herbs and steep for one-half hour in one pint of distilled water. Strain, drink two ounces every two hours.

B. *Internal:* For severe bleeding:

> 1 part marshmallow root
> 1 part buchu
> 2 parts white oak bark
> 1 part hydrangea
> ½ part ginger

Simmer one ounce of herbs in one pint of distilled water for one-half hour. Strain, drink two ounces every two hours until bleeding stops.

Note: Once the bleeding has stopped, drink two ounces of the above three times a day for one week.

White oak bark or tormentilla tinctures, decoctions or extract are excellent for this problem. The dosage of the tinctures should be twenty drops three to four times daily. Yarrow, shepherd's purse and geranium are other fine herbs for this condition.

HEMORRHAGES (See Bleeding)

HEMORRHOIDS

Principal Therapy - blood purification, dietary.

Hemorrhoids are a protrusion of the mucus membrane of the rectum which can occur at any age. The causes may be overuse of constipating protein and starchy foods, excessive use of milk and dairy products, sluggish liver function, constricted blood vessels in that area, obesity, lack of sufficient exercise, overuse of purgatives and putrification of old wastes.

Do a short fast using fresh carrot juice to relieve the pain. Clean the bowels with an enema to keep the gas and waste from causing internal pressure. The feces should be kept soft by using plenty of fruits such as raisins, figs, prunes, peaches and melons. Soak the dried fruits in distilled water or juice for four hours before eating them. Use leafy, green vegetables and sprouts. If nuts are to be used, powder them first and add them to salads or mix them with a little water before eating them. Use short fasts along with rest.

The prolapse can be replaced with the finger ·and then apply ice packs to the area immediately. Hanging upside down and slant board exercises are beneficial. These should be done daily.

Drink a decoction of white oak bark one-half cup three times daily between meals. Make a decoction of tormentil root and inject four ounces into the lower bowel and retain as long as possible. Keep dabbing the anus throughout the day with a cotton swab which has been soaked in tormentil.

Make a decoction with equal parts witch hazel and red raspberry. Soak a tampon with it and insert it up the rectum to remain overnight.

1. Mix the following:

   2 parts bayberry
   1 part wild alum root
   1 part shepherd's purse
   1 part licorice root
   1/8 part cayenne

   Powder the herbs and put in #00 gelatin capsules. Take two every two hours during pain. When relieved, take two or three times daily until the condition clears up.

   If the stomach can take it, drink one-half cup three times daily of this combination.

   Drink plenty of red raspberry leaf tea daily.

2. Saturating the rectal area with witch hazel is also excellent. You can soak a piece of cotton in witch hazel, insert into the rectum for overnight treatment. It will be ejected in the first morning bowel movement.

3. Possible calcium and rutin supplements are indicated when the vessel walls are weak anywhere in the body. Calc. fluor. 6x or 12x (cell salts) are excellent for this. Take five tablets every two hours until relieves.

   Wild leeks eaten daily and a tea of mistletoe also helps to regenerate the arteries. Horsetail grass, lobelia, comfrey and oat straw are herbs that increase body calcium.

4. Take enemas with witch hazel bark or bayberry bark decoctions. Take enemas in a slant board or knee position.

5. Mullein, wild alum root, catnip and bloodroot is a good tea combination to drink.

   2 parts mullein
   1 part catnip
   ½ part bloodroot
   1 part wild alum root

   Mix the herbs thoroughly and use one teaspoon to a cup of boiling water. Let it steep for one-half hour. Drink one-half cup four times daily.

6. An injection of bloodroot tea alone has cured piles and prolapses of the anus. Inject four to six ounces and retain as long as possible. Dab the outside of the anus with the tea.

7. Inject one pint of cold water in the lower bowel. Retain overnight or as long as possible. This should be done immediately after a bowel movement. Placing ice over the area after a bowel movement is also good.

8. Raw pulverized onions used as a poultice applied to the area has cured the worst cases.

9. Cut a red potato into a cigar-shaped suppository and insert it for overnight use.

10. Insert a clove of garlic before bed.

11. Mix the following:

> 2 parts dandelion
> 1 part cascara sagrada
> 1/2 part licorice root
> 1 part oregon grape root
> 1/8 part cayenne

Use one ounce of these herbs to one pint of water and simmer for fifteen minutes. Strain and drink one-half cup three to four times daily. Cayenne is excellent, but if the stomach is weak, substitute ginger.

12. Stoneroot tincture taken internally, one teaspoon three times a day is excellent. Swab the tincture on prolapsed areas.

HICCOUGHS

Principal Therapy - tranquilization.

Stop all food intake and apply a hot water fomentation over the stomach and chest. The fomentation can be made from a tea of lobelia or other antispasmodic herb. Sometimes drinking a glass of warm water or small amounts of lemon and lime juice will benefit this condition. Another fast remedy is a tablespoon of raw onion juice given every one-half hour.

Tincture of chestnut leaves, ten drops in warm water whenever needed is a specific for this condition. A tea made from skunk cabbage given in teaspoonfuls every ten minutes, or the tincture (fifteen drops in one-half cup of warm water) is a specific remedy.

The bowels should immediately be cleaned with a warm water enema or a tea made from chamomile, lobelia or catnip. Retain water for as long as possible while lying in a slant position. The water used in the enema should be as warm as possible. Thirty drops of an antispasmodic tea can also be added to two quarts of water injected into the bowels.

Hiccoughs are usually caused by a deranged stomach. An emetic is one of the fast cures. Read about emetics in this book.

A. *Hydrotherapy:* Soak both feet in hot water for ten to twenty minutes, then massage them with a stimulating massage oil.

HERPES (See Acne and Skin Diseases)

HOARSENESS

Principal Therapy - tranquilization (demulcent).

Whatever the cause may be, eliminate it. Eat fruit or fruits and vegetables for a few days to help remove excess mucus. An infusion of eyebright, one cup three or four times a day is good for this condition, along with a gargle made from a tea of goldenseal, and used several times daily. If the tincture of eyebright is used, fifteen to twenty drops every three or four hours may be taken. Smoking powdered licorice root is another remedy. Linden flowers made into an infusion, using a tablespoon every hour or fifteen to twenty drops of the tincture every three hours may be used.

A decoction of marshmallow root is another good remedy. Pimpernell root chewed or made into a decoction taken in cupfuls three times a day is good for a throat and vocal cord condition. Other herbs are coltsfoot, skunk cabbage, lobelia, mullein and lungwort.

A. *Internal:* Make a syrup out of wild cherry bark.

B. *Internal:* Mix together the following:

> 2 tablespoons flaxseed
> 1 tablespoon horehound

> Boil in one pint of water for ten minutes; strain. Squeeze one fresh lemon in the tea and add a pinch of ginger. Dosage: take one tablespoon every one-half hour.

C. *Internal:* Horseradish syrup (see formula A under Asthma).

> Garlic syrup: take one pound of peeled, minced garlic cloves and put them in a jar. Cover with three parts apple cider vinegar and one part distilled water. Shake well and let stand for four hours. Strain and add equal amounts of honey. Cap and keep in a cool place. Take one tablespoon three to eight times daily for asthma, bronchitis, coughs, colds, catarrhal condition, mucus, weak heart, sluggish digestion, poor circulation and high cholesterol.

> See also the formulas under Spasmodic Coughs and Lung Congestion.

D. *External:* Keep the throat warm with hot towels.

HIVES

Principal Therapy - blood purification.

In order to remove the cause of this condition, the poisonous matter must be removed from the body. A three day fast using just water or diluted fruit juices along with an enema every morning during fast will usually clear out the blood toxins. After the fast, use the cleansing diet in this book for seven days. Avoid the use of strong spices, meats, refined foods, fried foods, dairy products, tobacco, coffee and alcohol.

A. *Internal:* Give an emetic using one teaspoon of lobelia tincture or ipecac every ten minutes until vomiting is induced followed by a cup of mint tea. See emetics in this book. Many times poisons in the stomach are causing this problem. If an emetic is not acceptable, give a strong tea of one tablespoon of myrrh in a pint of boiling water. One tablespoon dose every fifteen minutes will neutralize stomach poisons.

Thirty drops of echinacea tincture taken four to five times daily is another good remedy. A tea made from burdock, sassafras, red raspberry, and red clover combined in equal parts given in cupful doses two or more times daily will clean the blood. Read the section on blood purification.

Digestive tonics should be used to tone the stomach, while easily digestible foods like spirulina, bee pollen, seaweeds, raw juices and vegetable broths should be the major part of the diet.

B. *External:* Read the section under Poison Oak and Ivy, and Acne and Skin Problems.

C. *Hydrotherapy:* Take a hot bath with one pound of baking soda or epsom salts added to the water.

HYPOGLYCEMIA

Principal Therapy - tonification.

Hypoglycemia is a disorder of too little blood sugar, which supplies the fuel for the cells, hence is unavailable for energy.

Avoid alcohol, tobacco, high protein diet, sugar and flour products, all other stimulating foods and habitual excesses. The sugar level is monitored by the ductless glands, especially the pituitary and adrenals (which command the blood sugar level to rise).

All carbohydrates (starch, sugar) are converted into glucose. During a meal, increased sugar level causes the pancreas (Islands of Langerhans) to produce insulin. The liver, under the stimulation of insulin, stores glucose as glycogen, thus keeping the blood sugar balance at a proper level. After the meal, the adrenal glands (cortical hormones) monitor the liver on how much sugar to release to satisfy the energy requirements of the body. In hypoglycemia, due to excesses of stress, starches, sugar, etc., the pancreas is forced to produce large amounts of insulin. This excess insulin removes too much sugar causing the liver to store large amounts of glycogen. This results in an inadequate sugar supply (energy) to the body. The brain is nourished exclusively by glucose and oxygen. A drop in sugar causes depression, anxiety, anger, etc.

The adrenal glands in time become exhausted and cannot bring the blood sugar concentration back to normal. Sugar is present in the blood after a meal in large amounts. The pancreas secretes insulin which reduces the blood sugar level too far. The weakened adrenals fail to react to bring the blood sugar back up. The body senses a lack of energy and symptoms result. Caffeine and uric acid are both stimulants that produce a false high by stimulating the adrenal glands to induce the liver to break down glycogen (sugar storage). The pancreas secretes insulin to store the excess again and a depressed feeling results. Another high is needed. Excess food, coffee, alcohol, subconscious desires, etc. are then craved. The whole body and consciousness are thrown out of balance.

The diet is centered around removing all stimulating spices, foods, and refined carbohydrates and is planned in such a way as to prevent the drop in the sugar level. Fruits, grains (low heated or sprouted), seeds, nuts, vegetables and all kinds of sprouts should make up the diet. Grains that are sprouted and low heated digest slower than meat, which results in a slower release of sugar and nutrients into the bloodstream without the uric acid by-product which is resultant after meat digestion.

Animal products are not easily digested. The body uses the protein it needs and the remainder is transformed into sugar and burned as energy, increasing blood sugar levels. Meat, with its uric acid by-product also acts as a false stimulant to the adrenals, raising blood sugar and adding stress to the liver and kidneys.

Sprouts and fruits (small amounts if symptoms are felt) have a positive influence in hypoglycemia. They are low in protein and do not have the uric acid by-product.

Nuts can be powdered, which will assist in digestion and will provide adequate protein. Spirulina, dulse and kelp can be used to maintain proper mineral balance and regulate the thyroid gland. Green drinks and chlorophyll are excellent as tonics to the whole body and will speed up the healing process. Parsley juice or tea is a specific to help rebuild the adrenals and blood. Wheatgrass should be taken in small amounts at first—one ounce daily, diluted in distilled water. Smaller meals should be eaten, well chewed, using the mentioned juices between meals.

The bowel should be kept clean at all times. Clean the lower intestines with an enema, then keep them regulated with laxative foods such as soaked raisins, figs, and prunes. Use herbal laxatives occasionally, if needed.

For more information on proper diet, see books by Dr. Ann Wigmore and Viktoras Kulvinskas.

A. *Internal:* A cup of dandelion tea one-half hour before meals acts as a tonic to the liver and stomach and helps to regulate blood sugar levels. The first line of defense is to tone up the digestive system.

> 1 part dandelion root
> 1 part calamus root
> 1 part gentian
> ¼ part ginger
> ¼ part cinnamon

Simmer one ounce of mixed herbs in one pint of water for twenty minutes. Strain and take two tablespoons immediately before meals and one hour before bed on an empty stomach.

B. *Internal:* The following is a specific formula for hypoglycemia and diabetes.

> 1 part goldenseal
> 1 part juniper berries

1 part uva ursi
1 part cedar berries
1 part dandelion root
1 part bistort
1 part licorice root powder
1 part huckleberry leaves.

Powder the herbs and put them into #00 capsules. Take two capsules three times a day between meals. This can also be taken as a decoction in doses of two ounces twice daily on an empty stomach. More can be taken if needed.

C. *External:* Dry brush the skin several times daily. Sleep in the open air. Get plenty of exercise daily.

D. *Hydrotherapy:* Use cool, whole baths if the body is warm. Alternate hot and cold packs morning and night for ten minutes over the kidney area, pancreas and adrenals (especially during Addison's Disease).

HYSTERIA (See Convulsions)

IMPETIGO (See Herpes under Acne and Skin Diseases)

INFECTIONS

Principal Therapy - blood purification, heat dispelling.

Use short two day fasts on carrot or citrus juices and a vegetarian diet for all infections. Avoid meat, dairy, coffee, hot spices, tea, high protein diets and the like.

To be effective in treating infections, the herb used as the alternative to antibiotics must be chosen properly according to the symptoms and the organs involved. This chart will provide specific information.

COMMON HERBS TO TREAT INFECTIONS

Common Name	Methods of Application	Specific Action
Buchu	Tincture/tea	Urinary tract
Burcock	Tincture/tea	Blood purifier
Calendula	Poultice/salve	Wounds
Chaparral	Tincture/capsules/douche	Anti-viral
Dandelion	Tea	Blood purifier
Echinacea	Tincture/capsules	All infections
Elecampane	Tincture/capsules	Bile stimulant
Garlic	Fresh oil/poultice	All infections
Goldenseal	Tincture/capsules/salve/douche	All infections
Juniper	Tincture	Urinary tract
Kava kava	Tincture/tea/poultice	Urinary tract, wounds
Myrrh	Tincture/capsules/salve	Wounds

Oregon grape	Tincture/tea	Bile stimulant
Plantain	Poultice/salve	Wounds
Thyme	Poultice/salve	Fungal infection
Uva ursi	Tincture/tea	Urinary tract
White oak	Tea/capsules/poultice/douche	All infection
Witch hazel	Extract	Acne
Yellow dock	Capsules/poultice/douche	Vaginal infection

A. *Internal:* Use chaparral and echinacea capsules. Take two every two hours and drink red clover tea.

B. *Internal:* Liquid chlorophyll and wheatgrass juice are excellent for a toxic blood condition. Take one tablespoon four to six times daily in water or juice.

C. *Internal:* Take two garlic capsules every four hours.

D. *External:* Use fomentations, plaster or poultices from:

  2 parts plantain
  2 parts echinacea
  1/8 part cayenne
  1 part slippery elm bark

ITCHING (See Hives and Poison Oak and Ivy)

INSOMNIA

The attitude of the mind is of great importance in following the natural regimen of living and of treatment of insomnia. By our habitual thoughts we create in our brains the actual centers which make either for health or disease.

Some people on account of a tense nervous condition spend more vital energy while resting and sleeping than others do while at work. In most instances, nerve exhaustion in its many different manifestations is brought about not through overwork, but through the tense, fretful, impatient, irritable, hurrying way in which the work is performed.

The following rules, if closely followed, will help to induce sound sleep:

1. Sleep in a well ventilated and not overheated room.

2. Never sleep in the garments worn during the day. Wear a night garment of light, porous material, so that the poisonous exhalations of the skin may easily escape; or better still, wear none.

3. Let the covering be neither too warm nor too heavy.

4. Avoid excitement or extraordinary strain just before bedtime, if possible.

5. Do not eat three hours before bedtime.

6. After going to bed, practice relaxation before sleeping.

A walk in the fresh air before bed or walking in the grass barefoot may be helpful to induce sleep.

A.   *Internal:* Drink teas of equal parts hops and chamomile before retiring.

B.   *Internal:* Mix equal parts of the following and make an infusion. Drink one cup before bed or when needed:

Wood betony   Chamomile   Valerian
Peppermint   Catnip

C.   *Internal:* Refer to formula A under the section on Nervousness.

KIDNEY AND BLADDER INFECTIONS

Principal Therapy - blood purification, heat dispelling.

Do a three day apple juice fast using an enema every morning adding one tablespoon of apple cider vinegar to two quarts of warm water. Then use the cleansing diet in this book for seven days with the addition of two ounces of parsley juice or liquid chlorophyll morning and night mixed in eight ounces of apple juice.

A.   *Internal:* Pipsissewa tincture twenty drops and echinacea tincture twenty drops taken together in one cup of water three to four times daily is a good remedy for kidney and bladder infections.

B.   *Internal:* Take chaparral and echinacea capsules. Alternate them two every hour until pain stops.

C.   *Internal:* Mix the following together:

1 part plantain   2 parts goldenseal
1 part slippery elm   1 part uva ursi
½ pat ginger

Make an infusion. Drink one-half cup every one to two hours.

D.   *External:* See Arthritis, Gout, Rheumatism formula C for ginger fomentation over the kidneys.

E.   *External:* See Appendicitis formula B for castor oil packs.

Note: Fast on vegetable broths and herb teas until the pain is gone.

KIDNEY STONES

Principal Therapy - deobstruent (lithotriptics) (demulcent).

Use the same dietary and cleansing suggestions mentioned under Kidney and Bladder Infections. Drink two ounces of lemon juice in water morning and night.

A.   *Internal:* Mix together the following herbs:

1 part gravel root
1 part parsley root
1 part marshmallow root

¼ part lobelia
¼ part ginger root

Take one ounce of herbs and simmer for twenty minutes in one and one-half pints of distilled water. Drink one-half cup three times daily. Add honey if needed.

Note: Use castor oil packs (see Appendicitis formula B) or hot fomentations over the kidneys. Fast until the pain is gone.

Note: If there is pain, twenty drops of a tincture made from kava kava every hour is good. Also see antispasmodic tinctures in this book with the all purpose liniment.

LACTATION

Principal Therapy - tonification, blood purification.

The most important thing during breast feeding is diet and blood purification. Foods that are high in calcium like cabbage and carrots should be eaten raw daily. Raw juice from green plants and carrots will aid in calcium absorption and blood cleansing.

The bowels should be kept clean with high fiber, bulk producing foods like seaweeds, seeds and nuts. One teaspoon of agar agar in one cup of warm water three times daily will add iodine, trace minerals and bulk to the diet. Try to make the diet at least 75% raw foods. Concentrate on vitamin A and D, calcium foods and sunbathing.

A. *Internal:* Drinking herb teas high in silica and calcium can be used daily. Comfrey, nettle, oat straw and horsetail grass are a few. A good combination to assure having enough healthy milk is:

1 part anise seed
1 part fennel
1 part red raspberry
1 part marshmallow root

Simmer one ounce of herbs for five minutes in one pint of distilled water. Strain, drink one-half cup three times daily.

Note: Do not go on long fasts or harsh cleansing diets during pregnancy and lactation.

LIVER PROBLEMS, INDIGESTION, JAUNDICE, HEPATITIS

Principal Therapy - blood purification, deobstruent (hepatic).

Do a three to seven day carrot and apple juice fast. Use an enema for three consecutive days with a castor oil pack four consecutive evenings before bed. Follow this with the cleansing diet in this book for one week.

A. *Internal:* Tincture of oregon grape root. Take twenty drops in warm water three times daily.

B. *Internal:* Mix the following together:

> 1 part barberry root
> 1 part wild yam
> 1 part dandelion
> ½ part licorice root

Simmer one ounce in a pint of water for ten minutes; strain. Drink two ounces three to four times daily.

MEASLES (See Chicken Pox and Smallpox)

Principal Therapy - blood purification, diaphoresis.

In addition or as an alternative treatment for measles or chicken pox, a hot fomentation of thyme tea applied to the affected area several times daily will help draw out the toxins through the skin pores. During the fever, diluted juices (50% distilled water) of orange, lemon, lime or carrot can be taken. Vegetable broths are also very good. Make an infusion out of one or more of yarrow, marigold, elderflowers or catnip sweetened with a little honey to increase perspiration (diaphoresis).

If the gums are infected, rub them with tinctures of lobelia, echinacea or goldenseal. Half and half apple cider vinegar and water will also disinfect the gums.

The following homeopathic remedies can be given. Aconitum 3x or 4x (five drops in water every half hour); when sweating is induced, reduce the duration to every two hours. For babies, Ferr. Phos. 6x or 12x, one tablet every one or two hors. Belladonna 4x: use this remedy when the blood flushes to the head or when there is conjunctivitis or ear infections.

Calcium in liquid or powder form is always good to take during fevers and infections.

MENIERE'S DISEASE AND VERTIGO

Principal Therapy - blood purification, tonification (stomach, nerves, kidneys).

Clean the bowels for five consecutive days, then once a week with a catnip tea enema. Follow the cleansing diet in this book and do 48-hour fasts once a month. Avoid nerve damaging foods like coffee, tea, meat, excessive protein and dairy products and salt. Keep relaxed as much as possible.

Get spinal adjustments or acupuncture. Acupuncture is a very successful treatment along with the proper diet for problems affecting balance, nerves and infections. Get plenty of exercise to stimulate circulation. Eat whole grains and foods that are high in calcium and B vitamins.

A. *Internal:* Drink three cups of blessed thistle tea daily. Take chaparral and gotu kola tablets. Alternate these two every two hours. One ounce of bee pollen morning and night is a good nerve and systematic tonic.

Panax ginseng extract (twenty drops daily) or ten drops morning and night is excellent for this condition.

B. *Hydrotherapy:* Hot and cold packs over the upper spine, and alternating hot and cold showers in the morning and evening will aid circulation. Then dry skin brush the whole body, brushing toward the heart. Skin brushing is one of the best lymphatic stimulants there is.

Note: The diet must be kept vegetarian style. This problem can be overcome with perseverance. Any therapy that is good for the nerves will help to overcome this condition.

FEMALE PROBLEMS

LEUKORRHEA AND VAGINITIS

Principal Therapy - blood purification.

Use the dietary suggestions found under Menopause.

A. *Internal:* Take myrrh/goldenseal capsules two every two hours.

B. *Internal* (Douche)*:* Mix together equal parts of the following:

Goldenseal
Red raspberry
Echinacea
Slippery elm

Make a strong infusion using one ounce to a pint of distilled water; strain. Add one teaspoon of apple cider vinegar. Douche in morning and try to retain liquid for five minutes (incline position).

Other douches: Use just bayberry bark or white oak bark.

MENOPAUSE

Principal Therapy - blood purification, tonification.

Menopause is the period at which the menstrual activity ceases. This usually occurs between the ages of forty and fifty. Hot flashes, disturbed calcium metabolism, irritability and nervous derangements are some of the typical symptoms. The course of preventitive treatment should be based in nutrition and blood cleansing. Excellent results can be obtained by exercising out of doors, deep breathing and skin brushing.

The diet should be simple, easy to digest and mainly vegetarian, avoiding all dairy, meat, coffee, tea, alcohol, nicotine and so forth. Eat whole grains, sprouts, green leafy vegetables, raw fruit and vegetable juices, garlic, figs, dates, cabbage, all seaweeds, dulse, bananas, avocados, grapes, pecans, walnuts, almonds, black and white sesame seeds, sunflower seeds, beets, bee pollen, spirulina and green juices. Use the cleansing diet in this book for seven days, four times yearly with the use of enemas every morning during the cleanse.

A. *Internal:* Many times the kidneys are found to be weak. Buchu, parsley, goldenrod, uva ursi and oat straw teas will help in kidney activity and tone the kidneys. Only use these teas if suspected kidney problems are present. Otherwise a good diet, distilled water and juices will help the cleansing of the blood and kidneys.

Take two or three kelp tablets daily which will aid in providing iodine and trace minerals for proper thyroid activity. Take this formula six days a week, which will tone the female reproductive system.

Note: Do not use this formula during pregnancy.

> 1 part ginger
> 1 part black haw
> 1 part helonias root
> 1 pat siberian ginseng
> 1 part squaw vine
> 1 part licorice root
> 1 part dong quai

Combine all these powdered herbs or as many that can be found. Put them in #00 capsules and the dose is usually two capsules two times daily between meals or whenever symptoms occur.

Liquid chlorophyll, with the fat soluble chlorophyllins left in the liquid is an excellent tonic. Two tablespoons twice daily or two ounces twice daily is adequate. Take calcium tablets between meals or use plenty of foods high in calcium.

B. *External:* Hot and cold fomentations over the lower spine and abdomen will help relieve symptoms. If the body is hot, take cool, whole baths. If the body is cold, use warm, whole baths morning and evening for ten minute durations.

Note: If the ovaries are lacking and there is a history of menstrual irregularities, raw ovary may be taken two consecutive weeks out of every month for four to six months. Raw glandulars are strong medicines and a qualified practitioner should be consulted before their use.

MENORRHAGIA (Profuse menstruation)

A short one or two day fast should be used during the worst times of this disease. A warm water enema should be administered immediately and daily if needed. Cool water douches or douches made from a decoction of white oak bark or bayberry or other astringents should be taken. The douches can be administered several times a day if necessary. If there is pain during douching, use just cool water or delete them entirely.

During eating periods, follow the diet suggested under menopause. The blood has to be purified and the diet corrected during all systemic diseases such as this one. Avoid all stimulants.

A. *Internal:* Tinctures from tormentil root, white oak bark or cinnamon may be used, fifteen to twenty drops every half-hour. Cinnamon tincture is a specific for this problem. A decoction of two ounces taken every hour made from alum root or bethroot is excellent.

> 2 parts bethroot
> 1 part yarrow
> 1 part blue cohosh
> 1 part slippery elm
> ½ part ginger

Simmer one ounce of these combined herbs in one pint of water for twenty minutes. Strain, drink one-fourth cup hot every two hours.

If the menses are extremely profuse, take large cotton balls and soak them in white oak bark tea. Tie a string around the middle of the cotton ball and insert in the vagina. Remove this every eight hours and douche with cool water or an astringent tea.

Bed rest is most important during menorrhagia. For toning the female organs, use the suggested tonic mentioned under menopause or amenorrhea.

B. *Hyrdotherapy:* Cool, whole baths taken in the evening will act as a tonic to the whole body. Only take them if the body is warm. Dry skin brush the body morning and evening to strengthen the nerves and internal organs.

MENSTRUAL CRAMPS

Principal Therapy - tranquilization.

Fast until all symptoms subside. Give a warm water enema. Catnip and chamomile tea enemas are specific for this problem. Usually a warm fomentation following the enema will give quick relief. Take two calcium tablets every hour until cramps subside. It is good to check for calcium deficiencies if constant cramping and spasms continue.

A. *Internal:* Mix the following together:

> 1 ounce cramp bark
> 1/2 ounce scullcap
> 1 teaspoon cardamon seeds
> 1/8 teaspoon cayenne

Pour one pint of boiling water over two tablespoons of this herb mixture. Cover and let steep for twenty minutes. Drink one-fourth cup every one-half hour until cramps stop.

B. *Internal:* Mix the following herbs together:

> 4 parts squaw vine
> 2 parts cramp bark
> 1 part false unicorn root

Simmer one ounce of herbs in a pint of water for twenty minutes; strain. Drink three tablespoons four times daily (preventative). Drink two ounces every hour during cramping, then reduce to three times daily. This formula is also good for after birth pains.

Also see Antispasmodic Formula under Spasmodic Coughs and Lung Congestion, formula B.

C. *Internal:* Mix together the following as a menstrual cramp and nerve tonic.

> 1½ ounces mistletoe
> 1 ounce wild yam
> ¼ ounce black cohosh
> 1 ounce scullcap
> ¼ ounce ginger
> 1 ounce valerian

Boil two ounces of this mixture in one quart of water down to one pint. Strain, and while warm, add two ounces of honey or vegetable glycerine. Take one teaspoon every one-half hour during cramping or one teaspoon three times a day as a tonic.

D. *Internal:* Mix together the following to soothe cramping:

> 1 part ginger root
> 2 parts cramp bark
> 1 part fennel

Pour one cup of boiling water over one teaspoon of combined herbs. Steep for fifteen minutes. Strain and drink immediately. Add ten to twenty drops of antispasmodic tincture or five drops of lobelia tincture to the tea just before drinking.

E. *External:* Use castor oil pack over the ovaries and pelvic area. Refer to Appendicitis formula B.

F. *External:* Use ginger fomentations. Refer to Arthritis, formula C.

G. *External:* Refer to Cramps and Spasms, formulas B and C.

H. *External:* Use hot baths and reflexology.

INFLAMMATORY DYSMENORRHEA

Follow the treatment suggested above but douche with equal parts of red raspberry leaf, slippery elm and goldenseal tea. Take goldenseal and myrrh capsules internally two every two hours. Fast until inflammation is gone.

Drink carrot juice and plenty of slippery elm tea, flaxseed, or other demulcents. Read demulcent therapy under heat-dispelling.

MECHANICAL DYSMENORRHEA

The term applied to that form which is supposed to arise from stricture of the canal of the cervix. The treatments mentioned above are good for this condition, although a correct diagnosis should be made to determine the proper treatment.

METRORRHAGIA

This condition is bleeding between menstrual periods. Be sure to obtain the correct diagnosis. The suggested treatment under menorrhagia is usually sufficient during times of bleeding.

OVARIAN CYSTS (Endometriosis)

A. *Internal:* Cut cotton in pieces two inches by four inches. Lay them on top of each other until you have a small pile about one inch high. Tie a string tightly around the middle and leave one end about ten inches long loosely hanging.

Go to a drug store or herbal pharmacy and purchase "ichthammol", (a black salve) and vegetable glycerine. Health food stores will usually carry the glycerine. Mix two teaspoons of ichthammol and two teaspoons of glycerine together in a cup or small pan. (Use more of this mixture if needed.) Soak the cotton in this mixture thoroughly and insert it into the vagina up to the cervix, leaving the long end of the string hanging out. Wear a heavy cotton cloth or sanitary napkin over the vaginal opening so the mixture will not leak on your bed clothing.

Follow this procedure five nights weekly before bed and remove it each morning by pulling slightly on the string. This will draw out the infection and help shrink fibroid tumors and ovarian cysts, or other growth that are in the uterus. I have seen a fibroid tumor completely disappear in one month that was so large it blocked the colon and inhibited bowel movements.

Douche in the morning with an infusion made from equal parts goldenseal and myrrh. Make a quart of this tea and add one teaspoon of apple cider vinegar.

This procedure is also good for chronic vaginitis, and other vaginal and uterine infections.

Note: If ichthammol black salve cannot be found, make a poultice out of equal parts of slilppery elm powder, white oak bark powder and enough water and french clay to make it of thin consistency. Mix the cotton layers in this and follow the above directions.

B. *Internal:* Mix the following:

   1 part licorice root
   1 part prickly ash bark
   2 parts chaparral
   2 parts pipsissewa

1 part cramp bark
1 part helonias root (false unicorn)
1 part saw palmento
1 part red clover

Mix the powdered herbs in a blender and put them in #00 capsules. Take two, three times a day.

C. *External:* Put a castor oil pack over the ovaries four consecutive nights per week. Before applying the castor oil pack, rub poke root oil over the ovary that is affected, then apply the pack.

It is important to use a cleansing diet, followed with a short fast and a vegetarian diet, deleting meats, fish, fowl and all dairy products.

MORNING SICKNESS

Principal Therapy - carminitive.

Many dietary experts have noticed a decrease in morning sickness when the diet is regulated and a vegetarian diet is used. A clean stomach, bowel and bloodstream will reduce this problem if not eliminate it entirely.

Keep the bowels clean by using one teaspoon twice daily of powdered flaxseed in a cup of juice or water. Agar agaar will also regulate the bowels used in the same way. Eat plenty of raw fruits and vegetables and drink carrot and apple juice with small amounts of cabbage mix together daily. The ratio of amounts of these freshly squeezed juices can be determined by each individual. Usually cabbage is one-quarter the amount of the carrot and apple.

Berries of all kinds are excellent for morning sickness. Strawberries can be used in small amounts if no allergic response to them has been noticed.

A. *Internal:* A tea made from ginger is excellent for this condition with a little honey added to it. Many times just warm water, lemon and honey will handle the problem. Alfalfa tea or capsules and red raspberry teas are excellent. All mint teas with the addition of calcium, vitamin B and vitamin B^6 have eliminated the problem.

Sometimes adding just a pinch of powdered goldenseal to any of the suggested teas will help. Tincture of cinnamon taken alone five to ten drops in water or added to the tea of your choice is another remedy for this problem.

See the combination of herbs under Gastritis, Indigestion and Gas formula A.

B. *Hydrotherapy:* Whole, warm baths taken morning and evening will relax the stomach and nervous system.

MUMPS (See Adenoids)

NEPHRITIS (See Hematuria and Kidney and Bladder Infections)

NERVOUSNESS

Principal Therapy - tranquilization.

Study and use the dietary and cleansing suggestions under Neuralgia and Arthritis.

A. *Internal:* Mix together equal parts of the following:

> Valerian
> Spearmint
> Lemon Balm
> Lady's slipper
> Scullcap

> Drink as an infusion when needed using one ounce to a pint of boiling water. Steep for twenty minutes.

B. *External:* Use ginger foot baths. Refer to formula B under Headaches.

C. *External:* See Antispasmodic formula under Spasmodic Coughs and Lung Congestion.

NEURALGIA AND TIC DOULOUREUX

Principal Therapy - tranquilization, blood purification.

Follow the diet, hydrotherapy and herbal suggestions that are listed under Arthritis. This condition usually is caused by deposits and congestion putting pressure on the nerves causing sharp stabbing pains. Acupuncture, chiropractic adjustments and massage will relieve the pain and help balance the flow of energy through the nervous system and circulation. Use foods especially high in all B vitamins like whole grains, nutritional yeast, bee pollen, millet, rice, bran syrup and so on.

A. *Internal:* Lobelia tincture, ten to forty drops, in warm water or in a good nervine tea is a specific for neuralgia. Study the use of the castor oil pack in this book and apply it directly to the area. The use of fomentations made from lobelia, hops, wood betony and mistletoe are also very good several times a day.

The herb combination under Nervousness made from valerian root, spearmint, lemon balm, lady's slipper and scullcap is excellent for this condition.

Taking two capsules of valerian root every four hours along with calcium tablets every two hours is a good remedy. Under the section on Spasmodic Coughs and Lung Congestion is an antispasmodic tincture. This tincture used thirty drops every twenty minutes during painful times has been a marvelous compound for this problem.

Apply volatile oils to pain and swelling and cover with an electric heating pad or wet, hot towels several times a day. The all purpose liniment in this book is good for this. Camphor, Tiger Balm, Fu-sho oil and others can also be used.

TIC DOULOUREUX

Acupuncture is a specific for this problem. Along with it, use hot, wet fomentations over the area after the painful part (face) has been rubbed with camphor or other suggested volatile oils.

A. *Internal:* Drink a tea made from equal parts wood betony and plantain. Three cups daily may be used, adding one drop of wintergreen oil to each cup.

Study nervine and antispasmodic herbs to help make a proper choicce of other teas.

B. *External:* Use warm, whole baths or fomentations several times a day if needed.

NIGHTMARES

Principal Therapy - blood purification.

Do not eat four hours before bed. Use the cleansing diet in this book for seven days with the use of an enema every morning. Study the section on proper food combinations.

If the problem is emotional, then see a qualified counselor to assist you.

A. *Internal:* Drink nervine teas. A cup of hops tea one-half hour before bed is excellent. Tinctures made from hops, valerian or others can be added to teas or fifteen to thirty drops can be taken in a cup of warm water one-half hour before bed.

B. *External:* Take whole, warm baths before bed. Anything relaxing will help. Try to create a harmonious environment. Get plenty of fresh air and exercise and dry brush skin morning and night.

If the blood is clean and the mind positive, the problem will not exist. Try to find the cause. Many times we don't give ourselves enough time to recuperate from our activities. Recuperation will balance most life styles and secure good sleeping habits. We all need to get away from our daily routines.

NIGHTSWEATS

Principal Therapy - heat dispelling, blood purification, stimulation.

Sweating is a sign that the body is eliminating poisons through the skin. It can be causd by a toxic system, hormone imbalance or blockages in the body.

Use the cleansing diet in this book with an enema every morning, then return to a diet of fruits, vegetables, whole grains, seeds and nuts. Avoid meats, salt, tobacco, nicotine, poultry and so forth. Drink two ounces of liquid chlorophyll morning and night diluted with four to six ounces of apple juice. Do not eat four hours before bedtime. Fast one day weekly on distilled or purified water.

A. *Internal:* Drink teas that will stimulate the circulation like ginger and prickly ash. Get plenty of exercise and fresh air daily. Dry brush the skin morning and evening.

If the body is continuously warm, use cooling herbs like alfalfa, plantain, and others (see heat dispelling therapy). Sometimes eating fruit for one week will eliminate this condition. Two cups of goldenseal, sage or strawberry leaves in tea form taken two hours before bed will help. I have seen elderly people drink yarrow or sage tea cold daily and at night to alleviate this condition.

Most bitter herbs like goldenseal, wormwood, gentian, etc. will tone the digestive system and will help prevent nightsweats.

B. *External:* Warm, whole baths with two cups of epsom salts taken nightly, with alternating hot and cold showers in the morning is excellent. After nightsweats are over, use cool, whole baths ten minutes in the morning to help tone the system.

Note: See women's diseases if hormone imbalance is the problem. The female tonic formulas are excellent for this malady.

NOSEBLEEDS (Epistaxis)
Bleeding from the nose can be caused by injury, hemophilia, fevers, lung, heart or kidney disease. Tumors can also be present in the mucus membrane.

Keep the person quiet while lying down. Have him snuff cold water with a little salt or lemon juice added to the water. This can be done several times a day. The nose is then plugged with cotton, leaving the person lying flat on their back with the head hanging slightly lower than the body.

Ferrum phosphoricum, (phosphate of iron) 12x can be taken every hour, usually five tablets are sufficient until bleeding stops. Then continue five tablets three times daily for 48 hours. It will help tone and equalize circulation.

Apply ice or very cold water to the forehead just above the nose and also on the nape of the neck while the person is lying down with the head tilted back. Make a decoction of white oak bark or bayberry or ephedra sinica. When these cool, they can be snuffed up the nose, then soak a cotton ball in the tea and insert into both nostrils. Repeat until relief is obtained.

If nosebleeds happen quite often, it is a good suggestion to take daily supplements with calcium and rutin, which will help build and tone fragile capillaries. Taking liquid chlorophyll internally and diluting it with 25% water and snuffing it up the nostril is also good. Wheatgrass juice is excellent for this condition.

Cayennne tincture ten drops in one-half cup of water every twenty minutes will equalize circulation. Taking cayenne capsules or cayenne and goldenseal together will also produce positive results. The dose is two capsules every hour until relief is obtained.

The eclectic physicians would use tincture of cinnamon from ten to thirty drops in one-half cup of warm water every one-half hour to stop bleeding of all types.

OBESITY

Principal Therapy - nutritional, stimulation.

There can be many causes of obesity: negative emotions, fear, overeating, glandular and nutritional deficiencies and ill health. One should see a nutritionally-educated doctor who does not use a high protein diet but teaches a low fat, low protein, high naural complex carbohydrate eating style.

Exercise daily and it is advisable to live primarily on a fruit and vegetable diet. Use small quantities of seeds, nuts and sprouted grains. I have seen diet alone improve the worst conditions in less than a year as the bloodstream and tissues become more alkaline, the glands begin functioning properly and the weight is reduced. Patience is required and remember, this is a chronic condition and it takes time to heal these illnesses.

The thyroid gland and gonads work together and when plant iodine supplements are given, the whole metabolism is improved. Kelp and dulse tablets take with meals daily will improve thyroid activity. Watercress and all other seaweeds are excellent also. The pituitary, thyroid and gonads are the main concern during obesity. Extracts from animal glands are helpful if used properly in appropriate dosages. Bee pollen (one-half ounce daily), carrot, beet and apple juice can be taken daily to assist glandular output.

Omit the use of all stimulation in the diet like hot spices, coffee, tea, tobacco, salt, sugar and so forth. These will cause a false appetite. Vitamins should be taken after meals because they also have a tendency to stimulate appetite.

Here are some suggested foods: lemons, green leafy vegetables, carrots, apples, cantaloupe, celery, tomatoes, all citrus fruits, melons, berries, plums, almonds, sesame seeds, garlic, seaweeds, figs, asparagus, cabbage, chives, ginseng tea or extract, wheat germ and grapes.

Avoid water reducing medications and high protein diets which are very harmful.

A. *Internal:* Chickweed, burdock root and nettle herb teas taken between meals will help reduce fat and appetite. A teaspoon of powdered psyllium or flaxseed in a warm cup of water or juice before meals will also stop excessive food cravings. Taking digestive enzymes before meals will aid digestion. Follow the food combining suggestions in this book.

For women who might have glandular deficiencies, the female tonic under Menopause is excellent. Men can take siberian or panax ginseng for glandular problems. The dose is twenty drops of extract or two capsules twice daily on an empty stomach, morning and evening. Sarsparilla tea for men and women, three cups daily is excellent for purifying the blood and glandular stimulation.

B. *Hydrotherapy:* Cool, whole baths or sitz baths taken in the mornings for ten minutes before exercising can be taken daily. These baths will stimulate gonad secretions. Two cups of epsom salts added to warm, whole baths with the addition of steam baths can be taken three times a week to promote sweating to reduce water held in the tissue and to promote proper circulation. Diaphoretic and stimulating teas can be taken before baths to assist in elimination. After the baths, dry the body with brisk towel rubbing.

PARALYSIS

Principal Therapy - stimulation.

Use the cleansing diet in this book with the use of enemas daily until the condition improves. If this has been a long term condition, a nutritious vegetarian diet should be used, using easily digestible foods. Raw, freshly prepared vegetable and fruit juices, bee pollen, spirulina, green, leafy vegetables, all raw seeds and nuts should be included. Take calcium supplements.

A. *Internal:* Nervine teas and tinctures should be taken. See the antispasmodic tincture in this book. A tincture made from avena sativa (oats) fifteen to twenty drops four times daily, will stimulate the brain and spinal cord. Equal parts scullcap and mistletoe, used as a tea, taken daily is excellent. Use teaspoonsfuls if the patient is a child. The formula under the section on Nervousness is also excellent.

B. *External:* Most important is acupuncture treatments. At home, hot and cold fomentations over the spine can be used several times a day, allowing for rest periods in between. After the fomentations, rub the affected area with stimulating liniments. See the all purpose liniment in this book. Spinal manipulations and massage will also help bring the nerves back to transporting energy impulses.

Do not let the body get chilled. Use warm baths or hot packs if this occurs.

PARASITES (See Convulsions)

PERITONITIS

Principal Therapy - tranquilization and heat dispelling (demulcent).

Take a slippery elm retention enema every morning if there is pain. A short three day carrot juice fast is indicated or a diet using oatmeal gruels, barley and lentil soups, parsley tea and other potassium fruits and vegetables. During the inflammatory stage, eating should be avoided and drink as much slippery elm tea as possible, sipping it constantly.

A. *Internal:* Aconite is one of the best remedies for inflammations, homeopathic (3x or 4x). Take five drops in a glass of water at hour intervals until the pain is gone. Ferrum phox. 12x, five tablets every hour is also good. Once the pain is gone, discontinue these remedies.

Bryonia is a specific remedy for bronchitis, pneumonia, neuritis, appendicitis, pancreatitis, endocarditis, and peritonitis. Take ten to twenty drops of the tincture every hour in water along with five tablets of ferrum phos. 12x or mag. phos 6x - 12x, until the pain is gone. If there is fever, use the therapy under Pleurisy and Pneumonia. Pleurisy root is excellent for this condition. Once the condition is under control, make a decoction out of comfrey root and drink two ounces every three to four hours, along with echinacea tablets two to three times a day or the tincture fifteen drops three times daily.

B. *Hydrotherapy:* Use warm, whole baths or warm, wet packs over the abdomen. A castor oil pack is also good.

PHLEBITIS (See Varicose Veins)

PLEURISY AND PNEUMONIA

Principal Therapy - diaphoresis, stimulation, deobstruent (expectorants).

See formulas under Asthma. They are all excellent for these conditions. The water cure using whole baths and diaphoretics is a specific for these two feverish conditions.

Another good treatment is to immediately give an enema and use them twice daily during the acute symptoms. A fast is indicated until all symptoms pass. Then use the cleansing diet in this book for seven days.

A. *Internal:* When the patient is in bed sweating, possibly after a cool bath is given, to promote sweating, the best remedy I have had experience with is the following:

> 1 ounce pleurisy root powder
> ½ ounce boneset
> 2 tablets freshly grated ginger

Simmer all ingredients for ten minutes in one and one-half pints of water. Drink one-half cup hot every hour or two tablespoons every one-half hour. Hot lemon juice taken between times will promote sweating.

Pleurisy root taken alone every hour in one-half cup doses can be used if this combination cannot be used. Coltsfoot, angelica and prickly ash can be added to pleurisy root or other diaphoretics as a substitute. Comfrey root, yerba santa and horehound with added stimulants can also be used.

Five drops of lobelia tincture or cayenne tincture can be added to the teas just before drinking.

B. *External:* Be sure to rinse the body off occasionally with water and apply apple cider vinegar as suggested under the section on Colds, Fevers and Flu.

While sweating in bed, apply cool water fomentations to the chest. When they become warm, change them immediately. Rub liniments over the chest area after the fomentations are removed and let the patient rest.

After recovery, study the section under Colds, Fevers and Flu on recovery from acute illness and tonification therapy.

Note: If there is infection or a history of infections, take goldenseal, echinacea or garlic capsules, two every two hours.

POISON OAK AND POISON IVY

Principal Therapy - blood purification, tranquilization.

Do a three day carrot juice fast or use the cleansing diet in this book for seven days. During the inflammatory stage a short two day fast drinking three cups of slippery elm tea daily along with carrot juice will relieve the symptoms.

A. *Internal:* Take chaparral or echinacea capsules internally every two hours or alternate them.

B. *External:* Take slippery elm powder and mix with a little water to make a paste. Spread on the skin.

C. *External:* To reduce itching, apply moistened baking soda or epsom salts. Epsom salt baths of three pounds to one tub of cool water will relieve itch. Apply cool damp cloths to the area.

Note: Do not eat during the most infected period.

D. *Hydrotherapy:* Use whole, cool baths several times a day if necessary to stop itching. Read the section on hives for further suggestions.

PROSTATITIS, BRIGHT'S DISEASE, ENLARGED PROSTATE

Principal Therapy - blood purification.

Use the hydrotherapy and dietary suggestions given under the treatment for Herpes.

A. Internal: Pipsissewa tincture, twenty-five drops three times a day is an excellent remedy for this condition, while drinking three cups of slippery elm tea daily. Make sure to use cool water enemas daily until the inflammation subsides. Adding three ounces of liquid chlorophyll or two cups of slippery elm tea to your retention enema water will reduce inflammations and swelling.

B. *Internal:* Mix together the following:

    1 part gravel root
    1 part plantain
    1 part echinacea
    1 part parsley root

¼ part ginger root
1 part buchu
½ part lobelia

Use one ounce of the herbs to a pint of water. Make a decoction and drink one-half cup three times daily, add honey to taste, or put powdered herbs in #00 capsules and take two, three times a day.

C. *Internal:* Drink two ounces of fresh parsley juice daily, morning and evening. It can be mixed in apple juice.

D. *Internal:* Take echinacea and chaparral capsules. Alternate them two every two hours during inflammation. Then reduce to two every four hours when inflammation subsides.

E. *External:* Sit in a cool (80 degrees or below) tub of water one-half hour morning and night. Add a strong infusion of uva ursi to the bath water. See formula C under Acne and Skin Diseases.

Another good remedy is saw palmetto. The tincture can be taken in doses of fifteen to twenty drops or the extract five to ten drops taken in water four times daily is an excellent remedy. It can be taken every hour during inflammatory stages.

PSORIASIS (See Eczema)

PYELITIS (See Hematuria)

Pyelitis is an inflammation of the mucus membrane of the pelvis of the kidney.

PYORRHEA AND GINGIVITIS

Principal Therapy - blood purification, dietary.

This problem is usually caused by lack of exercise for the teeth, hyperacidity of the system and the corroding action of mineral deposits on the teeth.

Use the cleansing diet in this book, then a three day fruit fast using apples, pears, oranges, melons, ripe lemons and two cups of carrot juice daily. An enema should be taken for three consecutive days in the mornings. Drink two to four ounces of liquid chlorophyll daily.

This diet will clean the blood and remove the neutralize excess acid from the system. Avoid excessive starches, meats, poultry, coffee, tea, alcohol, cigarettes, etc. Eat 60% of your diet raw, especially raw celery, carrots, beets, spinach, seeds, almonds, bee pollen, green leafy vegetables and sprouts. Add different seaweeds to the diet. Remain on a vegetarian diet.

Another cause of this problem is the swallowing of hot or cold foods or drinks. This causes the enamel to crack and weaken the structure to overactive acids in the blood.

A. *Internal:* Take myrrh/goldenseal capsules, two every three hours until inflammation stops, then two, three times daily for fourteen days.

Echinacea or the combination under Acne and Skin Problems can also be used. Rub the gums inside and outside with your fingers after dipping them in cold water. Then rinse the mouth with a tea made from goldenseal root or myrrh. Tincture of these can be used for this also. A tea made from white oak bark or bayberry will tone the gums.

Take calcium fluor. 6x or 12x and silica for all teeth and gum problems, three tablets five times daily during painful times.

Get the teeth and gums cleaned by a dentist every six months if needed.

If the kidneys are weak, drink buchu or uva ursi tea and vegetable broths to help neutralize the acids. Study food combinations and the diet and treatment under Arthritis.

QUINSY (See Adenoids)

RINGWORM (See treatment for parasites under Convulsions)

Principal Therapy - blood purification.

A three day citrus fruit fast is excellent, while cleansing the bowels with an enema on all three days. Then use the cleansing diet in this book for seven days.

A. *Internal:* Take chaparral or wormwood capsules daily, two tablets or capsules three times a day. Black walnut tincture (twenty-five drops) in one-half cup of warm water three times daily is excellent. Eat plenty of garlic, onions and other foods that are high in sulfur.

B. *External:* The affected area can be washed several times daily with diluted (25%) apple cider vinegar, garlic oil or juice, wormwood or thyme tea. Ointments made from these suggested herbs or calendula can be used. If good sour whey is handy, it is excellent as an external wash for this problem and most other skin diseases.

A salve made from wormwood, burdock root, chaparral and chickweed in equal parts is very good. This can be put into tea form and taken internally and used as a wash.

C. *Hydrotherapy:* Take cool, whole baths with one-half cup of apple cider vinegar added to the bath water. Soak for one-half hour two to three times daily.

SINUSITIS (Sinus Infection)

Principal Therapy - blood purification, heat dispelling.

Thoroughly clean the colon with an enema daily until the infection is gone. Go on a five day fruit fast using ripe oranges, lemons, apples, melons and pears. Then go on a vegetarian cleansing diet as suggested in this book.

During times of pain, hot and cold water fomentations over the forehead and sinus area or just cold water fomentations will ease the pain. Use which works best for the patient. The sinus area can be rubbed with the all purpose liniment.

A. *Internal:* Make a tea out of goldenseal or mullein and snuff a teaspoonful up each nostril several times a day but not to irritate the condition. Take garlic, chaparral or echinacea tablets, two tablets every two hours of one of these, or alternate them until the infection is gone. Twenty drops of echinacea tincture every two hours is excellent. A tincture made from horseradish is excellent for all sinus and upper congestive problems. See also horseradish syrup.

B. *Hydrotherapy:* A very effective treatment is to boil two quarts of water, then turn the stove off and add fifteen drops of eucalyptus, peppermint or some other volatile oil to the water. Cover your head and the pot of water with a towel and inhale through the nose and mouth several times. Do this two or three times daily.

SORES (Mouth, Thrush)

Principal Therapy - blood purification.

This condition is usually caused by poor eating, wrong food combinations, high protein diet, too much citrus and overeating.

A 48-hour fast on carrot juice and distilled water will clean the stomach of excessive acids. Then continue with the cleansing diet in this book for seven days. Gargle with a strong tea made from one or more of these herbs: thyme, myrrh, goldenseal or echinacea. Take goldenseal or myrrh capsules (two every two hours) until the sores begin to heal, then two capsules three times daily for fourteen days.

The sores can be painted with lobelia or black walnut tincture several times a day. Avoid cooked meats, fish, poultry and acid drinks like coffee, tea, etc. Use proper food combinations and never combine more than five different foods at a meal.

If the digestion is weak, drink two ounces of a decoction of gentian or goldenseal tea, twenty minutes before meals. Red raspberry and chickweed tea are good to neutralize acid and to aid digestion. Digestive enzymes can be used but do not depend on enzymes; tone the whole body so the pancreas, liver and spleen produce their own digestive juices and enzymes.

SPASMODIC COUGHS AND LUNG CONGESTION

Principal Therapy - tranquilization, blood purification.

Use the dietary, cleansing suggestions and remedies under Coughs, Sore Throat and Lung Congestion. See also the remedies mentioned under Asthma.

The following are also excellent remedies.

A. *Internal:* Cough Syrup

> 3 teaspoons ginger
> 1 teaspoon licorice

Simmer in two cups of water for ten minutes. Remove from heat; add two teaspoons of coltsfoot and horehound. Cool and strain. Add four tablespoons of honey or vegetable glycerine.

Dose: Two tablespoons when needed.

B. *Internal:* Antispasmodic Formula

> 1 part scullcap
> 1 part mistletoe, American
> 1 part lobelia
> 1 part valerian
> 1 part black cohosh
> 1 part lady's slipper
> ½ part ginger

Mix four ounces of the powdered, combined herbs in one pint alcohol (vodka, brandy, gin or rum—apple cider vinegar may be substituted). Keep it corked and in a dark place. Let it sit for fourteen days and shake it daily. Strain, put in a dark bottle with a tight cap.

Dose: Fifteen to thirty drops as needed.

SPERMATORRHEA

Principal Therapy - blood purification, tonification.

Abnormal involuntary emissions of semen is caused by a poor diet and stress which leads to sexual weakness, impotence and overstimulation of the sexual organs.

Use the cleansing diet in this book for ten days, then remain on a vegetarian diet. Take one teaspoon of powdered flaxseed three times a day mixed in water or fruit juice until the condition is cleared up. The bowel must be kept clean so use enemas every other day during the ten days on the cleansing diet. Take two ounces of freshly squeezed parsley juice morning and evening, mixed in six ounces of apple juice.

Avoid meats, large amounts of seeds and nuts, poultry, coffee, alcohol, stimulating spices, tobacco and all other stimulants and toxic foods. Steamed vegetables, sprouts, bee pollen, beet juice (two ounces every other day), seaweed, raw green vegetables, baked potato skins, celery juice (excellent) and all ripe fruits. The object of this diet is to use low protein, low fat, high natural carbohydrate foods like sprouted grains, wild rice, millet, brown rice and rye.

Keep the bowels moving with laxative herbs for two weeks. Study the section under Constipation in this book.

A. *Internal:* The combination of herbs under Prostatitis are excellent for this condition. Pipsissewa tincture, twenty drops three times a day will help clean the kidneys, prostate and bladder. Other herbs for this condition are buchu, plantain, goldenseal, uva ursi and juniper berries.

Alternate echinacea and chaparral tablets, two every four hours.

Tonification. To tone this body part, use panax ginseng extract ten drops morning and evening. Kelp, siberian ginseng, saw palmetto berries, damiana or gota kola are all good to strengthen the system. The whole lifetyle and diet should be considered to improve this problem.

If the nerves are weak, use nervines and calcium to strengthen them. See Nervousness in this book.

B. *Hydrotherapy:* Take cool sitz baths or whole baths morning and night. Add fifteen drops of juniper berry oil to the bath.

Note: Acupuncture and spinal manipulations are excellent therapies for this condition.

STYE

Principal Therapy - blood purification.

Do a five day fruit fast with the addition of carrot and celery juice. Clean the bowels with an enema every morning of the fast. To relieve eyestrain, inflamations and styes, beat fresh eggwhites and spread on a linen. Apply over the eye for fast relief. Chopped and diced carrots or mashed potato (raw or cooked) made into poultices are also very good. They can be left on for one hour and repeated three times a day.

Drink three cups of goldenseal tea or eyebright, fennel or myrrh to help clean the blood and liver. These herbs can also be taken in capsule form, two capsules three times daily.

Take silica (6x or 12x) five tablets three times a day for one week to aid the healing process. Use ferrum phos. 12x, three tablets every hour during inflammatory stages. Put one drop of castor oil in the eye morning and night. This will reduce the swelling.

Avoid refined, fried and processed foods, meats, salt, oils, alcohol, tobacco, dairy products, and white flour. They should be given up entirely. Switch to a vegetarian diet and use the cleansing diet in this book four times yearly.

A. *Hydrotherapy:* Warm, wet packs will relieve pain and bring the stye to a head. Hot and cold will also do the same and help draw the pus to a head. Use hot poultices to break the stye open once the pus has surfaced (see eye baths under hydrotherapy).

SYPHILIS (See Gonorrhea)

Principal Therapy - blood purification, heat dispelling.

Use the herbs and diet suggestions as mentioned under Gonorrhea. There is a specific formula mentioned for syphilis. If the herbs cannot be found, the exact procedures mentioned under Gonorrhea are indicated.

TOOTHACHE (See Pyorrhea and Gingivitis)

Principal Therapy - tranquilization, blood purification.

Follow the blood purification and dietary suggestions under Pyorrhea. Usually very few toothaches can stand a 48 hour water fast. This should be done at the onset of the pain, then switch to the cleansing diet in this book.

A. *Internal:* Take myrrh/goldenseal capsules or echinacea, two capsules every two hours. Echinacea tincture is excellent, fifteen to forty drops four times a day during the infectious stages. Eat plenty of garlic, drink chlorophyll juice (four ounces daily) and use an enema every morning until the pain is gone. Celery juice is very good to rid the body of acid and clean the blood and kidneys.

B. *External:* Oil of cloves or oil of sassafras can be applied to the painful area. Saturate a cotton ball with these oils and apply to the affected area. A very successful poultice is made from slippery elm, lobelia tincture and cayenne tincture. Mix the tinctures with slippery elm, roll into a ball and apply to the area. Clay is excellent when mixed with the oils mentioned or the tinctures, and applied externally. Kava kava in tincture form has an analgesic effect to the nerves. It can be substituted for one of the above.

To prevent breaking apart, these poultices can be wrapped in gauze in the shape of a small cigarette and applied directly.

Drink pennyroyal, hops and chamomile tea daily. Mix them together in equal parts or use one separately.

C. *External:* Cool water packs applied externally several times daily will ease the pain and help normalize blood flow. Ten minute durations are sufficient.

TUBERCULOSIS

Principal Therapy - blood purification (lymphatic system).

The blood, bowels and lymphatic system are the major areas to consider during this disease. Use the cleansing diet in this book for one week along with enemas every morning. Avoid the foods that cause congestion like milk, eggs, fried foods, high protein foods, refined sugar and starches. Eat mostly green vegetables, sprouts, seeds, nuts (avoid peanuts and roasted salted nuts), whole grains and fruits in season, or dried fruits, reconstituted. Calcium is a very important mineral to consider during tuberculosis. Use cabbage and carrots raw. Take calcium supplements between meals on an empty stomach.

Get plenty of fresh air and deep breathing exercise. To relax the chest, use a castor oil pack and warm fomentations made from lobelia or hops.

A. *Internal:* Use the formulas under Asthma or the section under Coughs, Sore Throats and Lung Congestion.

    To help clear lymphatic congestion, poke root tincture, five to ten drops, three times a day and echinacea, fifteen to thirty drops three times daily are excellent remedies. If these remedies cannot be found, use chaparral or goldenseal, two capsules four times daily of either one or alternate them. Liquid chlorophyll (four ounces daily) is excellent for all congestive and infectious diseases.

B. *Hydrotherapy:* Water therapy will increase circulation if done properly. Alternating warm and cold baths or showers morning and night is good. When the patient gets strong, use whole, cool baths in the evenings.

TUMORS AND CANCER

Principal Therapy - blood purification.

Cancer cells are abnormal cells that invade healthy tissues. They migrate through the system, and deposit themselves in areas of the body causing growths or tumors.

Harry S. Hoxsey in his book: "You Don't Have To Die" states:
"In the 1920s Dr. Otto Warburg, a Nobel Prize winner, demonstrated that the metabolism (chemical changes incidental to life and growth) of cancerous tissue differs radically from that of normal tissue. The latter acquires its nourishment from oxidation, and usually dies if deprived of oxygen. But cancerous tissue subsists by a process in which cell-nutritive substances are broken down by specialized chemicals much as food is broken down in ordinary digestion, and so needs little or no oxygen to exist. Subsequent experiments established that normal animal tissue may become cancerous if deprived of oxygen at long intervals.

"Since the blood provides cells of the body with oxygen, Warburg's discovery indicated that the condition of the blood stream must play an important part in the development of cancer. This is substantiated by the fact that malignant tumors frequently are found in or near scars, at the side of ulcers, in atrophied organs and in other places where the blood supply is poor."

Avoid all inorganic foods. Excessive protein will cause a build up of toxins and ultimately cause metabolic imbalances. Stay away from meat products and synthetic foods. A pure 100% organic vegetarian diet must be used, high in vitamins A, C and E. Most of the food should be raw, especially fruits, green leafy vegetables and sprouts. Proteins must come in the form of seeds and nuts. Almonds are excellent, others are sesame and sunflower seeds. Use high potassium foods. Cancer cells cannot live in a high potassium environment. Use only cold-pressed oils. Olive and safflower oils are examples. It is better not to use oils at all—oils are found naturally in vegetable seeds and nuts. Breakfast should consist only of fresh fruit and fruit juices. Never use protein foods in the morning; this will slow down elimination. Use lemon, orange, grape, carrot, beet and apple juice daily.

The bowels must be kept active. Use plenty of soaked figs, prunes and raisins. If constipation is a problem, use laxative herbs. Take one teaspoon of flax-seed or psyllium seed in water or juice one hour after meals. It has been proven that chlorophyll is an anti-cancer agent that slows the growth of cancerous tumors. It creates an environment unfavorable to bacterial growth. A rectal implant of chlorophyll (enema with the solution held for thirty minutes) taken daily after the bowel is cleaned, will help to detoxify the system. Coffee enemas are also good; they can be alternated with chlorophyll implants (see nutrient implants).

Directions for coffee enema: Take three tablespoons of ground (drip) coffee (not instant) to one quart of water; let it boil three minutes and then simmer fifteen minutes more. Strain and use at body temperature. The daily amount can be prepared at one time. Retain in an inclined position for twenty minutes. During painful periods, it can be done every two to four hours.

A high chlorophyll diet has proven therapeutically effective for both external and internal infections such as sinusitis, osteomyelitis, pyorrhea, cancer, peritonitis, ulcers, arteriosclerosis, etc. Wheatgrass juice is the best. It can be grown at home and juiced very inexpensively. See "Survival Into the 21st Century" by Viktoras Kulvinskas for further information on wheatgrass and chlorophyll.

Move to a warm, unpolluted climate where fresh air and sunshine is a constant. Exercise lightly. If the individual is strong enough, salt baths can be used to draw out the toxins. Soak in a warm tub of water. Add to it three pounds of epsom or kosher salt. Soak for only fifteen to twenty minutes. Rinse, rub natural oils in the skin to prevent drying.

A. *Internal:* If tumors are present, use cabbage leaf poultices or castor oil packs. When pain is present, wild lettuce and valerian tincture, ten drops in warm water every hour is necessary.

Mix in equal parts:

Chaparral
Bloodroot
Red clover
Echinacea
Dandelion root
Violet leaves
Santicle
Buckthorn bark
Burdock root
Ginger
Licorice root

Mix these powdered herbs together and put them in #00 capsules. Take two capsules four to six times daily. Along with this, garlic, wheatgrass juice and beet juice could be taken daily. Fluid is needed to neutralize and flush out the poisons.

This treatment might seem to be too much work. Cancer is usually a fatal disease. It takes 100% of an individual's time to be effective. It is most important to keep the liver, lungs, skin, bowels and kidneys in good condition. Cancer is a wasting disease which affects these organs. Plenty of rest is needed. Avoid stressful situations.

Metabolic Therapy

1. Get a hair analysis to determine minerals that are needed and what heavy metals may be causing a toxic effect.

2. Keep the bowels moving using enemas, colonics, nutrient implants and other suggestions indicated above.

3. Poly-ZYM-023 are enzymes that will break down the protective shield around the tumor. They can be purchased from General Research Laboratories, Inc., 139 Illinois Street, El Segundo, California 90245.

4. Amygdalin, two 500 milligram tablets are taken three times a day.

5. Vitamin A in emulsified form to minimize liver involvement. Start off by taking 100,000 units daily. Take twice daily, morning and evening. Alternate using two weeks on and one week off. Blurred vision and a soapy feeling in the mouth are signs that the body has too much vitamin A.

6. Take three raw thymus gland, three times a day to help increase lymphocytes. Make sure three are taken in the evening with vitamin A to increase immunity response.

7. Take six to twelve raw glandular tissue of the affected gland. For example, if the adrenals are involved, use raw adrenals.

8. Drink four 8-ounce glasses of freshly squeezed juice daily. For more information on metabolic therapy write to Metabolic Research Foundation, 518 Zenith Drive, Glenview, Illinois 60025.

9. Use chlorophyll enema implants to increase red blood cells and to decrease pain (see nutrient implants).

10. Use foods that are high in iodine and potassium, low in sodium, protein and fat. Drink potassium broths daily. Carrot and apple juice freshly squeezed should be taken in eight ounce quantities two to three times daily.

High Potassium Foods

Apricot, dried	Lentils, dry or sprouted
Asparagus	Limes, fresh
Banana	Mushrooms, raw
Barley, pearled	Nectarines
Bean, Navy (dried)	Okra, fresh
Lima (fresh)	Onions
Beets, raw	Oranges
Bread, sprouted, no salt	Parsley, fresh
Broccoli, fresh	Peaches, dried or raw
Brussel sprouts, fresh	Pears, Bartlett
Cabbage	Peas, dry or fresh
Cantaloupe	Persimmons
Caraway seed	Pineapple, raw
Carrots, raw	Plums, raw
Cauliflower (fresh, raw)	Prunes, dried or raw
Celery seeds	Quince, raw
Chard (small leaves)	Raisins
Cherries (dark, raw)	Rhubarb, raw
Dandelion greens	Rice, wild or brown
Dill seeds	Rolled oats
Endive	Sage
Figs, dried or raw (unsulphured)	Spinach, raw
Garlic	Squash, raw Acorn, Hubbard
Grapes, concord, emperor	White and yellow summer
Grapefruit, fresh	Tangerines
Horseradish, freshly prepared	Tapioca, raw
Kale, leaves	Turnips, raw leaves
Lemons, fresh	Watermelon

11. Read "You Don't have To Die" by Harry S. Hoxsey and "A Cancer Therapy" by Max Gerson M.D.

12. Take four chaparral tablets (15 grain) and nine red clover combination tablets daily.

URINE RETENTION (Burning urine, backache, dropsy)

Principal Therapy - blood purification.

Use the dietary and herbal suggestions under Spermatorrhea and the suggestions under Kidney and Bladder Infections.

A. *Internal:* Mix together the following herbs:

    2 parts fenugreek
    2 parts juniper berries
    1 part celery seed
    ½ part anise seed
    ¼ part ginger

Take one ounce of mixed herbs and bring to a boil for five minutes in one pint of distilled water. Cover and turn stove off. Steep for twenty minutes; strain. Drink one cup three times daily.

B. *External:* Use castor oil packs or hot ginger fomentations.

C. *External:* Alternate hot and cold water fomentations over the kidneys for fifteen minutes to one-half hour, two to three times a day.

D. *Hydrotherapy:* Use warm, whole baths for one-half hour, morning and evenings.

ULCERS

Principal Therapy - tranquilization, dietary.

Study the treatment under Gastritis. Use the same dietary, herbal and hydrotherapy treatments.

A. *Internal:* Mix together the following:

> 1 part slippery elm bark
> ½ part licorice root
> 1 part marshmallow root
> 1 part comfrey root
> 1 part goldenseal

> Use as a decoction and drink two ounces every two hours until the condition clears. Then reduce to three times daily for one week. Or, put powdered herbs in #00 gelatin capsules and take two to three times daily after meals and before bed on an empty stomach. Take two comfrey tablets or capsules every hour during inflammation and burning; then reduce to two every four hours.

B   *Internal:* Drink herb teas made from slippery elm, red raspberry, comfrey and marshmallow.

Clean the bowels with an enema; adjust the diet, use proper food combinations and fast three consecutive days a month on carrot and cabbage juice.

VARICOSE VEINS

Principal Therapy blood purification, tonification.

Bed rest until relief is noticed to relieve the pressure on the weak vessel walls is indicated. Use short two day fasts on fruit or vegetable juices, then use the cleansing diet in this book for one week. The diet for people with weak veins and arteries should be vegetarian, using seeds, nuts, fruits, whole grains or sprouted and green, leafy vegetables.

Keep the bowels moving twice daily using enemas if needed. Soaked figs, raisins and flaxseed will assure proper movements (see Constipation).

A. *Internal:* Mix together the following:

> 2 parts St. John's wort
> 1 part arnica flowers
> 1 part yarrow
> 1 part comfrey leaves
> 1 part prickly ash bark

Take an ounce of these herbs and steep in one pint of boiling water for twenty minutes. Strain, drink one cup three times daily.

Yarrow and red raspberry, equal parts, is also a good tea to drink three cups of daily if the above compound cannot be made.

Take calcium and rutin tablets daily. Rub St. John's wort oil into the affected area. Also make a strong decoction from white oak bark and foment the area. Wrap another cloth over the fomentation and leave on for several hours.

Drink red clover tea daily or the red clover combination in tablet form to clean the blood. Vegetable broths are excellent when leeks, onions and garlic are added to it.

WEAK DEBILITATED CONDITIONS

The following is an excellent vitamin and mineral tonic to take any time. Use after acute and chronic illnesses to help rebuild vitality. Good for goiter and thyroid diseases.

Mix together the following:

> 1 ounce alfalfa
> 1 ounce parsley root
> ½ ounce dandelion root
> ½ ounce burdock root
> ½ ounce comfrey root
> ½ ounce yellow dock root
> ½ ounce nettles leaves
> ½ ounce dulse

Simmer for twenty minutes in a quart of water in an uncovered pot. Let cool and strain. Return liquid to a pot and simmer uncovered for one hour until it is reduced to one cup. Stir in one cup of unsulphured blackstrap molasses and store in the refrigerator. Take one tablespoon three times daily. The above combination (powdered) can be put into #00 capsules and two to four can be taken with every meal.

REFERENCES

BACK TO EDEN, by Jethro Kloss, 1939, (Woodbridge Press Publishing Company, Santa Barbara, California).

COMMON HERBS FOR COMMON ILLNESSES, by William McGrath, 1977, (NuLife Publishing, Inc., Provo, Utah).

THE HERB BOOK, by John Lust, 1974, (Benedict Lust Publications, 25 Dewart Road, Greenwich, Connecticut 06830).

MEDICINAL PLANTS OF THE MOUNTAIN WEST, by Michael Moore, 1979, (The Museum of New Mexico Press, Santa Fe, New Mexico 87503).

NATURAL MEDICINE, by Robert Thomson, (McGraw-Hill Book Company), 1977.

NATUREA MEDICINA, by Dr. A.W. Kuts-Cheraux, B.S., M.D., N.D., Editor-in-Chief, 1953, (American Naturopathic Physicians and Surgeons Association, Des Moines, Iowa).

OWN YOUR OWN BODY, by Stan D. Malstorm, M.D., (Keats Publishing, Inc., New Canaan, Connecticut), 1977.

SCHOOL OF NATURAL HEALING, by Dr. John R. Christopher, 1976 (BiWorld Publishers, Inc., Provo, Utah).

SCIENCE OF HERBAL MEDICINE, by John Heinerman, 1979, (BiWorld Publishing, Inc., Provo, Utah).

TEXTBOOK OF MATERIA MEDICA, 4th Edition, by A.S. Blumgarten, M.D., F.A.C.P., 1926, (The Macmillan Company, New York).

UPDATE ON HERBS, Quarterly publication of the Association for the Promotion of Herbal Healing (APHH) since 1982, (1009 Third Street, Santa Cruz, California 95060).

THE WAY OF HERBS, by Michael Tierra, C.A., N.D., 1980, 1983, (Washington Square Press, New York, New York).

GENERAL INDEX

INDEX OF HERBS

INDEX OF DISEASES

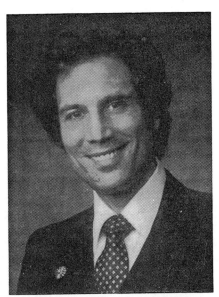

ABOUT THE AUTHOR

Mr. Santillo was born and raised in Lockport, New York and received his B.S. degree from Edinboro State Teachers' College in Pennsylvania, attending on football and track scholarships.

Following graduation from Edinboro, Mr. Santillo developed thirty-three different allergies and signs of rheumatoid arthritis. After enduring three years of traditional medical treatment, and taking prescription drugs to no avail, Mr. Santillo began his search for a real solution to his problems. Over the course of many years he obtained the following degrees: Doctor of Naturopathy (Anglo-American Institute of Drugless Therapy), Health Practitioner (Hippocrates Health Institute of Boston, Mass. under Dr. Ann Wigmore and Victor Kulvinskas), Iridology Certificate of Merit (under Dr. Bernard Jensen), Master Herbalist (from Dr. John R. Christopher at the school of Natural Healing in Utah). Continuing his education, Mr. Santillo has attended many courses and seminars including: Oriental Herbal Medicine (with Sabhuti Dharmananda, Ph.D., Director of the Institute for Traditional Medicine and Preventative Health Care), Myopractic Therapy (with Dr. Jym Marinakas, N.D.), Medical Botany (from the Platonic Herbal Academy in Santa Cruz, California, with Ed Smith and Michael Tierra), and eight years of study under Dr. Phil Zimmerman and Dr. Thurman Fleet earning his Doctor's degree from the Concept-Therapy Institute, San Antonio, Texas.

NATURAL HEALING WITH HERBS CORRESPONDENCE COURSE INFORMATION

This correspondence course has been written by the author for both the layperson and the physician. It is a course that will help prepare an individual to conduct his or her own herbal practice. The instruction presented in the course is unique in that it is coordinated with the material in the book, "Natural Healing With Herbs", which helps to make it simple for all to understand. Therapies utilizing nutritional foods, and both Chinese and American herbs (including their philosophies), are thoroughly discussed to furnish an understanding of both Eastern and Western medicine.

The course is divided into separate sections with questions and answers at the end of each section. Upon completion of the course, a final examination will be provided for the student to be completed and then mailed back to the author for correction. The student, upon satisfactorily completing the course, will receive his or her Master Herbalist Degree. There is no time schedule on completing the course; students may take six months, others one year. The student may proceed at his own pace.

The course is available for only $375.00 and an additional $16.25 if you have not purchased the book, "Natural Healing With Herbs." It is essential that the student purchase the entire course plus the book, "Natural Healing With Herbs" at the same time. (If two or more courses are ordered at the same time, you pay only $350.00 each.) If an individual prefers, he may make two payments. The first payment is $275.00 and includes only the first part of the course. A preliminary lesson preview is available for $7.00. The second part of the course will be mailed to the student upon receipt of the second payment of $100.00, which will be due within 30 days of the mailing date of the first part. (This includes shipping and handling charges.) A special price is offered to retail health food store owners or managers. Please write to the address below for more information. Make all checks or money orders (in U.S. funds only), payable to Humbart Santillo. Allow 3 - 4 weeks for delivery for courses paid by money order and 7 - 8 weeks for delivery for courses paid by check.

To assist the student, there are tapes available for purchase recorded live at herbal seminars given internationally by the author. They include further instruction of the proper use of herbs, diet, and the role the mind plays in healing.

Hundreds of people have been satisfied with this information. If within a two week trial period you find you are not satisfied with the material you have received, return the course for your refund minus $25.00 processing fee. This is a wonderful opportunity for the true seeker of herbal knowledge to receive proper, factual instruction.

To order courses or for more information, please write (no phone calls will be accepted): Herbal Correspondence Course, P.O. Box 468, East Amherst, New York, 14051.

This course of study includes the following subjects:

ANATOMY AND PHYSIOLOGY
-Body Systems
-Pathology and Herbal Remedies

THE CAUSE OF DISEASE
-The Cell
-Elimination
-Acute and Chronic Diseases

THE PROPERTIES OF HERBS

THE CHEMICAL CONSTITUENTS OF PLANTS

HERBAL PREPARATIONS

HERBAL FORMULATIONS

METHODS OF APPLICATION

DIAGNOSIS
-Pulse Diagnosis
-Questioning
-Yin Yang Theory
-Five Element Theory

THE TEN HERBAL THERAPIES

PHYSIO-MEDICAL APPROACH TO HEALING

TREATMENT OF INFLAMMATION AND PAIN

MONITORING THE HEALING PROCESS
-Using the Temperature, Pulse, Blood Pressure, Urine and Saliva

HERBS FOR PREGNANCY AND FEMALE DISEASES

HERBS FOR MALE DISEASES

CHINESE HERBS

VITAMINS AND MINERALS IN PLANTS

FOOD AS MEDICINE

HERBAL SEMINAR TAPES

These tapes are a live recording of an Herbal Seminar given to laymen, doctors, and other professionals by Mr. Santillo. The information begins with the basics of herbology and extends into a comprehensive coverage of therapies used in clinics throughout the world. It correlates historical herbology with the most recent in American and Chinese herbal philosophies. The tapes can be purchased with or without "Natural Healing with Herbs" Herbal Correspondence Course. Below is a description of the information available on each tape.

TAPE #1: Side A — This side explains the role that the mind plays in healing — how ideas and thoughts effect the body, and when negative, will result in dis-ease (disease). An interesting discussion is given explaining the parts of the brain and how they relay thought energy throughout the body, causing tension, stress, and other psychosomatic disorders. Once one understands this material, he or she is in a position to improve their mental attitude and avoid the negative effects of stress. The physical cause of disease is explained on this side along with other subjects such as acid-alkaline balance, cleansing diets, detoxification, enervation (lowered nerve energy), and toxemia. These subjects lead into a complete discussion on acute and chronic diseases and the difference between a healing crisis and a disease crisis. Then the dosages of herbs are discussed in the treatment of acute and chronic diseases.

Side B — The information here explains the three functions of herbs: eliminating, maintaining (balance), and building, and coordinating these with the healing properties of herbs, such as demulcents, laxatives, expectorants, etc. There are eight major therapies used to treat disease which are also discussed on this side, continuing to Tape #2, Side A.

TAPE #2: Side A — This tape explains therapies such as stimulation therapy, tranquilization therapy, blood purification and tonification therapies.

Side B — This side continues with more therapies such as sweating, emesis, diuresis, and purging. Herbs are listed under each therapy with a full discussion of what herbal properties are and their definitions.

TAPE #3: Side A — This tape gives a complete explanation of how to prepare and use herbal infusions, decoctions, boluses, douches, electuaries, pills, enemas, tinctures, and oils.

Side B — This side continues the discussion of the previous side with explanations of how to prepare and use poultices, plasters, castor oil packs (for the treatment of tumors), capsules, salves, and concentrates.

TAPE #4:Side A — In Chinese medicine, diseases are categorized as being either hot or cold. A discussion of this subject is presented along with suggested symptoms to look for help in determining illnesses of these two types. Dietary suggestions are given along with a cleansing diet and transition diet. Primary and secondary symptoms are discussed, along with how to determine one's major weaknesses and strengths. This gives the herbalist a basis to determine which part of the body to treat.

Side B — A thorough explanation is given on how to treat colds, fevers, and flus using cold sheet treatments, hydrotherapy, and the herbs fenugreek, catnip, fennel, comfrey, and thyme. Most important on this tape is an explanation of how to build proper herbal formulas for both acute and chronic illnesses. The final part of this side deals with how each disease goes through five stages of development from the onset to the cure. Symptoms are discussed so a therapist can recognize which stage the disease is in so that proper herbs can be chosen for that particular stage.

This is just an overview of some of the exciting subjects on these tapes. One can see how valuable this information is and also how difficult knowledge like this is to find. These tapes include concentrated, easy-to-understand information which can be of assistance to anyone who has the interest. These tapes are invaluable for laymen, doctors, or students who want to increase their own health or who want to help others.

Humbart D. Santillo, B.S., M.H.

The cost of this four-tape seminar, "Herbs, Nutrition and Healing," is $45.00 postpaid (U.S. funds only). Make checks payable to Hohm Press, P.O. Box 2501, Prescott, AZ 86302.

Please send _____ copies of the book *NATURAL HEALING WITH HERBS* at $16.25 postpaid.

Please send _____ copies of the tape series, *HERBS, NUTRITION AND HEALING* at $45.00 postpaid.

Name _____

Address _____

City _____ State _____ Zip _____

FOOD ENZYMES; THE MISSING LINK TO RADIANT HEALTH
By Humbart Santillo/New from Hohm Press

For Your Convenience On Cassette

FOOD ENZYMES:
The Missing Link to Radiant Health

by Humbart Santillo

Also included on cassette tape is information on:
- Enzymes as a foundation to health
- Enzymes and immunity
- Enzymes and weight loss

PLUS a copy of the book **FOOD ENZYMES: The Missing Link to Radiant Health**
by Humbart Santillo $41.00 post paid

Quantity	Item	Cost	Total
	FOOD ENZYMES: The Missing Link to Radiant Health by Humbart Santillo	$5.20 pp	
	FOOD ENZYMES: The Missing Link to Radiant Health by Humbart Santillo (cassette package includes book)	$41.00 pp	
		Total	

☐ check   ☐ money order

Name _____

Address _____

City _____ State _____ Zip _____

Send check or money order to:
Hohm Press, P.O. Box 2501, Prescott, Arizona 86302

*Hohm Press publishes books
on contemporary spirituality and health:
We make available publications of only the highest quality
and expertise. Subject matter is selected
not by commercial appeal but by the value and elegance
offered to the reader.
For a complete brochure write Hohm Press.*

P. O. 2501, Prescott, Arizona 86302

*This book was set by Hohm Press on a
Compugraphic MCS and run out on a Compugraphic 8400.
The face used is English Times, 10 point on an 11 point set.
It was printed and bound by the George Banta Company
of Menasha, Wisconsin. The paper is a 55 lb. Butte des Morts.*

NOTES

NOTES

NOTES

NOTES

NOTES

NOTES

NOTES

NOTES